DERMATOLOGY
MADE EASY

OTHER TITLES FROM SCION

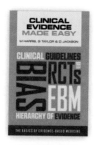

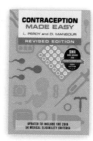

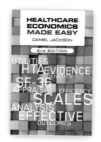

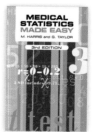

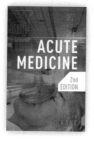

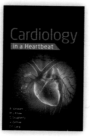

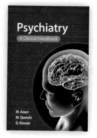

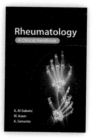

For more information see www.scionpublishing.com

DERMATOLOGY
MADE EASY

AMANDA OAKLEY

Founder and Editor in Chief of DermNet New Zealand

Dermatologist at Waikato Hospital, Hamilton, New Zealand

Adjunct Associate Professor, Department of Medicine, Faculty of Medical and Health Sciences, The University of Auckland, New Zealand

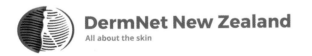

© **Scion Publishing Ltd, 2017**

First published 2017

All rights reserved. No part of this book may be reproduced or transmitted, in any form or by any means, without permission.

A CIP catalogue record for this book is available from the British Library.

ISBN 978 1 907904 82 0

Scion Publishing Limited

The Old Hayloft, Vantage Business Park, Bloxham Road, Banbury OX16 9UX, UK

www.scionpublishing.com

Important Note from the Publisher

The information contained within this book was obtained by Scion Publishing Ltd from sources believed by us to be reliable. However, while every effort has been made to ensure its accuracy, no responsibility for loss or injury whatsoever occasioned to any person acting or refraining from action as a result of information contained herein can be accepted by the authors or publishers.

Readers are reminded that medicine is a constantly evolving science and while the authors and publishers have ensured that all dosages, applications and practices are based on current indications, there may be specific practices which differ between communities. You should always follow the guidelines laid down by the manufacturers of specific products and the relevant authorities in the country in which you are practising.

Typeset by Medlar Publishing Solutions Pvt Ltd, India

Printed in the UK

Contents

About the author

Dr Amanda Oakley is Adjunct Associate Professor for the Department of Medicine at the University of Auckland. She lives in Hamilton, New Zealand, where she is a Dermatologist for Waikato District Health Board and in private practice at the Tristram Clinic. She diagnoses for MoleMap New Zealand, writes a monthly column for the general practice magazine, *New Zealand Doctor*, and is frequently called upon to speak at conferences and deliver workshops on dermatological matters. Professor Oakley is actively engaged in clinical research with many publications in peer-reviewed medical journals in print and online. Her main areas of professional interest are vulval diseases, dermatoscopy and the early diagnosis of melanoma, teledermatology, and education of consumers and health professionals.

Professor Oakley has been President of Waikato Postgraduate Medicine, the New Zealand Dermatological Association and the Australian and New Zealand Vulvovaginal Society. She is a Trustee of the Waikato Medical Research Foundation and of DermNet New Zealand and is actively involved with several other medical organisations.

Professor Oakley has received many awards for her efforts, including Honorary Memberships of the American Academy of Dermatology, the American Dermatological Association, the Skin Cancer College of Australasia and MelNet New Zealand.

Her greatest joy is the success of DermNet New Zealand (www.dermnetnz.org), from which this book, *Dermatology Made Easy*, is derived.

Preface

Dermatology Made Easy, the title of this book, is an oxymoron. Dermatological diagnosis is frequently challenging; the specialty has more than 3000 named acute and chronic diseases. The barrier function of the skin and its interaction with the external environment and the cutaneous immune system contribute to the complexity. Every patient presents with a unique combination of signs and is anxious or distressed by their symptoms. Treatment may be complicated, or not required, depending on diagnosis and individual patient factors. Specialist dermatologists are scarce and are often difficult or expensive to access.

I prepared this book to complement the DermNet New Zealand website (www.dermnetnz.org), which aims to be *All about the skin*. Launched by the New Zealand Dermatological Society in 1996, when the worldwide web was only 3 years old, DermNet NZ has become the most popular English language resource on dermatological matters, with up to 4 million pages viewed each month. Now owned by a charitable trust, you will find more than 2000 titles and 15 000 images on skin diseases, conditions, procedures and treatments – far more than we could include in the book. Our online readership includes dermatologists, general practitioners, medical students and other health professionals, researchers, scholars, patients, their relatives and friends.

First learn the terminology of dermatology. Then use this book to help diagnose a skin disease or condition. Take a history and examine your patient. Document the location or distribution of a lesion or eruption, and the arrangement and morphology of individual lesions.

The first chapter, *Differential diagnosis*, helps you make a diagnosis according to symptoms, morphology, and/or the affected body site(s). Don't forget to consider patient age and gender, the onset and behaviour of the presenting complaint, past medical history and medications.

You can review information about common infections (Chapter 2), inflammatory rashes (Chapter 3) non-inflammatory conditions (Chapter 4), and skin lesions (Chapter 5), and formulate a plan for further investigations and treatment (Chapter 6).

In this book I have tried to cover most common drugs used in the UK, USA and Australasia; however, you should be aware that although the drugs detailed will all be appropriate for treatment, not all will be available on prescription in all territories. Please refer to your local prescribing guidelines and datasheets. In dermatology, be aware that many treatments are used off-licence.

Still stuck? Go online to www.dermnetnz.org for more information.

Enjoy!

Amanda Oakley
March 2017

If you notice errors or omissions, don't forget to tell us by using the feedback form at
www.dermnetnz.org/contact-us/

Acknowledgements

Tēnā koutou katoa ("greetings").

I am hugely grateful to past and current trustees, sponsors and supporters of the DermNet New Zealand Trust, a New Zealand registered charity. The 2017 Trustees are New Zealand dermatologists Marius Rademaker, Anthony Yung, Sandra Winhoven, Victoria Scott-Lang, and myself.

The pages in this book are adapted from the material on www.DermNetNZ.org. They are derived from online pages published over the last 21 years that were originally written by dermatologists, dermatology registrars, other medical practitioners, students and professional science writers – many of whom volunteered their time and effort to improve the largest online resource *All about the skin*. These authors live in New Zealand, Australia, the United Kingdom, the United States of America and elsewhere, making our online library and this book truly international.

I would like to thank Anne Maloney (GP in Berkshire, UK, with a special interest in dermatology) and Karen McKoy (dermatologist based at the Lahey Clinical in Burlington, USA) for their advice on the different treatment options used in the UK and USA.

The list of DermNet New Zealand authors is long, and rather than inadvertently leave anyone out, I offer sincere thanks to you all.

The book includes more than 1000 clinical images. I would like to express my gratitude to the dermatologists, pathologists and their patients that willingly consented to having their skin conditions used for education and publication purposes – in print and online. I am particularly grateful to The Medical Photography team at Waikato Hospital, and for the generous support of the Waikato District Health Board. Thank you.

Ngā mihi nui ("thanks very much").

Abbreviations

AC	alternating current	INR	international normalised ratio
ACE	angiotensin-converting enzyme	IPL	intense pulsed light
ACTH	adrenocorticotrophic hormone	IUD	intrauterine device
AGEP	acute generalised exanthematous pustulosis	IV	intravenous
		LDH	lactic acid dehydrogenase
AIDS	acquired immune deficiency syndrome	LE	lupus erythematosus
		LFT	liver function test
ANA	antinuclear antibody	LH	luteinising hormone
ANCA	anti-neutrophil cytoplasmic antibodies	LS	lichen sclerosus
		MASI	Melasma Area and Severity Index
BCC	basal cell carcinoma	MDM	multidisciplinary meeting
BMI	body mass index	MMP	matrix metalloproteinase
BP	blood pressure	MMR	measles, mumps, rubella
BSA	body surface area	MRI	magnetic resonance imaging
CBC	complete blood count	MSH	melanocyte-stimulating hormone
CCCA	central centrifugal cicatricial alopecia		
		NSAID	non-steroidal anti-inflammatory drug
CNS	central nervous system		
CPC	clinicopathological correlation	PCR	polymerase chain reaction
CRP	C-reactive protein	PDT	photodynamic therapy
CT	computerised tomography	PET	positron emission tomography
DC	direct current	PLE/PMLE	polymorphic light eruption
DEET	diethyltoluamide	PUVA	photochemotherapy
DEXA	dual-energy X-ray absorptiometry	RAST	radioallergosorbent test
DIHS	drug-induced hypersensitivity syndrome	RNA	ribonucleic acid
		SC	subcutaneous
DNA	deoxyribonucleic acid	SCAR	severe cutaneous adverse reaction
DRESS	drug reaction with eosinophilia and systemic symptoms	SCC	squamous cell carcinoma
		SDRIFE	symmetrical drug-related intertriginous and flexural exanthema
EBV	Epstein–Barr virus		
ECG	electrocardiograph		
ED	exfoliative dermatitis	SIL	squamous intraepithelial lesion
ENA	extractable nuclear antigen	SJS	Stevens–Johnson syndrome
FBC	full blood count	SK	seborrhoeic keratosis
FDA	Food and Drug Administration	SLE	systemic lupus erythematosus
FSH	follicle-stimulating hormone	SPF	sun protection factor
GA	granuloma annulare	SSSS	staphylococcal scalded skin syndrome
H&E	haematoxylin and eosin		
HFM	hand, foot and mouth	TB	tuberculosis
HHV	human herpes virus	TEN	toxic epidermal necrolysis
HIV	human immunodeficiency virus	TIA	transient ischaemic attack
HLA	human leucocyte antigen	TNF	tumour necrosis factor
HPA	hypothalamic–pituitary–adrenal	UV	ultraviolet
HPV	human papillomavirus	UVR	ultraviolet radiation
HSV	herpes simplex virus	VIN	vulval intraepithelial neoplasia
IEC	intraepidermal carcinoma	VZV	varicella-zoster virus

Terminology

The following terms have been agreed by the International League of Dermatological Societies for the description of cutaneous lesions (Br J Dermatol, 2016;174:1351). *Table 1* provides the basic definitions for cutaneous lesions and *Table 2* provides additional detail including terms for distribution, shape, topography and palpation. Between the tables are photographs which help to identify the differences between terms.

Table 1. Basic descriptive terms for cutaneous lesions.

Term	Definition	Comments
Macule	A flat, circumscribed, nonpalpable lesion that differs in colour from the surrounding skin. It can be any colour or shape.	The average diameter, shape, colour and border should be described. In North America, a macule (≤1 cm) is distinguished from a patch (>1 cm).
Papule	An elevated, solid, palpable lesion that is ≤1 cm in diameter.	The average diameter, shape, colour, topography (surface characteristics, e.g. flat topped) and border should be described; degree of elevation and consistency or feel can be included.
Plaque	A circumscribed, palpable lesion >1 cm in diameter; most plaques are elevated.[a] Plaques may result from a coalescence of papules.	The average diameter, shape, colour, topography and border (e.g. well demarcated vs. ill defined) should be described; degree of elevation and consistency or feel can be included.
Nodule	An elevated, solid, palpable lesion >1 cm usually located primarily in the dermis and/or subcutis. The greatest portion of the lesion may be exophytic or beneath the skin surface.	The average diameter, shape, colour, topography and border should be described; degree of elevation and consistency or feel can be included.
Weal	A transient elevation of the skin due to dermal oedema, often pale centrally with an erythematous rim.	There are no surface changes.
Vesicle	A circumscribed lesion ≤1 cm in diameter that contains liquid (clear, serous or haemorrhagic).	'Small blister'.
Bulla	A circumscribed lesion >1 cm in diameter that contains liquid (clear, serous or haemorrhagic).	'Large blister'.
Pustule	A circumscribed lesion that contains pus.	
Crust	Dried serum, blood or pus on the surface of the skin.	
Scale	A visible accumulation of keratin, forming a flat plate or flake.	Types of scale: ■ Silvery (micaceous), e.g. psoriasis. ■ Powdery (furfuraceous), e.g. pityriasis (tinea) versicolor. ■ Greasy, e.g. seborrhoeic dermatitis.

Table 1. (*continued*)

Term	Definition	Comments
		▪ Gritty, e.g. actinic keratosis. ▪ Polygonal, e.g. ichthyosis. Collarette of scale: fine white scale at the edge of an inflammatory lesion or resolving infectious process, e.g. pityriasis rosea, resolving folliculitis, resolving furunculosis.
Erosion	Loss of either a portion of or the entire epidermis.	It may arise following detachment of the roof of a blister, e.g. bullous impetigo.
Excoriation	A loss of the epidermis and a portion of the dermis due to scratching or an exogenous injury.	It may be linear or punctate.
Ulcer	Full-thickness loss of the epidermis plus at least a portion of the dermis; it may extend into the subcutaneous tissue.	The size, shape and depth should be described as well as the characteristics of the border, base and surrounding tissue.

ªThere is ongoing discussion as to whether nonelevated, but palpable, lesions such as those of morphoea should be termed plaques; the authors included such lesions as plaques, hence the statement that most, but not all, plaques are elevated.

Reproduced from the *British Journal of Dermatology* 2016;174:1351, with permission from John Wiley & Sons Ltd.

Papules

On the whole, papules are oval or round. They can also be described as:

- Acuminate (pointed, pityriasis rubra pilaris; left)
- Dome-shaped (rosacea; right)

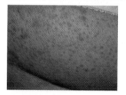 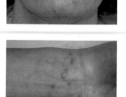

- Filiform (thread-like, viral wart; left)
- Flat-topped (lichen planus; right)

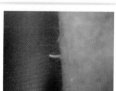

- Pedunculated (with a narrow stalk, skin tag; left)
- Sessile (without a stalk, arising from a wide base, syringomas; middle)
- Umbilicated (central dell, molluscum contagiosum; right)

  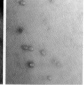

Plaques

Can be any shape, for example:

- Round (ecthyma; left)
- Oval (psoriasis; right)

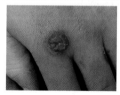 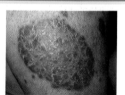

- Linear (lichen striatus; left)
- Arcuate (half-circle or part of a circle, annular erythema; right)

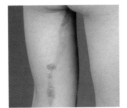 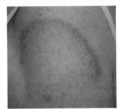

- Annular (ring, granuloma annulare; left)
- Polygonal (many sided, lichen planus; right)

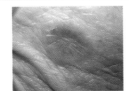 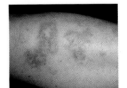

- Polycyclic (overlapping rings, subacute lupus erythematosus; left)
- Polymorphic (various shapes, lichen planus; right)

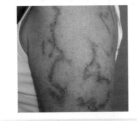 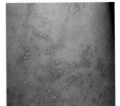

- Serpiginous (snake-like line, cutaneous larva migrans; left)
- Targetoid (two or more concentric rings like a bull's eye or rosette, urticarial vasculitis; right)

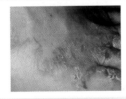 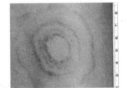

- Irregular (seborrhoeic keratosis, left; basal cell carcinoma, right)

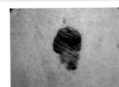 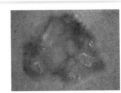

Surface signs

The surface of a papule or plaque may be smooth, dry, scaly or crusted. Scale can be described in various ways, for example:

- Central, peripheral (pityriasis rosea herald patch; left), scattered
- Desquamation or exfoliation (peeling; right)

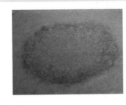 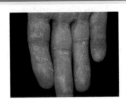

- Maceration (wet, athlete's foot; left)
- Psoriasiform (psoriasis-like; right)

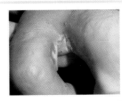 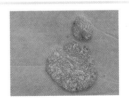

- Verrucous (wart-like, erythropoietic protoporphyria; left)
- Pityriasiform (bran-like powder, seborrhoeic dermatitis; right)

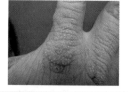
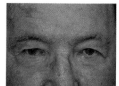

- Mica-like (layered, attached at the centre but not at the periphery, (pityriasis lichenoides; left)
- Hyperkeratotic or keratotic (thick, hyperkeratotic actinic keratosis; right)
- Silvery or yellowish

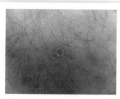
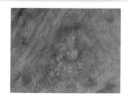

- Crust-scale (scale mixed with serous ooze; left)
- Lichenoid (adherent, lichen planus; right)

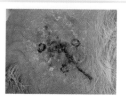
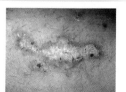

- Adherent (not necessarily lichenoid, e.g. when describing actinic keratosis; left)
- Minimal
- Trailing scale or collarette of scale (scale arising just inside the border of a plaque, pityriasis rosea; right)

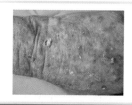
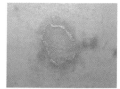

Secondary changes

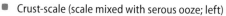

- Excoriation (superficial broken areas of skin due to scratching; left)
- Prurigo (picked or excoriated firm papule; right)

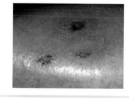
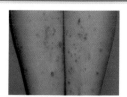

- Erosion (loss of epidermis; left)
- Ulcer (complete loss of epidermis, dermis +/– subcutis (subcutaneous fat); right)

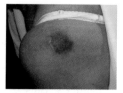
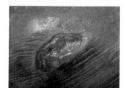

- Fissure (linear crack in the epidermis; left)
- Lichenification (papules or plaques due to epidermal thickening due to rubbing and scratching, causing prominent skin markings. Surface is often dry; right)

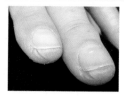
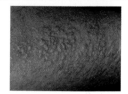

Table 2. Additional terms for cutaneous lesions: distribution, shape, topography and palpation.

Term	Definition	Clinical example(s)
Distribution of cutaneous lesions		
Acral	Lesions of distal extremities, ears, nose, penis, nipples.	Acral type of vitiligo, acrocyanosis.
Asymmetrical	Lesion or distribution pattern that lacks symmetry along an axis (e.g. the midline).	Acute allergic contact dermatitis, herpes zoster, lichen striatus; in the case of a single lesion, melanoma.
Dermatomal (zosteriform)[a]	Lesions confined to one or more segments of skin innervated by a single spinal nerve (dermatomes).	Herpes zoster, segmental neurofibromatosis.
Disseminated ▪ Generalised/widespread ▪ Within an anatomical region (e.g. the back, an extremity)	Lesions distributed randomly over most of the body surface area (generalised/widespread) or within an anatomical region.	Varicella, disseminated zoster, morbilliform drug eruption, viral exanthems. Folliculitis (buttocks), Grover disease (trunk).
Exposed skin ▪ Exposed to the environment ▪ Exposed to sunlight or other forms of radiation (e.g. photodistributed)	Areas exposed to external agents (chemical allergens, irritants or physical agents).	Allergic contact dermatitis to plants, airborne contact dermatitis. Polymorphic light eruption, phototoxic drug eruption, radiation dermatitis.
Extensor sites (of extremities)	Areas overlying muscles and tendons involved in extension, as well as joints (e.g. extensor forearm, elbow, knee).	Psoriasis, keratosis pilaris, frictional lichenoid dermatitis.
Flexural sites	Areas overlying muscle and tendons involved in flexion of joints or the inner aspect of joints (e.g. antecubital or popliteal fossae).	Atopic dermatitis.
Follicular and perifollicular	Lesions located within or around hair follicles.	Folliculitis, pityriasis rubra pilaris, keratosis pilaris.
Generalised/widespread	Distributed over most of the body surface area (see above).	Viral exanthems (e.g. rubeola, rubella), morbilliform drug eruption.
Grouped ▪ Herpetiform ▪ Agminated ▪ Satellitosis	Clusters of papulovesicles. Solid papules within a cluster. Smaller papules surrounding a larger lesion.	Herpes simplex. Agminated melanocytic naevi, leiomyomas. Melanoma metastases, pyogenic granulomas.
Interdigital	Area between the fingers or toes.	Tinea pedis, erythrasma.
Intertriginous	Present in major body folds (axilla, submammary, inguinal crease, beneath pannus, intergluteal fold).	Inverse psoriasis, intertrigo, cutaneous candidosis (candidiasis), Langerhans cell histiocytosis.

Table 2. (*continued*)

Term	Definition	Clinical example(s)
Distribution of cutaneous lesions		
Linear	Linear arrangement of lesions.	
▪ Köbner phenomenon	Lesions induced by physical stimuli (e.g. trauma, scratching, friction, sunburn).	Psoriasis, lichen planus, vitiligo.
▪ Dermatomal (zosteriform)[a]	See 'Dermatomal' above.	See 'Dermatomal' above.
▪ Sporotrichoid	Lesions along lymphatic vessels.	Sporotrichosis, *Mycobacterium marinum* infection.
▪ Along Blaschko lines	Lesions due to mosaicism.	Epidermal naevus, linear lichen planus, lichen striatus.
Localised	Lesions confined to one or a few areas.	Leiomyomas, scalp psoriasis.
Palmar, plantar, palmoplantar	Lesions on the palms and/or soles.	Keratoderma, pustulosis palmaris et plantaris.
Periorificial (e.g. periocular, periorbital, perianal)	Lesions around body orifices.	Vitiligo, periorificial dermatitis.
Seborrhoeic regions	Areas with the highest density of sebaceous glands (e.g. scalp, face, upper trunk).	Seborrhoeic dermatitis, Darier disease.
Segmental		
▪ Block-like	Lesions along embryonic growth lines[a].	Pigmentary mosaicism.
▪ Along Blaschko lines	Lesions along embryonic growth lines[a].	Pigmentary mosaicism, incontinentia pigmenti.
▪ Dermatomal (zosteriform)[a]	See 'Dermatomal'.	Herpes zoster.
Symmetrical	Lesions or pattern with symmetry along an axis (e.g. the midline).	Psoriasis, atopic dermatitis.
Unilateral	Lesions confined to either the left or the right half of the body.	Herpes zoster, CHILD syndrome,[b] segmental vitiligo.
Universal	Involving the entire body.	Alopecia universalis.
Zosteriform (dermatomal)[a]	See 'Dermatomal'.	See 'Dermatomal'.

Form (top view)	Definition	Clinical example(s)
Shape and topography of cutaneous lesions		
Circumscribed		
▪ Well circumscribed	Distinct demarcation between involved and uninvolved skin.	Psoriasis, vitiligo.
▪ Poorly circumscribed	Indistinct demarcation between involved and uninvolved skin.	Atopic dermatitis.
Digitate	Resembles fingers.	Digitate dermatosis, a form of parapsoriasis.
Figurate	A shape or form with rounded margins.	
▪ Annular	Shape of a ring (clear centrally).	Tinea corporis, granuloma annulare, erythema annulare centrifugum.
▪ Arciform	A segment of a ring; arch-like.	Urticaria, erythema annulare centrifugum.
▪ Polycyclic	Coalescence of several rings.	Subacute cutaneous lupus erythematosus.

Table 2. (continued)

Form (top view)	Definition	Clinical example(s)
Shape and topography of cutaneous lesions		
■ Serpiginous	Wavy pattern, reminiscent of a snake.	Cutaneous larva migrans.
Geometric		
■ Artefactual	Lesions induced by trauma are often angulated or have linear edges; the configuration can reflect sites of exposure to irritants or allergens.	Trauma (including self-induced and factitial).
■ Block-like	Embryonic pattern resembling rectangular blocks whose size can vary (see 'Segmental').	Pigmentary mosaicism, chimerism.
■ Checkerboard	See 'Block-like'.	Pigmentary mosaicism, chimerism.
Guttate	Small, with a shape that often resembles a droplet.	Guttate psoriasis, idiopathic guttate hypomelanosis; often multiple similar-appearing lesions.
Oval	A round shape with slight elongation, resembling that of an ellipse or egg.	Pityriasis rosea.
Polygonal	A lesion whose shape resembles a polygon with multiple angles.	Lichen planus.
Polymorphic	Variable sizes and shapes as well as types of lesions.	Polymorphic light eruption, Kawasaki disease.
Reticulate	Net-like or lacy pattern.	Livedo reticularis, erythema ab igne, oral lichen planus.
Round (discoid)	Circular or coin-shaped.	Discoid lupus erythematosus, nummular eczema, fixed drug eruption.

Form (profile/side view)	Definition	Clinical example(s)
Acuminate	Elevated with tapering to a sharp point(s).	Filiform wart, cutaneous horn.
Depressed	Surface below that of normal adjacent skin.	Dermal atrophy: atrophoderma. Lipoatrophy: antiretroviral therapy, corticosteroid injections.
Domed	Hemispherical form.	Intradermal melanocytic naevus, fibrous papule of the nose, molluscum contagiosum.
Flat-topped	Elevated with a flat top.	Lichen planus, lichen striatus, condylomata lata.
Papillomatous	Multiple projections resembling a nipple.	Papillomatous intradermal melanocytic naevus, epidermal naevus.
Pedunculated	Papule or nodule attached by a thinner stalk.	Skin tag (acrochordon).
Raised edge	Elevated peripheral rim.	Porokeratosis.
Umbilicated	Small central depression.	Varicella, herpes simplex, molluscum contagiosum.
Verruciform	Multiple projections resembling a wart.	Verrucae.

Table 2. (continued)

Texture or feel	Definition	Clinical example(s)
Palpation of cutaneous lesions		
Atrophy	A diminution of tissue, divided into epidermal, dermal and subcutaneous.	Epidermal: lichen sclerosus. Dermal: anetoderma. Subcutaneous: lipoatrophy.
Compressible	Pressure leads to reduction in volume.	Venous lake.
Firm	Feels solid and compact.	Cutaneous metastasis, dermatofibroma.
Fixed	Is not mobile.	Osteoma, Heberden nodes, tumour attached to deep soft tissue.
Fluctuant	Compressible, implying liquefaction.	Inflamed epidermoid cyst, abscess.
Induration	Firm texture in the absence of calcification or bone formation.	Morphoea, systemic sclerosis.
Mobile	Can be moved over deeper soft tissue structures.	Lipoma, epidermoid inclusion cyst, dermatofibroma.
Pulsatile	Throbs.	Arteriovenous malformation.
Rock hard	Very hard.	Calcinosis cutis, osteoma cutis.
Rope-like	Feels like a rope within the skin.	Thrombophlebitis.
Rough	Lesion with an uneven and coarse surface.	Actinic keratosis.
Rubbery	Resembles rubber: firm but with some compressibility.	Epidermoid inclusion cyst, reactive lymph nodes.
Smooth	Even, uniform surface.	Fibrous papule of the nose.
Soft	Compressible, shape easy to change or mould.	Skin tag, intradermal melanocytic naevus, neurofibroma.
Warm	Temperature higher than normal surrounding skin.	Arteriovenous malformation, erysipelas, cellulitis.

[a]Some clinicians also use the term segmental for a zosteriform/dermatomal distribution pattern.
[b]CHILD, congenital hemidysplasia with ichthyosiform erythroderma and limb defects.
Reproduced from the *British Journal of Dermatology* 2016;174:1351, with permission from John Wiley & Sons Ltd.

Chapter 1

Differential diagnosis

1.1 Introduction

When faced with a patient with an undiagnosed dermatological problem, start by returning to the basics of medical consultation, as follows.

Take a history

- What are the symptoms (cutaneous and non-cutaneous: itch, pain, fever)?
- How bad is the itch/pain? Use rating scale: 0 (none) to 10 (very severe).
- Do symptoms interrupt sleep? Use rating scale: 0 (sound sleep) to 10 (no sleep at all).
- When did symptoms begin?
- Is there a rash?
- If so, did it arise before or after itch/pain/fever began?
- Are any close contacts affected by similar symptoms?
- Any new drugs including over the counter products?
- Any recent surgical procedures or injuries?
- General medical, surgical, allergy and drug history.
- History of eczema in childhood, asthma or hay fever?
- Relevant family history?

Examine the patient

- Entire skin.
- If itchy, be sure to examine finger and toe webs for burrows.
- Mucosal surfaces.
- In an unwell patient, record temperature, pulse, blood pressure. Conduct a full medical examination.

Then work through the appropriate diagnostic tables which provide, by symptoms, morphology and body site, the possible causes of the problem.

As you can see from the contents list on page 1, alphabetical order has been used to simplify your access to the appropriate section.

1.2 By symptoms

1.2.1 Fever and a rash – acute presentation of an unwell patient

Fever most commonly indicates bacterial or viral infection. If there is no systemic sepsis, localised rashes associated with infection tend to cause fewer systemic symptoms than generalised rashes associated with infection. Mucosal involvement is common. There are some acute auto-inflammatory disorders that mimic infection due to neutrophil activation.

Consider performing the following tests:
- Swab for bacterial and viral culture if blisters, erosions, pustules or crusts.
- Blood culture if high fever.
- CBC, CRP.
- Coagulation screen if purpura or very sick patient.
- PCR and serology for specific bacteria or viruses.
- Echocardiography if emboli suspected.
- Skin biopsy of fresh skin lesions for histology and culture.

Treatment depends on the cause. Consider referral to emergency department if you are suspicious of serious infection or the patient is very unwell.

Differential diagnosis

Consider:
- Is the rash localised or generalised? What is its distribution? Are mucosal sites involved?
- Severity of symptoms?
- Predominant morphology: erythema, blisters/erosions, pustules/crusts, purple/black areas?

Fever and localised rash ▶ PAINFUL RED, HOT SKIN

- **Cellulitis** – see Section 2.1.2
  - ☐ unilateral swelling/induration
  - ☐ spreads over hours to days
  - ☐ may have associated wound or skin disease

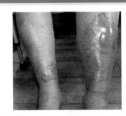

- **Erysipelas** – see Section 2.1.2
  - ☐ unilateral or bilateral large plaques with sharp, stepped edge
  - ☐ large blisters
  - ☐ face, lower legs or anywhere
  - ☐ spreads over hours to days
  - ☐ may have associated lymphangitis (red streak to local lymph nodes)
  - ☐ culture *Streptococcus pyogenes*

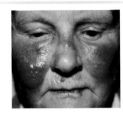

- **Erythema nodosum** – see Section 3.14
  - ☐ tender subcutaneous nodules
  - ☐ usually on lower legs

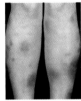

■ **Panniculitis – other** – see Section 3.14

    ☐ many causes

    ☐ often associated with underlying disease

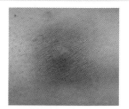

Fever and localised rash ▶ PROMINENT BLISTERS/EROSIONS

■ **Enteroviral vesicular stomatitis** (HFM in an adult) – see Section 2.3.3

    ☐ mainly young children

    ☐ symmetrical vesicles – mainly hands, feet and mouth

    ☐ can extend to limbs and buttocks

    ☐ culture/PCR enterovirus

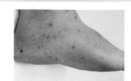

■ **Herpes simplex** – see Section 2.3.4

    ☐ monomorphic, umbilicated vesicles, erosions, crust

    ☐ culture/PCR *Herpes simplex*

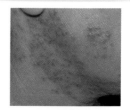

■ **Herpes zoster** – see Section 2.3.5

    ☐ dermatomal

    ☐ painful

    ☐ monomorphic vesicles (early), erosions, crust and ulceration (late)

    ☐ culture/PCR varicella-zoster virus

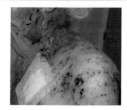

■ **Impetigo** – see Section 2.1.4

    ☐ crusted plaques, vesicles, bullae, pustules

    ☐ culture *Staphylococcus aureus* +/− *Streptococcus pyogenes*

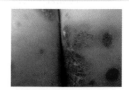

Fever and localised rash ▶ PUSTULES

■ **Folliculitis/furunculosis** – see Section 2.1.3

    ☐ based on hair follicle

    ☐ fever if multiple or secondary cellulitis

    ☐ culture *Staphylococcus aureus, Pseudomonas*

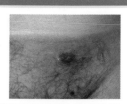

■ **Neutrophilic dermatosis of dorsal hands** – see www.dermnetnz.
org/topics/neutrophilic-dermatosis-of-the-hands/

    ☐ dorsum of hands

    ☐ culture negative

    ☐ biopsy confirmatory

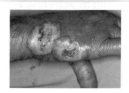

Fever and localised rash ▶ Purple/black areas

- **Ecthyma** – see Section 2.1.1
  - ☐ not very unwell
  - ☐ eschar
  - ☐ small deep ulcers
  - ☐ culture *Staph. aureus* +/– *Strep. pyogenes*

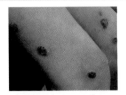

- **Meningococcal disease** – see www.dermnetnz.org/topics/meningococcal-disease
  - ☐ rapid deterioration in status
  - ☐ purpura of extremities and more generally in extremis (purpura fulminans, figure)
  - ☐ neck stiffness
  - ☐ eyes sensitive to light
  - ☐ obtunded
  - ☐ blood culture/PCR *Neisseria meningitidis*

- **Necrotising fasciitis** – see www.dermnetnz.org/topics/necrotising-fasciitis
  - ☐ very sick; septic shock
  - ☐ rapid spread of cellulitis with purpura/blistering (figure, Fournier gangrene)
  - ☐ anaesthetic areas in early lesions
  - ☐ bacterial culture essential

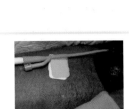

- **Necrotising spider bite** – see www.dermnetnz.org/topics/spider-bites
  - ☐ endemic venomous spiders
  - ☐ spider must be observed to make this diagnosis
  - ☐ central punctum with purpura/necrosis, surrounding erythema and induration

- **Vascular occlusion** – see www.dermnetnz.org/topics/vascular-skin-problems
  - ☐ cholesterol emboli
    - ▪ recent vascular/cardiac procedure
  - ☐ septic emboli (left)
    - ▪ endocarditis, arthritis
  - ☐ calciphylaxis (right)
    - ▪ renal dialysis, diabetes

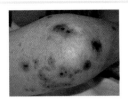
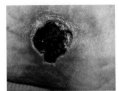

Fever and generalised rash ▶ Redness

- **Drug hypersensitivity syndrome** – see Section 3.5.2
  - ☐ morbilliform or other rash
  - ☐ drug within 8 weeks of onset
  - ☐ other organs affected (renal, hepatic, respiratory, haematological)
  - ☐ may have eosinophilia

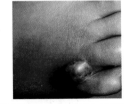
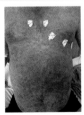

■ Erythema infectiosum/fifth disease – see Section 2.3.3

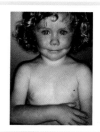

- ☐ child > adult
- ☐ slapped red cheek appearance
- ☐ relapsing reticulate rash on arms
- ☐ serology/PCR Parvovirus B19

■ Erythema marginatum – see www.dermnetnz.org/topics/rheumatic-fever

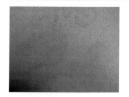

- ☐ rheumatic fever
- ☐ evanescent annular/polycyclic rash with elevated border with temperature spike
- ☐ evidence of streptococcal infection

■ Erythroderma (red rash affecting >90% body surface) – see Section 3.8

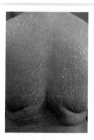

- ☐ pre-existing atopic eczema, psoriasis (right)
- ☐ new onset: drug eruption, pityriasis rubra pilaris, lymphoma

■ Kawasaki disease – see www.dermnetnz.org/topics/kawasaki-disease

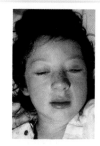

- ☐ young child with red skin and mucosal surfaces
- ☐ swollen hands and feet
- ☐ peeling a late feature
- ☐ lymphadenopathy
- ☐ cardiac artery aneurysms
- ☐ other organ involvement leads to a variety of signs
- ☐ no specific diagnostic test

■ Measles – see Section 2.3.3

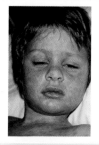

- ☐ red eyes, red tongue, Koplik spots
- ☐ coryza, cough
- ☐ rash has bronze hue
- ☐ serology/RT-PCR measles

■ Non-specific exanthem – see Section 2.3.4

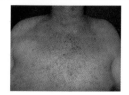

- ☐ upper respiratory symptoms

- **Rare infections** – see www.dermnetnz.org/topics/ skin-infections/
  - ☐ arbovirus (recent travel)
  - ☐ rubella (unvaccinated; image courtesy of Dr T. Evans)
  - ☐ typhoid fever

- **Rare inflammatory disorders** – see www.dermnetnz.org/topics/ autoinflammatory-syndromes
  - ☐ various auto-inflammatory syndromes
  - ☐ often, genetic markers present

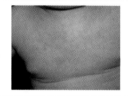

- **Roseola/erythema subitum** – see Section 2.3.3
  - ☐ infant
  - ☐ high fever + upper respiratory symptoms
  - ☐ rash is brief
  - ☐ serology for herpes virus 6 and 7 is not generally available

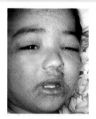

- **Scarlet fever** (*Strep. pyogenes*) – see Section 2.3.3
  - ☐ strawberry tongue
  - ☐ scarlatiniform rash: tiny red macules or rough papules
  - ☐ swollen then peeling hands
  - ☐ evidence of streptococcal infection

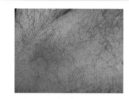

Fever and generalised rash ▶ BLISTERS/EROSIONS

- **Acute febrile neutrophilic dermatosis** – see www.dermnetnz. org/topics/acute-febrile-neutrophilic-dermatosis
  - ☐ neck, limbs, upper trunk
  - ☐ pseudovesicular plaques, blisters, pustules, purpura, or ulceration
  - ☐ disease associations: rheumatoid arthritis, inflammatory bowel disease, autoimmune arthritis, myeloid dysplasia
  - ☐ biopsy suggestive (neutrophils)

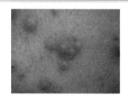

- **Bullous drug eruption** – see Section 3.5.2
  - ☐ blistering form of drug hypersensitivity syndrome
  - ☐ drug within 8 weeks of onset
  - ☐ other organs affected
  - ☐ may have eosinophilia

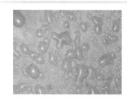

- **Enterovirus infection** – see Section 2.3.3
  - ☐ mild systemic symptoms
  - ☐ vesicular eruption
  - ☐ often followed by nail shedding
  - ☐ PCR/serology enterovirus

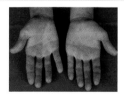

- **Erythema multiforme** – see Section 3.7
  - ☐ mainly hands, feet, face
  - ☐ target lesions
  - ☐ often preceded by herpes simplex, orf, vaccination, drug, etc.

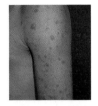

- **Mycoplasma** – see **www.dermnetnz.org/topics/mycoplasma-pneumoniae-infection**
  - ☐ erythema multiforme or Stevens–Johnson syndrome-like eruption
  - ☐ may or may not have pneumonia
  - ☐ serology *Mycoplasma pneumoniae*

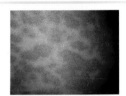

- **Staphylococcal scalded skin** – see **www.dermnetnz.org/topics/staphylococcal-scalded-skin-syndrome**
  - ☐ infant or elderly, diabetic or renal impairment
  - ☐ discomfort is mild
  - ☐ develops from localised bullous impetigo
  - ☐ culture *Staph. aureus*

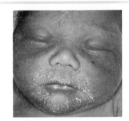

- **Stevens–Johnson/toxic epidermal necrolysis** – see Section 3.5.4
  - ☐ patient very unwell
  - ☐ nearly always drug-induced
  - ☐ red skin comes off in sheets

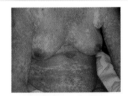

- **Varicella** (chickenpox) – see Section 2.3.3
  - ☐ more itch than pain
  - ☐ mainly scalp, face, trunk
  - ☐ culture/PCR varicella-zoster virus

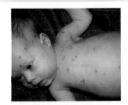

Fever and generalised rash ▶ Pustules/crusts

May involve mucosal surfaces.

- **Acute generalised exanthematous pustulosis** (AGEP) – see **www.dermnetnz.org/topics/acute-generalised-exanthematous-pustulosis**
  - ☐ drug eruption
  - ☐ biopsy suggestive

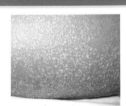

- **Eczema herpeticum** – see **www.dermnetnz.org/topics/eczema-herpeticum**
  - ☐ prior eczema or rarely, other skin disease
  - ☐ clustered monomorphic, umbilicated vesicles, pustules or crusts
  - ☐ culture/PCR *Herpes simplex*

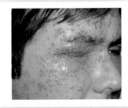

- **Generalised pustular psoriasis** (Zumbusch) – see www.dermnetnz.
  org/topics/generalised-pustular-psoriasis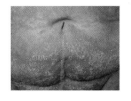
    - may or may not have history of plaque psoriasis
    - symmetrical eruption of numerous superficial pustules on red skin
    - often annular, flexural
    - associated with hypocalcaemia
    - biopsy suggestive

- **Varicella** – see Section 2.3.3
    - more itch than pain
    - mainly scalp, face, trunk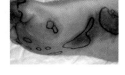
    - culture/PCR varicella-zoster virus

Fever and generalised rash ▸ WIDESPREAD PURPLE/BLACK AREAS

- **Purpura fulminans/disseminated intravascular coagulation** –
  see www.dermnetnz.org/topics/disseminated-intravascular-
  coagulation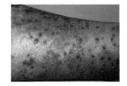
    - usually due to meningococcal disease (neck stiffness,
      photophobia)
    - rapid deterioration in mental status
    - purpura initially affects extremities
    - blood cultures/meningococcal PCR may reveal cause

- **Vasculitis** – see Section 3.23
    - palpable purpura
    - recent infection or drug or underlying chronic disease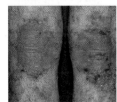
    - biopsy confirmatory

1.2.2 Itchy skin

Itch is defined by a desire to scratch. An acute
or chronic itchy rash is most often due to
dermatitis/eczema. Dermatitis can be primary,
or secondary to scratching.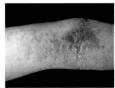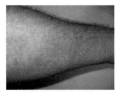
  Stages are as follows.
- **Acute dermatitis:**
    - red, oozy, swollen skin (top left)
- **Subacute dermatitis:**
    - red, dry skin (top right)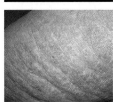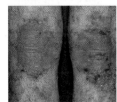
- **Chronic dermatitis:**
    - skin coloured
    - dark, dry, thickened skin with prominent
      lines (lichenification, bottom left)
- **Infected dermatitis:**
    - painful, swollen, pustules, crusting
      (bottom right).

If clinical diagnosis of an itchy skin problem is uncertain, consider performing the following tests:

- Dermatoscopic examination of hair shaft, if scalp affected (see fig.).

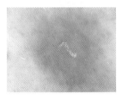

- Dermatoscopic examination of possible burrows, if hands affected (see fig.).

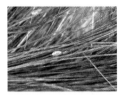

- Swab for bacterial and viral culture if pustules or crusting.
- Skin biopsy for histopathology, and if available, direct immunofluorescence (see fig.).

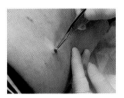

- If itch is generalised and no primary skin rash observed, check blood count, iron studies, renal, liver and thyroid function, chest X-ray.

General treatments for itchy skin conditions may include:

- Topical emollients, hydrocortisone cream.
- 1% menthol cream to cool localised itchy areas.
- Oral antihistamines.
- Tricyclic antidepressants such as amitriptyline.

Differential diagnosis

Consider:

- Is the itch localised or generalised? What is its distribution?
- Is there a primary rash or not?
- Erosions, crusting, bruising and infection can be due to excoriation and are of no help diagnostically.

Very itchy skin with localised rash

- **Contact dermatitis** – see Section 3.6.4
  - site depends on cause
  - irritant > allergen
  - asymmetrical, odd shapes
  - often intermittent

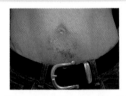

- **Head lice** – see Section 2.4.2
  - egg cases close to scalp
  - blood spots behind ears

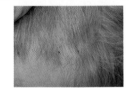

- **Insect bites/papular urticaria** – see Section 2.4.1
  - crops of urticated papules
  - central punctum or vesicle
  - favour exposed sites, depending on cause

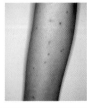

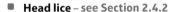

Lichen planus – see Section 3.11
- may be localised to any site
- grouped firm polygonal violaceous plaques
- biopsy confirmatory

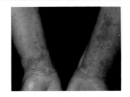

Lichen sclerosus – see Section 3.12
- vulva > penis > elsewhere
- white dry skin
- sometimes, purpura, blisters, resorption, scarring
- biopsy confirmatory

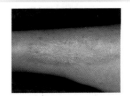

Lichen simplex – see Section 3.6.8
- localised lichenification
- common sites: wrist, ankle, neck, genitals
- sometimes bilateral

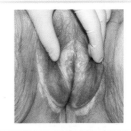

Pompholyx (dyshidrotic eczema) – see Section 3.6.11
- crops of vesicles along fingers, toes, palms, soles

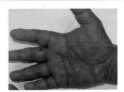

Venous dermatitis – see Section 3.6.13
- affects one ankle initially then may spread to other leg and can generalise (autoeczematisation)
- signs of venous disease: hardened, narrowed ankle (lipodermatosclerosis), orange–brown discoloration (haemosiderin)
- +/– varicose veins

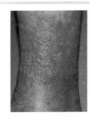

Mildly itchy skin with localised rash

Asteatotic eczema – see Section 3.6.2
- crazy paving, red cracked patches
- mainly lower legs

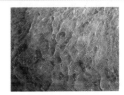

Psoriasis – see Section 3.19
- itch is sometimes severe
- localised variant affects scalp, elbows, knees; or palms and soles

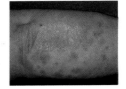

- **Seborrhoeic dermatitis** – see Section 3.6.12
  - ☐ in and around hair-bearing scalp, eyebrows, hairy chest
  - ☐ skin folds behind ears, nasolabial fold, axilla
  - ☐ salmon pink, flaky

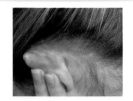

Very itchy skin with generalised rash

- **Atopic dermatitis** (eczema) – see Section 3.6.2
  - ☐ mainly flexural, symmetrical
  - ☐ may have dry skin

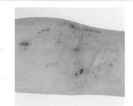

- **Bullous pemphigoid** – see Section 3.2
  - ☐ elderly, especially with brain injury
  - ☐ may start like eczema or urticaria
  - ☐ large blisters
  - ☐ biopsy confirmatory

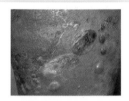

- **Dermatitis herpetiformis** – see www.dermnetnz.org/topics/dermatitis-herpetiformis
  - ☐ crops of tiny blisters, quickly scratched
  - ☐ biopsy confirmatory

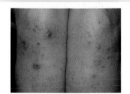

- **Discoid eczema** – see Section 3.6.5
  - ☐ bilateral, not symmetrical
  - ☐ roundish plaques

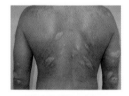

- **Disseminated secondary eczema** – see Section 3.6.6
  - ☐ non-specific dermatitis
  - ☐ initial site often venous dermatitis
  - ☐ can also follow localised dermatophyte infection, e.g. tinea pedis

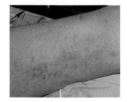

- **Erythroderma** – see Section 3.8
  - ☐ whole body (>85%) involvement
  - ☐ preceding eczema, psoriasis or *de novo*
  - ☐ also consider pityriasis rubra pilaris, lymphoma, drug

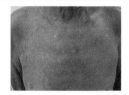

- **Lichen planus** – see Section 3.11
  - ☐ skin +/– mucosal surfaces
  - ☐ grouped firm polygonal violaceous plaques on wrists, shins, lower back
  - ☐ lacy white pattern in buccal mucosa
  - ☐ painful erosions on tongue, vulva, vagina, penis
  - ☐ biopsy confirmatory

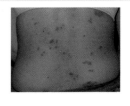

- **Mycosis fungoides** (cutaneous T-cell lymphoma) – see www.dermnetnz.org/topics/cutaneous-t-cell-lymphoma
  - ☐ slowly evolving slightly scaly annular and roundish patches, plaques and sometimes nodules
  - ☐ various morphologies
  - ☐ buttocks, breasts common initial sites
  - ☐ biopsy confirmatory

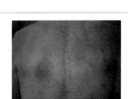

- **Neurodermatitis** – see Section 3.6.8
  - ☐ multiple lichenified plaques

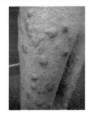

- **Nodular prurigo** – see www.dermnetnz.org/topics/nodular-prurigo
  - ☐ bilateral nodules on limbs resemble keratoacanthomas
  - ☐ papular variant

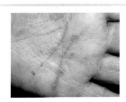

- **Scabies** – see Section 2.4.3
  - ☐ burrows between fingers, wrist creases
  - ☐ may be secondarily infected
  - ☐ papules in axillae, groin, penis
  - ☐ polymorphous rash on trunk
  - ☐ scale-crust between fingers, elbows, scalp in elderly or immune suppressed

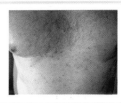

- **Transient acantholytic dermatosis** (Grover disease) – see Section 3.21
  - ☐ older male
  - ☐ red crusted papules on central trunk
  - ☐ may be precipitated by sweat
  - ☐ symmetrical on scalp, shoulders, elbows, buttocks, knees

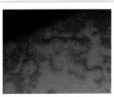

- **Urticaria** – see Section 3.22
  - ☐ acute <6 weeks
  - ☐ chronic >6 weeks
  - ☐ spontaneous or inducible weals
  - ☐ no blisters or dryness or scale
  - ☐ scratch skin to elicit linear weal in dermographism

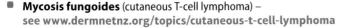
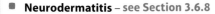
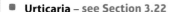

Mildly itchy skin with generalised rash

- **Psoriasis** – see Section 3.19
  - ☐ itch is sometimes severe
  - ☐ symmetrical well-circumscribed plaques with silvery scale
  - ☐ generalised large or small plaques

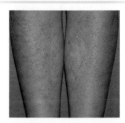

- **Xerotic eczema** – see Section 3.6.2
  - ☐ Generally dry skin

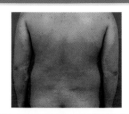

Localised itchy skin without rash

There may be secondary lesions due to scratching: erosions, purpura, lichen simplex and secondary infection. Localised itch is often neuropathic/neurogenic. If scalp is itchy, look carefully for head lice and their egg cases.

- **Brachioradial pruritus** – see www.dermnetnz.org/topics/brachioradial-pruritus
  - ☐ arms
  - ☐ figure shows purpura due to rubbing

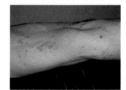

- **Meralgia paraesthetica** – see www.dermnetnz.org/topics/meralgia-paraesthetica
  - ☐ lateral thighs
  - ☐ figure shows secondary lichen simplex

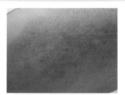

- **Notalgia paraesthetica** – see www.dermnetnz.org/topics/notalgia-paraesthetica
  - ☐ scapula
  - ☐ figure shows pigmentation due to rubbing

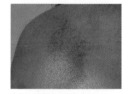

- **Scrotal pruritus** – see Section 3.6.8
  - ☐ figure shows severe lichenification

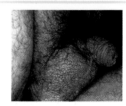

- **Vulval pruritus** – see Section 3.18
  - ▢ figure shows severe lichenification

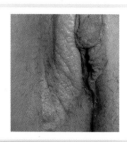

Generalised itchy skin without rash

Examine carefully for scabetic burrows.

- **Pruritus of pregnancy** – see www.dermnetnz.org/topics/
  skin-problems-in-pregnancy/
  - ▢ patient is pregnant

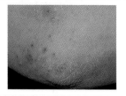

- **Systemic disease** – see www.dermnetnz.
  org/topics/itch-pruritus
  - ▢ chronic renal insufficiency
  - ▢ cholestasis
  - ▢ iron deficiency
  - ▢ polycythaemia vera
  - ▢ hyperthyroidism
  - ▢ lymphoma
  - ▢ diabetic neuropathy
  - ▢ drug-induced (e.g. opioid,
    vancomycin flushing)
  - ▢ unknown origin

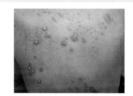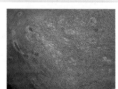

1.2.3 Painful skin conditions

The most common painful non-traumatic skin conditions are due to infection. Swab for bacterial and viral culture if there is any doubt as to the cause. Biopsy can be helpful in chronic conditions.

Painful localised rash with redness, blisters/erosions/pustules/crusting/fever

- **Cellulitis** – see Section 2.1.2
  - ▢ patient febrile, unwell
  - ▢ redness and swelling
  - ▢ CBC/FBC: neutrophil leucocytosis, raised CRP, *Strep. pyogenes*
    blood culture

- **Erysipelas** – see Section 2.1.2
  - ▢ patient febrile, unwell
  - ▢ spreading painful hot well-demarcated erythema, large thin
    blisters
  - ▢ CBC/FBC: neutrophil leucocytosis, raised CRP, *Strep. pyogenes*
    blood culture

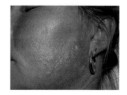

- **Furunculosis/boil** – see Section 2.1.3
  - ☐ based on hair follicle
  - ☐ may lead to abscess formation

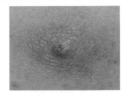

- **Herpes simplex** – see Section 2.3.4
  - ☐ primary or recurrent secondary disease
  - ☐ crops of tender vesicles, ulcers, swelling
  - ☐ may be within the distribution of a cutaneous nerve

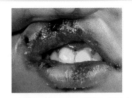

- **Herpes zoster** – see Section 2.3.5
  - ☐ unilateral vesicles
  - ☐ dermatomal

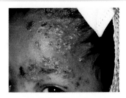

Painful ulcer

- **Arterial insufficiency** – see www.dermnetnz.org/topics/arterial-ulcer
  - ☐ cool periphery
  - ☐ absent or reduced pulses

- **Pyoderma gangrenosum** – see www.dermnetnz.org/topics/pyoderma-gangrenosum
  - ☐ often associated with underlying inflammatory bowel disease, rheumatoid arthritis, myeloid blood dyscrasia
  - ☐ irregular shape with overhanging purple edge

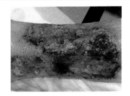

- **Vascular occlusion** – see www.dermnetnz.org/topics/vascular-skin-problems
  - ☐ stellate purpura
  - ☐ wound necrosis

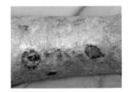

- **Vasculitis** – see Section 3.23
  - ☐ small or medium vessel inflammation
  - ☐ various causes

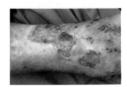

Painful tumour

- **Angioleiomyoma** – see www.dermnetnz.org/topics/leiomyoma

- **Angiolipoma** – see www.dermnetnz.org/topics/angiolipoma

- **Glomus tumour** (top) – see www.dermnetnz.org/topics/glomus-tumours

- **Perineural spread,** e.g. from basal cell carcinoma – see Section 5.4

- **Squamous cell carcinoma** (bottom) – see Section 5.12

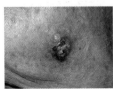
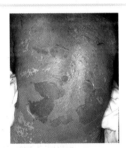

Generalised painful rash

- **Acute febrile neutrophilic dermatosis** – see www.dermnetnz.org/topics/acute-febrile-neutrophilic-dermatosis
  - neck, limbs
  - pseudovesicular plaques or bullae
  - may involve mucosal surfaces

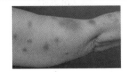

- **Stevens–Johnson/toxic epidermal necrolysis** – see Section 3.5.4
  - patient very unwell
  - severe adverse drug eruption
  - extensive mucosal ulceration (eyes, mouth, genitals, anus)
  - painful erythema, morbilliform eruption or diffuse extensive painful red skin which soon evolves to blistering, loss of epidermis

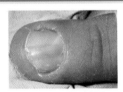

Pain and purple/black colour

- **Ecthyma** – see Section 2.1.4
  - eschar
  - small deep ulcers
  - culture *Staph. aureus*

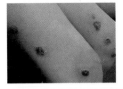

- **Necrotising fasciitis** – see www.dermnetnz.org/topics/necrotising-fasciitis
  - very sick
  - rapid spread
  - anaesthetic areas

- **Necrotising spider bite** – see www.dermnetnz.org/topics/spider-bites
  - endemic venomous spiders
  - spider must be observed to make this diagnosis
  - central punctum with purpura/necrosis, surrounding erythema and induration

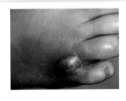

- **Vascular occlusion** – see www.dermnetnz.
  org/topics/vascular-skin-problems
  - ☐ cholesterol emboli (top left)
    - ▪ recent vascular procedure
  - ☐ septic emboli (top right)
    - ▪ endocarditis, arthritis
  - ☐ calciphylaxis (bottom left)
    - ▪ renal dialysis, diabetes

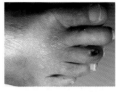
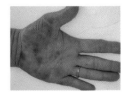
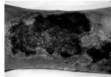

- **Vasculitis** – see Section 3.23
  - ☐ palpable purpura
  - ☐ recent infection or drug or underlying chronic disease

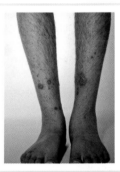

Pain without cutaneous signs

Name depends on body site, e.g.:
- Glossodynia (tongue).
- Meralgia paraesthetica (lateral thigh).
- Pudendal nerve entrapment (perineum).
- Scrotodynia.
- Vulvodynia.

1.3 By morphology

1.3.1 Introduction

See the *Terminology* section at the start of the book if you are unclear about any of the following terms. The primary eruptions commonly seen are as follows:
- Macules and patches.
- Nodules and tumours.
- Papules.
- Plaques.
- Purpura.
- Pustules.
- Telangiectasia.
- Ulcers.
- Vesicles and bullae.
- Weals.

In addition, the following secondary changes may be seen:
- Crusting.
- Erosion.
- Excoriation.
- Necrosis.
- Scaling.
- Sclerosis.
- Sinus formation.

1.3.2 Blistering diseases

- Vesicles are small blisters less than 5 mm in diameter.

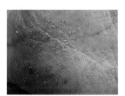

- A bulla is a larger blister. Note that the plural of bulla is bullae.

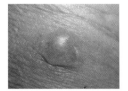

- Blisters may break or the roof of the blister may become detached forming an erosion.

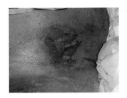

- Exudation of serous fluid forms a crust.

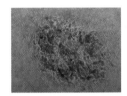

Acute blistering diseases

Acute blistering diseases can be generalised or localised to one body site, and are due to infection or inflammatory disorders. Although most commonly eczematous, generalised acute blistering diseases can be life threatening and often necessitate hospitalisation.

Acute blistering conditions should be investigated by taking swabs for bacterial and viral culture. Skin biopsy may be helpful in making a diagnosis.

Acute generalised blistering disease

Acute febrile neutrophilic dermatosis – see www.dermnetnz.
org/topics/acute-febrile-neutrophilic-dermatosis

- [ ] neck, limbs, upper trunk
- [ ] pseudovesicular plaques, blisters, pustules, purpura or ulceration
- [ ] disease associations: rheumatoid arthritis, inflammatory bowel disease, autoimmune arthritis, myeloid dysplasia
- [ ] biopsy suggestive

Atypical enterovirus infection – see Section 2.3.3

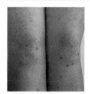

- [ ] widespread vesicular eruption
- [ ] clears in a few days

Chickenpox/varicella – see Section 2.3.3

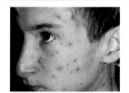

- [ ] childhood illness; more serious in adults
- [ ] scalp, face, oral mucosa, trunk
- [ ] culture/PCR varicella-zoster virus

Dermatitis – see Section 3.6

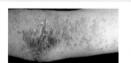

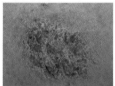

- [ ] atopic dermatitis (left)
- [ ] discoid eczema (right)

Drug hypersensitivity syndrome – see Section 3.5.2

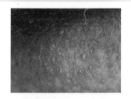

- [ ] drug started up to 8 weeks prior to onset
- [ ] morbilliform eruption that may blister (without necrolysis)
- [ ] often, mucosal involvement
- [ ] multiorgan damage (renal, hepatic, respiratory, haematological)
- [ ] often, marked eosinophilia

Eczema herpeticum – see www.dermnetnz.org/topics/eczema-herpeticum

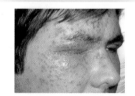

- [ ] history of atopic eczema
- [ ] momomorphic cluster of umbilicated vesicles
- [ ] culture/PCR Herpes simplex

Erythema multiforme – see Section 3.7

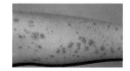

- [ ] reaction, e.g. to infection
- [ ] acute eruption of papules, plaques, target lesions
- [ ] acral distribution: cheeks, elbows, knees, hands, feet
- [ ] may have mucositis (lips, conjunctiva, genitals)

- **Polymorphic light eruption** – see Section 3.17
  - ☐ affects body sites exposed to sun, e.g. hands, upper chest, feet
  - ☐ papules, plaques, sometimes targetoid
  - ☐ may spare face
  - ☐ arises within hours of exposure to bright sunlight

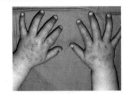

- **Staphylococcal scalded skin syndrome** – see www.dermnetnz. org/topics/staphylococcal-scalded-skin-syndrome
  - ☐ young child
  - ☐ miserable
  - ☐ red skin comes off in sheets
  - ☐ evidence of staphylococcal infection

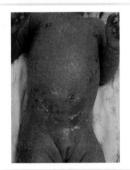

- **Stevens–Johnson syndrome/toxic epidermal necrolysis** – see Section 3.5.4
  - ☐ patient very unwell
  - ☐ mucosal involvement
  - ☐ nearly always drug-induced
  - ☐ rarely due to mycoplasma infection
  - ☐ painful red skin may come off in sheets or have multiple coalescing blisters

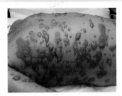

Acute localised blistering disease

- **Acute dermatitis** – see Section 3.6.1
  - ☐ contact dermatitis
  - ☐ plant dermatitis (left)
  - ☐ pompholyx (right)

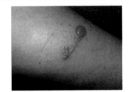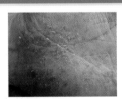

- **Bullous impetigo** – see Section 2.1.4
  - ☐ rapidly enlarging plaque
  - ☐ swab *Staph. aureus*
  - ☐ complicates wounds, scabies, etc.

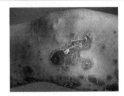

- **Chilblains** – see Section 3.3
  - ☐ fingers, toes
  - ☐ exposed to cold
  - ☐ purplish tender plaques

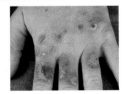

Enteroviral vesicular stomatitis – see Section 2.3.3
- hand, foot and mouth
- clears in a few days

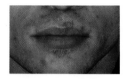

Erysipelas – see Section 2.1.2
- acute febrile illness
- swab *Strep. pyogenes*

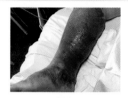

Fixed drug eruption – see www.dermnetnz.org/topics/fixed-drug-eruption
- recurring rash, often in same site
- due to intermittent drug taken within 24 hours of rash
- single or few lesions
- central blister

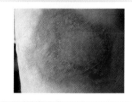

Herpes simplex – see Section 2.3.4
- monomorphic, umbilicated
- culture/PCR *Herpes simplex*

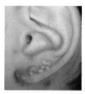

Herpes zoster (shingles) – see Section 2.3.5
- dermatomal
- culture/PCR varicella-zoster virus

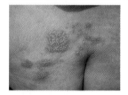

Insect bites and stings – see Section 2.4.1
- crops of urticated papules
- central vesicle or punctum
- favour exposed sites

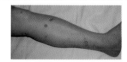

Miliaria – see www.dermnetnz.org/topics/miliaria
- central trunk
- sweat rash
- vesicles are very superficial

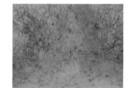

Necrotising fasciitis – see www.dermnetnz.org/topics/necrotising-fasciitis
- very sick; septic shock
- rapid spread of cellulitis with purpura/blistering
- anaesthetic areas in early lesions
- bacterial culture essential

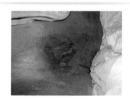

- **Transient acantholytic dermatosis** – see Section 3.21
  - ☐ acute or chronic
  - ☐ elderly males
  - ☐ itchy or asymptomatic
  - ☐ crusted papules

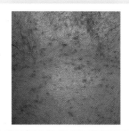

- **Trauma** – see www.dermnetnz.org/topics/reactions-to-external-agents
  - ☐ history of injury or neuropathy
  - ☐ friction, thermal, ultraviolet radiation, chemical, fracture

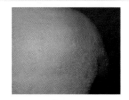

Chronic blistering diseases

Diagnosis of chronic blistering diseases often requires skin biopsy for histopathology and direct immunofluorescence. A blood test for specific antibodies (indirect immunofluorescence) may also prove helpful in making the diagnosis of an acquired immunobullous disease.

Blistering genodermatoses

- **Benign familial pemphigus** (Hailey-Hailey disease) – see www.dermnetnz.org/topics/hailey-hailey-disease
  - ☐ confined to flexures

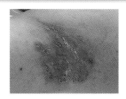

- **Epidermolysis bullosa** – see www.dermnetnz.org/topics/epidermolysis-bullosa
  - ☐ various types
  - ☐ onset at birth or early childhood

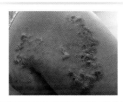

- **Mastocytosis** – see www.dermnetnz.org/topics/mastocytosis
  - ☐ various types
  - ☐ often, onset in childhood

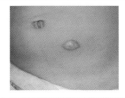

Chronic acquired blistering

- **Bullous pemphigoid** – see Section 3.2
  - ☐ mainly cutaneous (rarely mucosal)
  - ☐ mostly affects the elderly (rarely infants, children)
  - ☐ often associated stroke or dementia
  - ☐ subepidermal bullae
  - ☐ often eczematous or urticarial precursors

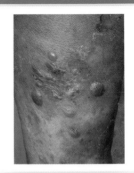

- **Dermatitis herpetiformis** – see www.dermnetnz.org/topics/
  dermatitis-herpetiformis
  - ☐ associated gluten sensitive enteropathy
  - ☐ intensely itchy; vesicles often removed by scratching leaving erosions
  - ☐ symmetrical on scalp, shoulders, elbows, knees, buttocks

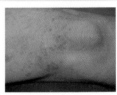

- **Other immunobullous diseases** –
  see www.dermnetnz.org/topics/
  blistering-skin-conditions
  - ☐ cicatricial pemphigoid
  - ☐ pemphigoid gestationis (left)
  - ☐ linear IgA dermatosis
  - ☐ epidermolysis bullosa acquisita
  - ☐ pemphigus vulgaris (right)
  - ☐ pemphigus foliaceus
  - ☐ paraneoplastic pemphigus

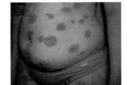 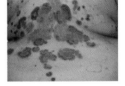

- **Porphyria cutanea tarda** – see www.dermnetnz.org/topics/
  porphyria-cutanea-tarda
  - ☐ metabolic photosensitivity
  - ☐ skin fragility, bullae, milia
  - ☐ dorsum of hands, face
  - ☐ onset in middle age

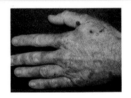

1.3.3 Macules and patches

Macules are strictly defined as flat or non-palpable areas of colour change less than 15 mm in diameter; patches are larger.

Non-febrile erythema: diffuse or generalised macules and patches

- **Acute, relapsing and chronic urticaria** – see Section 3.22
  - ☐ treatment may result in erythema without weals

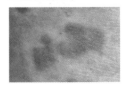

- **Drug eruption** – see Section 3.5.1
  - ☐ new drug (within a few days)

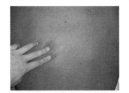

- **Secondary syphilis** – see www.dermnetnz.org/topics/syphilis
  - ☐ may also be febrile
  - ☐ often involves palms, soles, oral mucosa
  - ☐ lymphadenopathy

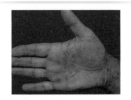

- **Urticaria-like rashes** – see www.dermnetnz.org/topics/urticaria-and-urticaria-like-conditions
  - ☐ weals last >24 hours
  - ☐ associated systemic symptoms
  - ☐ figure shows urticarial vasculitis

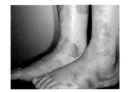

- **Viral exanthema** – see Section 2.3.1
  - ☐ non-specific toxic erythema

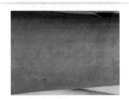

Non-febrile erythema: localised macules and patches ▶ ACUTE

- **Sunburn** – see www.dermnetnz.org/topics/sunburn
  - ☐ sun-exposed sites
  - ☐ consider photosensitising drugs

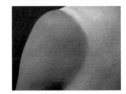

- **Thermal burn** – see www.dermnetnz.org/topics/thermal-burns
  - ☐ contact with hot item
  - ☐ consider neuropathy

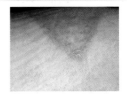

Non-febrile erythema: localised macules and patches ▶ CHRONIC

- **Erythematotelangiectatic rosacea** – see Section 3.20
  - ☐ mid-face
  - ☐ flushing

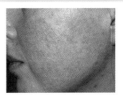

- **Erythromelalgia** – see www.dermnetnz.org/topics/erythromelalgia
  - ☐ feet, ankles
  - ☐ painful

Brown macules and patches: diffuse or generalised macules and patches

- **Addison disease** – see www.dermnetnz.org/topics/addison-disease
  - ☐ unwell patient

- **Capillaritis** – see Section 3.23
  - ☐ pigmented purpura
  - ☐ often: monomorphous macules
  - ☐ dermoscopy reveals red dots

- **Drug-induced pigmentation** (bleomycin) – see www.dermnetnz.org/topics/drug-induced-skin-pigmentation
  - ☐ sometimes photosensitive distribution

- **Haemochromatosis** – see www.dermnetnz.org/topics/haemochromatosis
  - ☐ bronze diabetes

- **Mastocytosis** (urticaria pigmentosa) – see www.dermnetnz.org/topics/mastocytosis
  - ☐ various kinds

- **Systemic sclerosis** (hyperpigmented compared to sister) – see www.dermnetnz.org/topics/systemic-sclerosis
  - ☐ patchy or diffuse
  - ☐ also, hypopigmented macules
  - ☐ scleroderma, sclerodactyly
  - ☐ systemic symptoms

Brown macules and patches: anywhere

- **Erythema ab igne** – see www.dermnetnz.org/topics/erythema-ab-igne
  - ☐ due to contact with local heat source
  - ☐ reticulate (vascular) pattern

- **Erythema dyschromicum perstans** – see www.dermnetnz.org/topics/erythema-dyschromicum-perstans
  - ☐ greyish hue
  - ☐ sharp margins
  - ☐ may start with inflammatory episode

Fixed drug eruption – see www.dermnetnz.org/topics/fixed-drug-eruption

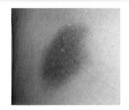

- usually, drug taken intermittently
- can involve mucosal surfaces

Melanoma *in situ* – see Section 5.9

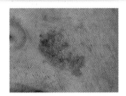

- slowly enlarging irregular macule
- asymmetry of colour and structure

Pigmented naevus – see Section 5.10

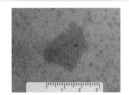

- café au lait macule
- junctional naevus
- ephilides, lentigines

Post-inflammatory pigmentation (acne) – see Section 4.9

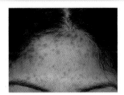

- preceding eczema, psoriasis, acne, etc.
- distribution depends on cause
- lichen planus has purplish hue

Brown macules and patches: site specific ▶ FACE

Melasma – see Section 4.7

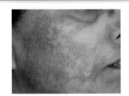

- blotchy symmetrical pigmentation
- cheeks, nose, forehead, chin, upper lip

Brown macules and patches: site specific ▶ NECK

Berloque dermatitis – see www.dermnetnz.org/topics/phytophotodermatitis

- contact dermatitis to fragrance

Brown macules and patches: site specific ▶ LOWER LEGS

Capillaritis – see Section 3.23

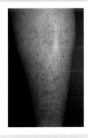

- often: monomorphous macules
- dermoscopy reveals red dots

- **Venous eczema** – see Section 3.6.13
  - ☐ haemosiderin deposition

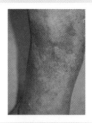

Brown macules and patches: site specific ▶ Flexures

- **Acanthosis nigricans** – see www.dermnetnz.org/topics/acanthosis-nigricans
  - ☐ symmetrical
  - ☐ also affects neck
  - ☐ velvety surface

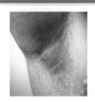

- **Erythrasma** – see www.dermnetnz.org/topics/erythrasma
  - ☐ spares vault of axilla, groin crease
  - ☐ slightly flaky

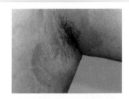

Brown macules and patches: site specific ▶ Trunk

- **Becker naevus** – see www.dermnetnz.org/topics/becker-naevus
  - ☐ unilateral
  - ☐ may have hypertrichosis

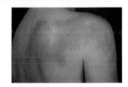

- **Pityriasis versicolor** – see Section 2.2.5
  - ☐ white, pink, brown macules
  - ☐ not always flaky

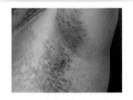

Blue/grey macules and patches: diffuse or generalised macules and patches

- **Drug-induced pigmentation** – see www.dermnetnz.org/topics/drug-induced-skin-pigmentation
  - ☐ sometimes photosensitive distribution
  - ☐ minocycline favours scars (figure)

- **Ochronosis** – see www.dermnetnz.org/topics/alkaptonuria-and-ochronosis
  - ☐ rare
  - ☐ site of hydroquinone application (figure)
  - ☐ alkaptonuria

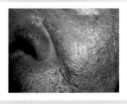

- **Postinflammatory pigmentation** – see Section 4.9
  - ☐ lichen planus

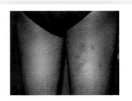

Blue/grey macules and patches: anywhere

- **Blue naevus** – see Section 5.10
  - ☐ scalp, face, hands, feet
  - ☐ spindle-cell melanocytic naevus

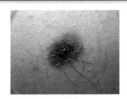

- **Dermal melanosis** – see www.dermnetnz.org/topics/lumbosacral-dermal-melanocytosis
  - ☐ rare except buttocks of neonates in dark skin

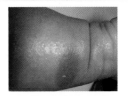

Purple macules and patches: any site

- **Livedo reticularis** – see www.dermnetnz.org/topics/livedo-reticularis
  - ☐ reticulate vascular pattern
  - ☐ various causes including vasculopathy, connective tissue disease, infection, malignancy

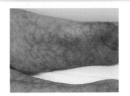

- **Purpura** – see www.dermnetnz.org/topics/purpura
  - ☐ bleeding into skin

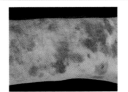

- **Venulectasia** – see www.dermnetnz.org/topics/telangiectasia/
  - ☐ blanches
  - ☐ dilated venules

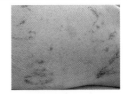

Purple macules and patches: distal distribution

- **Acrocyanosis** – see www.dermnetnz.org/topics/acrocyanosis
  - ☐ dusky discoloration of hands and feet
  - ☐ primary or secondary to malignancy, antiphospholipid syndrome, cold agglutinins, drugs

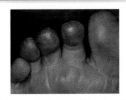

- **Cold injury** – see Section 3.3
  - ☐ chilblains
  - ☐ chilblain lupus (shown)
  - ☐ frostbite

- **Cryoglobulinaemia** – see www.dermnetnz.org/topics/ cryoglobulinaemia
  - ☐ petechiae in cooler body sites
  - ☐ essential (rare) or secondary to infection or autoimmune disease
  - ☐ systemic symptoms

White macules and patches: generalised pallor

- **Albinism** – see www.dermnetnz.org/topics/albinism
  - ☐ congenital

- **Anaemia or acute blood loss**
  - ☐ fatigue

- **Hypopituitarism**
  - ☐ systemic symptoms
  - ☐ decreased body hair

- **Systemic sclerosis** (salt and pepper hypo- and hyper-pigmentation) – see www.dermnetnz.org/topics/systemic-sclerosis
  - ☐ patchy or diffuse hypopigmentation
  - ☐ also, hyperpigmentation
  - ☐ scleroderma, sclerodactyly

White macules and patches: anywhere

- **Naevus anaemicus** – see www.dermnetnz.org/topics/ naevus-anaemicus
  - ☐ congenital
  - ☐ local variation in vascularity
  - ☐ vessels blanch on pressure

- **Naevus depigmentosus** – see www.dermnetnz.org/topics/ achromic-naevus
  - ☐ congenital
  - ☐ circumscribed area of hypopigmentation

- **Post-inflammatory hypopigmentation** – see Section 4.8
  - ☐ after injury, rash, infection, drug
  - ☐ shape and size depend on cause, e.g. psoriasis (figure)

- **Tuberous sclerosis** – see www.dermnetnz.org/topics/tuberous-sclerosis
  - ☐ ash-leaf macule
  - ☐ other signs, e.g. angiofibromas

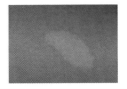

- **Vitiligo** – see Section 4.10
  - ☐ completely white patches or trichrome
  - ☐ bilateral, symmetrical
  - ☐ can affect sites of injury

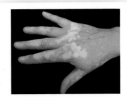

White macules and patches: face

- **Piebaldism** – see www.dermnetnz.org/topics/piebaldism
  - ☐ inherited and congenital
  - ☐ white forelock
  - ☐ white patches on face, trunk, knees

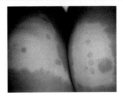

- **Pityriasis alba** – see Section 3.6.10
  - ☐ child or adolescent
  - ☐ cheeks or upper arms
  - ☐ oval dry pink or pale patches

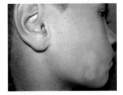

White macules and patches: limbs

- **Guttate hypomelanosis** – see www.dermnetnz.org/topics/idiopathic-guttate-hypomelanosis
  - ☐ sun-exposed sites

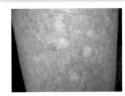

White macules and patches: trunk

- **Pityriasis versicolor** – see Section 2.2.5
  - ☐ mid–upper back and mid chest
  - ☐ pale, pink or brown macules, patches
  - ☐ diffuse bran-like scale
  - ☐ microscopy positive, culture negative

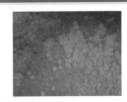

White distal digits

- **Vasospasm/Raynaud phenomenon** – see www.dermnetnz.org/topics/raynaud-phenomenon
  - ☐ intermittent attacks when cold

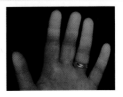

Yellow macules and patches: generalised

- **Carotenaemia** – see www.dermnetnz.org/topics/carotenaemia
  - ☐ most obvious on palms, soles
  - ☐ does not affect eyes

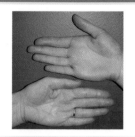

- **Jaundice**
  - ☐ greenish hue
  - ☐ corneal discoloration

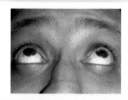

Yellow macules and patches: localised

- **Planar xanthomas** – see www.dermnetnz.org/topics/xanthomas
  - ☐ associated with hyperlipidaemia or paraproteinaemia in some patients

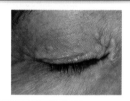

1.3.4 Papules and plaques

Very itchy papules, plaques

- **Dermatitis** (venous dermatitis) – see Section 3.6.1
  - ☐ various types of chronic dermatitis

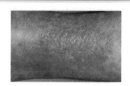

- **Insect bites/papular urticaria** – see Section 2.4.1
  - ☐ crops of discrete urticated papules
  - ☐ central vesicle or punctum
  - ☐ favour exposed sites

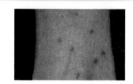

- **Prurigo mitis, nodularis** – see www.dermnetnz.org/topics/prurigo
  - ☐ intensely itchy papules and nodules
  - ☐ distal limbs

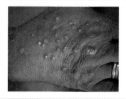

- **Scabies** – see Section 2.4.3
  - abrupt onset of symptoms
  - burrows in web spaces, lateral borders of fingers, wrist creases
  - may be impetiginised
  - papules in axillae, groin, penis
  - polymorphous rash on trunk
  - scale-crust between fingers, elbows, scalp in elderly or immune suppressed

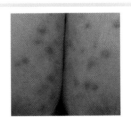

- **Transient acantholytic dermatosis** – see Section 3.21
  - sometimes, asymptomatic
  - older males
  - crusted papules
  - mid-trunk

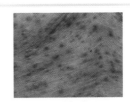

- **Urticaria** – see Section 3.22
  - evanescent weals
  - spontaneous and inducible types, e.g. dermographism (figure)

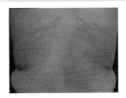

Follicular papules, plaques

- **Acne** – see Section 3.1
  - face, neck, upper trunk
  - comedones + inflammatory lesions

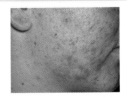

- **Follicular tumours: syndromes** – see www.dermnetnz.org/topics/hair-follicle-tumours
  - Birt–Hogg–Dubé (figure)
  - Cowden disease
  - Torre-Muir syndrome

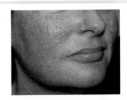

- **Folliculitis** (folliculitis keloidalis nuchae) – see Section 2.1.3
  - various types due to infection, occlusion, irritation and skin diseases

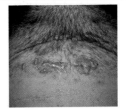

- **Keratosis pilaris** – see Section 4.6
  - non-inflammatory
  - upper outer arms, thighs
  - scaly central plug, often erythematous base
  - uncommon variants

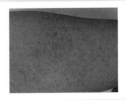

- **Pityriasis rubra pilaris** – see www.dermnetnz.org/topics/ pityriasis-rubra-pilaris
  - rare, various types
  - psoriasis-like with follicular prominence

- **Rosacea** – see Section 3.20
  - central-face
  - flushing

Non-follicular papules, plaques

- **Darier disease** – see www.dermnetnz.org/topics/darier-disease
  - genodermatosis
  - crusted papules scalp, trunk
  - flares with sun exposure

- **Eccrine/apocrine tumours** – see www.dermnetnz.org/topics/ sweat-gland-lesions
  - hidrocystoma
  - syringomas
  - poroma, and others

- **Miliaria** – see www.dermnetnz.org/topics/miliaria
  - mid-trunk
  - follows sweating

- **Milium/milia** – see Section 5.5
  - skin-coloured superficial sudoriferous papules

- **Pyogenic granuloma** – see Section 5.13
  - bleeding, soft growth

- **Vascular lesions: angioma** – see Section 5.13
    - ☐ compressible unless thrombosed

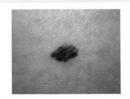

Scaly plaques: diffuse scale

- **Callus** – see www.dermnetnz.org/topics/corns-and-calluses
    - ☐ pressure site
    - ☐ localised hyperkeratosis
    - ☐ yellowish

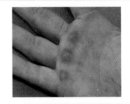

- **Cutaneous T-cell lymphoma** – see www.dermnetnz.org/topics/cutaneous-t-cell-lymphoma
    - ☐ irregular shape
    - ☐ poikiloderma
    - ☐ scale is usually mild

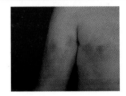

- **Discoid lupus erythematosus** – see Section 3.4
    - ☐ face, ears, scalp > upper trunk, hands
    - ☐ scale is due to plugged follicles
    - ☐ leads to scarring and dyspigmentation
    - ☐ can cause scarring alopecia

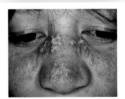

- **Lichen planus** – see Section 3.11
    - ☐ bilateral but often asymmetrical firm polygonal papules, plaques
    - ☐ adherent scale

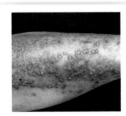

- **Lichen sclerosus** – see Section 3.12
    - ☐ white crinkled plaque
    - ☐ genital (90%)
    - ☐ most extragenital lichen sclerosus (10%) is on trunk

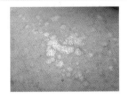

- **Pityriasis lichenoides** – see www.dermnetnz.org/topics/pityriasis-lichenoides
    - ☐ acute and chronic variants
    - ☐ mica scale

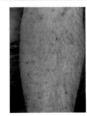

■ **Psoriasis** – see Section 3.19
  ☐ circumscribed erythematous plaques
  ☐ silvery scale

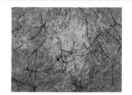

■ **Secondary syphilis** – see www.dermnetnz.org/topics/syphilis
  ☐ mainly trunk but involves palms, mucosa
  ☐ scale is usually mild

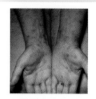

Scaly plaques: peripheral scale

■ **Annular erythema** – see www.dermnetnz.org/topics/erythema-annulare-centrifugum
  ☐ slow expanding rings
  ☐ peripheral trailing scale
  ☐ sometimes underlying systemic condition

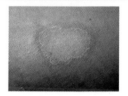

■ **Dermatophyte infection**: (tinea) – see Section 2.2.3
  ☐ irregular distribution and shape
  ☐ mycology microscopy and culture positive

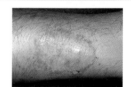

■ **Pityriasis rosea** – see Section 2.3.8
  ☐ herald patch
  ☐ oval 2–4 cm pink plaques on trunk
  ☐ peripheral trailing scale
  ☐ spares scalp, peripheries

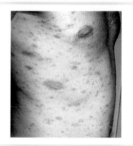

■ **Porokeratosis** – see www.dermnetnz.org/topics/porokeratosis
  ☐ non-inflammatory solitary or multiple lesions
  ☐ peripheral scaly rim around atrophic epidermis
  ☐ may be isolated, diffuse (distal limbs), dermatomal
    or linear in distribution

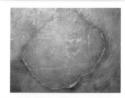

Papules, plaques with a smooth surface

■ **Granuloma annulare** – see Section 3.9
  ☐ often annular purplish plaques
  ☐ over hands, feet, elbows or anywhere

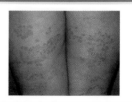

- **Insect bite/papular urticaria** – see Section 2.4.1
  - ☐ crops of urticated papules
  - ☐ central vesicle or punctum
  - ☐ favour exposed sites

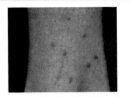

- **Keloid** – see www.dermnetnz.org/topics/keloids-and-hypertrophic-scars
  - ☐ excessive scar from minimal injury or acne
  - ☐ extends beyond site of injury/surgery

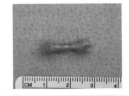
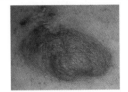

- **Lymphocytic infiltrate** – see www.dermnetnz.org/topics/jessner-lymphocytic-infiltrate
  - ☐ Jessner type or lymphocytoma cutis
  - ☐ erythematous irregular papule, plaque
  - ☐ most often face and upper trunk

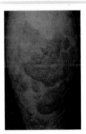

- **Lymphoma, leukaemia** – see www.dermnetnz.org/topics/leukaemia-cutis
  - ☐ erythematous irregular papule, plaque

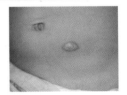

- **Mastocytoma** – see www.dermnetnz.org/topics/mastocytoma
  - ☐ urticated on rubbing
  - ☐ brownish plaque

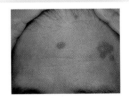

- **Other granulomas** – see www.dermnetnz.org/topics/granulomas/
  - ☐ sarcoidosis, granuloma faciale (face), erythema elevatum diutinum (trunk, limbs)
  - ☐ brownish irregular firm papule, plaque

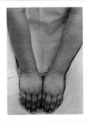

- **Polymorphous light eruption** – see Section 3.17
  - ☐ itchy papules on sun-exposed sites
  - ☐ appear a few hours after sun exposure

- **Urticaria** – see Section 3.22
    - ☐ weals
    - ☐ spontaneous and inducible types

- **Xanthoma** – see www.dermnetnz.org/topics/xanthomas
    - ☐ yellowish papule or plaque

Annular plaques

- **Annular erythema** – see www.dermnetnz.org/topics/erythema-annulare-centrifugum
    - ☐ slow expanding rings
    - ☐ peripheral trailing scale
    - ☐ sometimes underlying systemic condition

- **Dermatophyte infection** (tinea) – see Section 2.2.3
    - ☐ irregular distribution and shape
    - ☐ scaly; rarely blistered
    - ☐ mycology positive

- **Erythema chronicum migrans** – see www.dermnetnz.org/topics/lyme-disease/
    - ☐ slowly enlarging urticated erythema
    - ☐ follows tick bite
    - ☐ first stage of Lyme disease

- **Granuloma annulare** – see Section 3.9
    - ☐ usually, smooth surface
    - ☐ often, over joint

- **Psoriasis** – see Section 3.19
    - ☐ well-demarcated scaly plaque

- **Subacute lupus erythematosus** – see Section 3.4
  - ☐ upper trunk
  - ☐ provoked by sun exposure
  - ☐ ENA anti-Ro, La positive

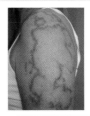

- **Urticaria** – see Section 3.22
  - ☐ weals
  - ☐ spontaneous and inducible types

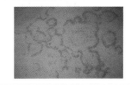

1.3.5 Purpura

What is purpura?

Purpura is the name given to discoloration of the skin or mucous membranes due to haemorrhage from small blood vessels.

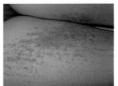
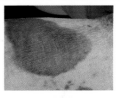

- Petechiae are small, purpuric lesions up to 2–3 mm across (top left).

- Palpable purpura are purpuric papules and plaques (bottom left).

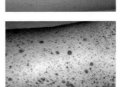
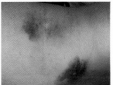

- Ecchymoses or bruises are larger extravasations of blood (top right).

- Extravasated blood usually breaks down and changes colour over a few weeks from purple, orange, brown and even blue and green (bottom right).

Classification of purpura – see www.dermnetnz.org/topics/purpura

There are many different types of purpura. Their classification depends on the appearance or cause of the condition.

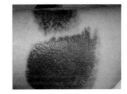

- **Thrombocytopenic purpura—due to destruction of platelets** (skin graft donor site in patient with thrombocytopenia)
  - ☐ primary thrombocytopenic purpura due to autoimmune or unknown reasons
  - ☐ secondary thrombocytopenic purpura due to external or internal factors, such as drugs, infections, systemic diseases

- **Other coagulation disorders**
  - ☐ dsseminated intravascular coagulation – clinical picture varies from a severe and rapidly fatal disorder (purpura fulminans, top) to a relatively minor disorder
  - ☐ heparin-induced thrombocytopenia – purpura and necrosis due to anti-platelet antibodies inducing platelet plugs that block blood vessels
  - ☐ warfarin-induced necrosis – purpura and necrosis due to blood clots related to relative protein C deficiency early in treatment
  - ☐ excessive anticoagulation (bottom; international normalised ratio 6.4)

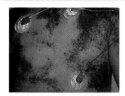

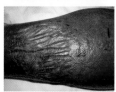

- **Vascular disorders—leakage of blood through the vessel wall**
  - ☐ damage to small blood vessels
  - ☐ increase in intraluminar pressure
  - ☐ deficient vascular support, as in aged and/or sun damaged skin especially in association with corticosteroid (senile or solar purpura)

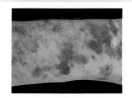

What are the signs and symptoms of purpura?

The signs and symptoms of purpura vary according to the type of purpura. The following broad generalisations may be made.

- Petechiae are usually present in thrombocytopenic purpura; there may be some external bleeding and bruising.

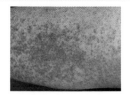

- Coagulation defects usually present as large ecchymoses and external bleeding; petechiae do not feature.

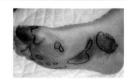

- Inflamed blood vessels (vasculitis) cause persistent and localised purpura with an erythematous inflammatory component – this may be palpable; ecchymoses and external bleeding are uncommon.

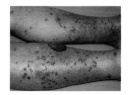

What is the treatment for purpura?

The underlying cause of purpura should be identified and treated accordingly.

1.3.6 Pustules

Pustules are small purulent vesicles, often less than 5 mm in diameter. Abscesses are larger ones.

- Pus can indicate bacterial, fungal or viral infection.
- Some pustules are sterile and are due to neutrophilic infiltrations in inflammatory skin disease.

Acute generalised pustular eruption

- **Acute generalised exanthematous pustulosis** – see www.
  dermnetnz.org/topics/acute-generalised-exanthematous-
  pustulosis
  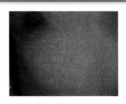
  - febrile illness
  - drug eruption
  - diffuse superficial pustules

- **Generalised pustular psoriasis** – see www.dermnetnz.org/
  topics/generalised-pustular-psoriasis
  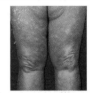
  - febrile illness
  - diffuse superficial pustules or annular plaques studded
    with pustules

Acute localised pustular eruption

- **Candidiasis** – see Section 2.2.2
  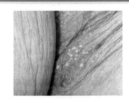
  - intertrigo, mucosal sites
  - superficial pustules that dry out easily; may erode
  - swab *Candida albicans*

- **Dermatophyte infection** – see Section 2.2.3
  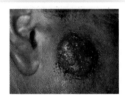
  - kerion: abscess formation
  - due to zoophilic fungus, e.g. *Microsporum canis*

- **Furunculosis** – see Section 2.1.3
  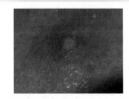
  - based on infection of hair follicle
  - may lead to abscess formation
  - swab *Staph. aureus*

- **Impetigo** – see Section 2.1.4
  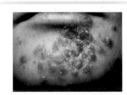
  - associated with head lice in young children
  - secondary to inflammatory seborrhoeic dermatitis
  - swabs: *Staph. aureus* +/– *Strep. pyogenes* I

Chronic generalised pustular eruption

- **Acne** – see Section 3.1
  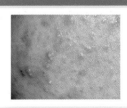
  - face, neck, upper trunk
  - comedones + inflammatory lesions
  - may scar if dermal inflammation

■ **Dermatophyte infection** – see Section 2.2.3
- ☐ irregular annular plaque with peripheral scale
- ☐ pustules of *Trichophyton interdigitale* on foot

■ **Erosive pustular dermatosis** – see www.dermnetnz.org/topics/
erosive-pustular-dermatosis
- ☐ sun damaged scalp
- ☐ often underlying squamous cell carcinoma
- ☐ greenish pus
- ☐ culture *Staph. aureus*

■ **Folliculitis** – see Section 2.1.3
- ☐ itchy or painful follicular pustules

■ **Localised pustulosis** – see www.dermnetnz.org/topics/
palmoplantar-pustulosis
- ☐ hands, feet
- ☐ sterile tender, itchy, pustules
- ☐ various types

■ **Miliaria** – see www.dermnetnz.org/topics/miliaria
- ☐ central trunk
- ☐ sweat rash
- ☐ pustules are very superficial

■ **Rosacea** – see Section 3.20
- ☐ mid-face
- ☐ erythema and flushing
- ☐ asymptomatic papules and pustules

■ **Scabies** – see Section 2.4.3
- ☐ irregular pustules on hands and feet
- ☐ burrows between fingers, volar wrists
- ☐ papules axillae, groin
- ☐ generalised polymorphous itchy rash, which may
  include pustules

1.3.7 Scaly rashes

Scale is surface keratin, a protein produced by keratinocytes. Skin diseases that have excessive scale or flaking (papulosquamous disorders) are due to epidermal inflammation or proliferation.

Scaly rashes have been present for weeks to months or longer.

Take a history

- What are the symptoms?
- When did the rash start?
- Do any family members have a similar problem?
- Record recent illness, past medical history and drugs.
- What is the effect of treatment?

Examine the patient

- Entire skin.
- Note distribution and morphology of lesions.
- Is the scale diffuse or peripheral, white or yellow, flaky or thick?

Diagnosis is generally clinical, but tests can be helpful when in doubt or for confirmation.

- Scraping for mycology (*Section 2.2.1 – fungal infections*).
- Dermoscopy for burrows (*Section 2.4.3*).
- Skin biopsy is often useful for confirmation, but close clinicopathological correlation is essential (*Section 6.2*).

Treatment depends on the cause.

Localised scaly rash present for <6 weeks

Irregular annular plaque with peripheral scale.

- **Dermatophyte infections** – see Section 2.2.3
    - tinea corporis – trunk, limbs
    - tinea cruris – groin
    - tinea pedis – feet
    - tinea manuum – hands
    - tinea faciei – face

Acute forms of tinea may also have follicular pustules.
Mycology positive.

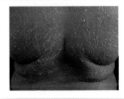

Generalised scaly rash present for <6 weeks ▶ WITH FEVER

- **Exfoliative dermatitis** – see Section 3.8
    - scaling form of erythroderma
    - starts as morbilliform or other pattern
    - often drug-induced

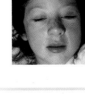

- **Kawasaki disease** – see www.dermnetnz.org/topics/kawasaki-disease
    - child
    - starts as morbilliform or erythematous rash
    - swelling of hands and feet
    - oral and ocular signs
    - lymphadenopathy

- **Scarlet fever** – see www.dermnetnz.org/topics/scarlet-fever
    - scarlatiniform rash (erythema then rough spots)
    - strawberry tongue
    - peeling starts after 5 days of illness
    - evidence of streptococcal infection

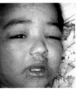

WITHOUT FEVER

- **Acute guttate psoriasis** – see www.dermnetnz.org/topics/guttate-psoriasis
  - ☐ round 0.5–3 cm red plaques with diffuse scale
  - ☐ trunk > limbs
  - ☐ may involve all body sites

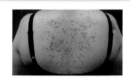

- **Pityriasiform or lichenoid drug eruption** – see www.dermnetnz.org/topics/lichenoid-drug-eruption
  - ☐ new drug (e.g. hydroxychloroquine)

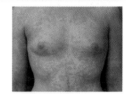

- **Pityriasis rosea** – see Section 2.3.8
  - ☐ herald patch
  - ☐ oval 2–4 cm pink plaques on trunk
  - ☐ peripheral, trailing scale
  - ☐ spares scalp, peripheries

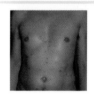

Localised scaly rash present for >6 weeks

- **Annular erythema** – see www.dermnetnz.org/topics/erythema-annulare-centrifugum
  - ☐ crops of slowly enlarging erythematous annular plaques on trunk
  - ☐ trailing scale

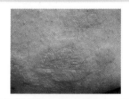

- **Dermatophyte infections** – see Section 2.2.3
  - ☐ tinea corporis – trunk, limbs
  - ☐ tinea cruris – groin
  - ☐ tinea pedis – feet
  - ☐ tinea manuum – hands
  - ☐ tinea faciei – face

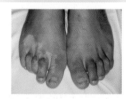

- **Discoid lupus erythematosus** – see Section 3.4
  - ☐ face, ears, scalp > upper trunk, hands
  - ☐ scale is partly due to plugged follicles
  - ☐ leads to scarring

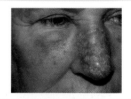

- **Keratosis pilaris** – see Section 4.6
  - ☐ upper arms > thighs > cheeks
  - ☐ hair follicles plugged with scale

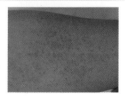

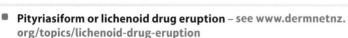

- **Palmoplantar keratoderma** – see www.dermnetnz.org/topics/
palmoplantar-keratoderma
    - ☐ thickened skin of palms and soles
    - ☐ congenital and acquired, punctate and diffuse variants

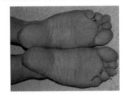

- **Pityriasis versicolor** – see Section 2.2.5
    - ☐ flaky rash on trunk
    - ☐ white, red, brown variants

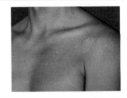

- **Psoriasis** – see Section 3.19
    - ☐ localised variant
    - ☐ scalp, elbows, knees or palms and soles

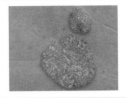

- **Seborrhoeic dermatitis** – see Section 3.6.12
    - ☐ in and around hair-bearing scalp, eyebrows, hairy chest
    - ☐ skin folds behind ears, nasolabial fold, axilla
    - ☐ salmon pink, flaky

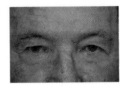

- **Subacute lupus erythematosus** – see Section 3.4
    - ☐ upper trunk, arms
    - ☐ photosensitive
    - ☐ annular, scaly plaques
    - ☐ leaves hypopigmented macules

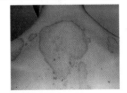

Generalised scaly rash present > 6 weeks

- **Chronic eczema/dermatitis** – see Section 3.6.1
    - ☐ itchy
    - ☐ lichenified

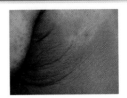

- **Chronic plaque psoriasis** – see Section 3.19
    - ☐ symmetrical well-circumscribed plaques with silvery scale
    - ☐ generalised large or small plaques

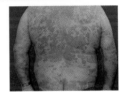

Crusted scabies – see Section 2.4.3
- scale is prominent between fingers, elbows, scalp
- may or may not be very itchy
- contacts have scabies

Ichthyosis – see Section 4.2
- dry skin

Lichen planus – see Section 3.11
- bilateral but asymmetrical firm papules, plaques
- polygonal shape
- itch and scale are variable

Tinea corporis, widespread – see Section 2.2.3
- irregular annular plaques
- peripheral scale

Uncommon disorders

Pityriasis lichenoides – see www.dermnetnz.org/topics/pityriasis-lichenoides
- trunk and limbs
- skin coloured or red, flat or indurated papules/small plaques
- mica scale (peels off in one sheet)

Pityriasis rubra pilaris – see www.dermnetnz.org/topics/pityriasis-rubra-pilaris
- psoriasis-like, symmetrical or erythrodermic scaly rash
- prominent keratoderma
- orange–red hue
- skip areas
- follicular prominence

Cutaneous T-cell lymphoma: cutaneous – see www.dermnetnz.org/topics/cutaneous-t-cell-lymphoma
- slowly evolving slightly scaly annular and roundish patches, plaques and sometimes nodules
- various morphologies including poikiloderma and erythroderma
- buttocks, breasts common initial sites

1.4 By body site

Some inflammatory skin conditions are recognised because of their primary localisation. Common acute and chronic conditions are listed together with some important uncommon or rare disorders.

It is important to take a full history, even when a disorder appears localised. A full skin examination can reveal the cause of a localised condition. Diagnosis is generally clinical, but tests can be helpful when in doubt or for confirmation.

- Painful, pustular, eroded, weeping, oozing or crusted rashes: swabs for bacteriology, virology (*Section 6.1*).
- Scaly rashes: scraping for mycology (*Section 6.1*).
- Chronic or recurrent dermatitis localised to specific sites: refer for patch tests (*Section 6.1*).
- Skin biopsy is often useful for confirmation but close clinico-pathological correlation is essential (*Section 6.2*).
- If considering lupus erythematosus (LE): CBC, ANA, ENA (*Section 6.1*).

The following specific sites are covered:
- Arms – see *Section 1.4.1*
- Ear – see *Section 1.4.2*
- Eyelid – see *Section 1.4.3*
- Face – see *Section 1.4.4*
- Flexures – see *Section 1.4.5*
- Genitalia – see *Section 1.4.6*
- Hands and feet – see *Section 1.4.7*
- Legs – see *Section 1.4.8*
- Lips – see *Section 1.4.9*
- Nails – see *Section 1.4.10*
- Oral mucosa – see *Section 1.4.11*
- Scalp – see *Section 1.4.12*
- Trunk – see *Section 1.4.13*

See also:
- *Fever and a rash (Section 6.1)*
- *Itchy skin (Section 1.2.2)*
- *Painful skin (Section 1.2.3)*
- *Morphology (Section 1.3)*
- *Pigmentary changes (Section 4.8)*
- *Solitary lesions (Chapter 5)*

Refer to DermNetNZ.org for rare disorders or rare presentations of common disorders.

1.4.1 Arms

Arms: bilateral, violaceous papules

- **Lichen planus** – see Section 3.11
  - ☐ volar wrists
  - ☐ firm, violaceous papules + white streaks
  - ☐ dusky post-inflammatory pigmentation
  - ☐ favour areas of earlier injury
  - ☐ also examine mouth

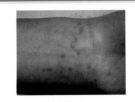

Arms: erosions/crusting

- **Herpes zoster** – see Section 2.3.5
  - ☐ acute pain
  - ☐ dermatomal distribution
  - ☐ erythema may precede vesicles
  - ☐ culture/PCR: varicella-zoster virus

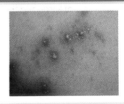

Arms: dry/scaly and very itchy

May also blister and swell.

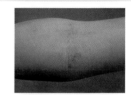

- **Allergic contact dermatitis** – see Section 3.6.4
    - acute flares on any site
    - asymmetrical, odd-shaped patches/plaques
    - patch tests positive

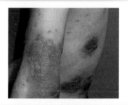

- **Atopic dermatitis** – see Section 3.6.3
    - antecubital fossa, wrists
    - acute flares are erythematous
    - chronic eczema is lichenified

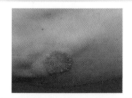

- **Discoid eczema** – see Section 3.6.5
    - coin-shaped crusted or dry plaques

Arms: dry/scaly with minimal itch

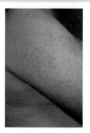

- **Keratosis pilaris** – see Section 4.6
    - follicular
    - extensor upper arms

- **Psoriasis** – see Section 3.19
    - extensor elbows
    - roughly symmetrical distribution
    - well-circumscribed erythematous scaly plaques
    - variable itch

Arms: multiple skin coloured papules

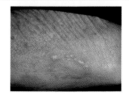

- **Granuloma annulare** – see Section 3.9
    - extensor elbows, dorsum of hands and fingers
    - arranged in rings

Arms: erythema without surface change

Erythema is less pronounced in dark skin.

- **Sunburn** – see www.dermnetnz.org/topics/sunburn
  - ☐ sun-exposed site

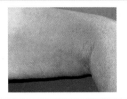

- **Urticaria** – see Section 3.22
  - ☐ weals can arise on any site
  - ☐ spontaneous and induced types

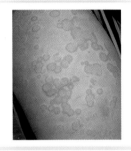

1.4.2 Ear

Ear: asymptomatic lesions

- **Comedones** – see www.dermnetnz.org/topics/comedones
  - ☐ acne (concha or anywhere)
  - ☐ discoid LE (concha)
  - ☐ solar comedones (lobe)

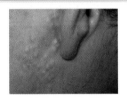

- **Gouty tophus** (photo courtesy of Dr Trevor Evans) – see www.dermnetnz.org/topics/gout
  - ☐ firm yellowish papules
  - ☐ often tender
  - ☐ hyperuricaemia

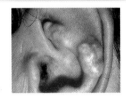

- **Keloid scar** – see www.dermnetnz.org/topics/keloids-and-hypertrophic-scars
  - ☐ posterior aspect of ear lobe
  - ☐ rubbery nodule
  - ☐ follows piercing

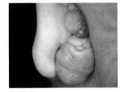

- **Weathering nodules**
  - ☐ elderly males
  - ☐ bilateral helices
  - ☐ fibrous 2–3 mm skin coloured papules
  - ☐ painless

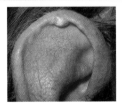

Ear: symptomatic lesions

- **Chondrodermatitis nodularis helicis** – see www.dermnetnz. org/topics/chondrodermatitis-nodularis-helicis
  - helix or antehelix
  - occasionally bilateral
  - on pressure site
  - scaly or crusted 3–8 mm papule
  - tender

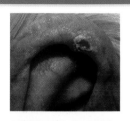

- **Contact dermatitis** – see Section 3.6.4
  - earring dermatitis due to nickel allergy
  - hair dye (paraphenylenediamine) allergy

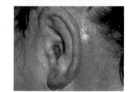

- **Juvenile spring eruption** – see www.dermnetnz.org/topics/ juvenile-spring-eruption
  - children
  - follows sun exposure a few hours earlier
  - itchy vesicles on helices

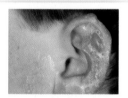

- **Otitis externa** – see www.dermnetnz.org/topics/otitis-externa
  - dermatitis involving ear canal
  - acute and chronic variants

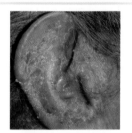

- **Relapsing polychondritis** (rare) – see www.dermnetnz.org/topics/ relapsing-polychondritis
  - may affect nose, trachea (hoarseness)
  - recurrent erythema and painful swelling ears, costochondral junctions
  - cartilage of trachea and larynx may collapse

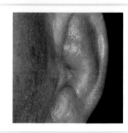

1.4.3 Eyelid

Eyelid: Asymptomatic lesions

- **Chalazion/meibomian cyst** (photo courtesy of Prof Raimo Suhonen) – see www.dermnetnz.org/topics/eyelid-skin-problems
  - eyelid margin papule

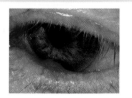

- **Hidrocystoma** – see www.dermnetnz.org/topics/
  cutaneous-cysts-and-pseudocysts
  - ☐ eyelid margin papule
  - ☐ translucent

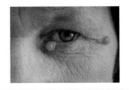

- **Syringomas** – see www.dermnetnz.org/topics/syringoma
  - ☐ upper and lower eyelids
  - ☐ eccrine origin

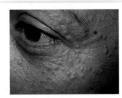

- **Xanthelasma** – see www.dermnetnz.org/topics/xanthomas
  - ☐ upper and lower medial eyelids
  - ☐ yellowish plaques

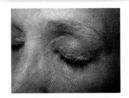

Eyelid: symptomatic lesions

- **Hordeolum/stye** – see www.dermnetnz.org/topics/
  eyelid-skin-problems
  - ☐ follicular infection

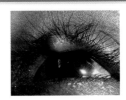

1.4.4 Face

Face: red papules/pustules

- **Acne vulgaris** – see Section 3.1
  - ☐ usually symmetrical appearance and onset often at puberty
  - ☐ open and closed comedones
  - ☐ inflammatory papules; nodules + cysts if severe

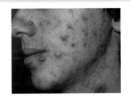

- **Periorificial dermatitis** – see Section 3.15
  - ☐ around mouth, nostrils, eyelids
  - ☐ spares 5–10 mm adjacent to orifice
  - ☐ inflammatory papules
  - ☐ may have erythema, flaking

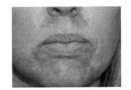

- **Pseudofolliculitis barbae** – see www.dermnetnz.org/topics/
  folliculitis-barbae
  - ☐ follicular papules
  - ☐ shaving rash – ingrown hairs

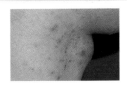

- **Rosacea** – see Section 3.20
  - ☐ inflammatory papules
  - ☐ flushing, erythema, telangiectasia
  - ☐ ocular rosacea/blepharitis
  - ☐ phymatous variants

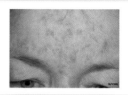

- **Tinea faciei** (chronic) – see Section 2.2.3
  - ☐ asymmetrical eruption
  - ☐ annular configuration is common
  - ☐ scaly edge
  - ☐ mycology positive

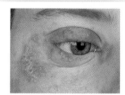

Face: erosions/crusting

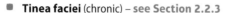

- **Herpes simplex** – see Section 2.3.4
  - ☐ monomorphic clustered vesicles or crusted papules
  - ☐ often locally recurrent in same site
  - ☐ swabs: *Herpes simplex*

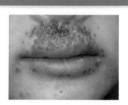

- **Herpes zoster** – see Section 2.3.5
  - ☐ dermatomal
  - ☐ painful
  - ☐ erythema may precede vesicles
  - ☐ culture/PCR: varicella-zoster virus

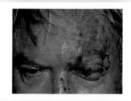

- **Impetigo** – see Section 2.1.4
  - ☐ irregular enlarging plaque
  - ☐ honey-coloured crusts
  - ☐ swabs: *Staph. aureus +/– Strep. pyogenes*

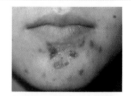

Face: dry/scaly and itchy

May also blister and swell.

- **Allergic contact dermatitis/eczema** – see Section 3.6.4
  - ☐ acute flares on any site
  - ☐ asymmetrical, odd-shaped patches/plaques
  - ☐ patch tests positive

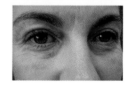

- **Atopic dermatitis/eczema** – see Section 3.6.3
  - ☐ eyelids, perioral sites including vermilion common
  - ☐ patchy or diffuse
  - ☐ intensely itchy
  - ☐ acute flares are erythematous
  - ☐ lichenification of eyelids with Dennie–Morgan folds (2 creases in lower eyelids)

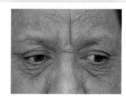

- **Irritant contact dermatitis** – see Section 3.6.4
  - ☐ common in atopics
  - ☐ provoked by cosmetics, cleansers, acne treatments, dust
  - ☐ dermatitis has sharp border

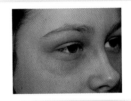

- **Photosensitive dermatitis** – see Section 3.16
  - ☐ exposed areas of face, arms, chest, legs
  - ☐ spares under hair, eyelids, creases
  - ☐ flares after exposure outdoors
  - ☐ may be drug-induced

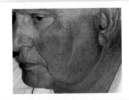

Face: dry/scaly with minimal itch

- **Actinic keratoses** – see Section 5.2
  - ☐ located on sun-exposed sites of temples, forehead, nose, cheekbones, angle of jaw, upper lip, lower vermilion lip
  - ☐ persistent small tender scaly papules, macules, plaques

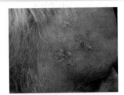

- **Discoid lupus erythematosus** (LE) – see Section 3.4
  - ☐ follicular plugging, hyperpigmentation, scarring
  - ☐ CBC, ANA, ENA often normal

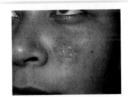

- **Psoriasis** – see Section 3.19
  - ☐ similar distribution to seborrhoeic dermatitis, + plaques in ears and preauricular sites
  - ☐ more pronounced and persistent than seborrhoeic dermatitis

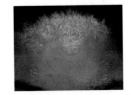

- **Seborrhoeic dermatitis** – see Section 3.6.12
  - ☐ hairline, eyebrows, skin folds, medial cheeks
  - ☐ blepharitis
  - ☐ erythema, flaking
  - ☐ skin rough on palpation

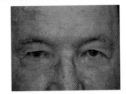

- **Tinea faciei** – see Section 2.2.3
  - ☐ young child or older adult
  - ☐ scaly edge
  - ☐ asymmetrical annular plaques
  - ☐ mycology positive

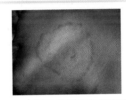

Face: skin coloured papules

- **Adnexal tumours** – see www.dermnetnz.org/topics/adnexal-tumours
  - various types and syndromes, e.g. Birt–Hogg–Dubé syndrome (figure)
  - follicular or eccrine origin

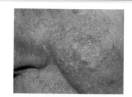

- **Comedones** – see www.dermnetnz.org/topics/comedones
  - acne (left) or
  - solar damage (right)

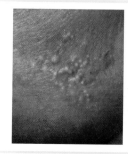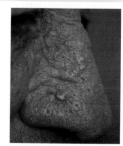

- **Milia** – see Section 5.5
  - periorbital or cheeks
  - superficial firm small papules

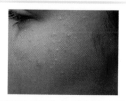

- **Sebaceous hyperplasia** – see www.dermnetnz.org/topics/sebaceous-hyperplasia
  - mostly >40 years
  - scattered on forehead, cheeks
  - yellowish with central dell

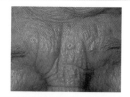

Face: plaques with smooth surface

- **Angioedema** – see Section 3.22
  - onset over minutes to hours; usually resolves within 24 hours
  - skin coloured soft to firm swelling

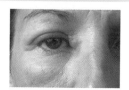

- **Basal cell carcinoma** – see Section 5.4
  - slowly enlarging destructive papule, nodule or plaque
  - early erosion, ulceration and bleeding

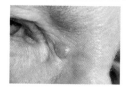

- **Granuloma faciale** – see www.dermnetnz.org/topics/granuloma-faciale
  - any site
  - yellowish brown to mauve infiltrated plaque

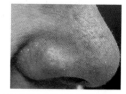

- **Sarcoidosis** – see www.dermnetnz.org/topics/sarcoidosis
  - yellowish brown to mauve infiltrated plaque
  - may arise within existing scar
  - lupus pernio affects nose and ears

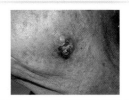

- **Squamous cell carcinoma** – see Section 5.12
  - enlarging tender scaly or crusted nodule

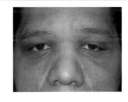

- **Tumid LE/Jessner lymphocytic infiltrate** – see Section 3.4
  - erythematous dermal plaques
  - check CBC, ANA, ENA

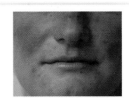

Face: erythema

Erythema is less pronounced in dark skin.

- **Dermatomyositis** – see www.dermnetnz.org/topics/dermatomyositis
  - violaceous eyelids – may be swollen
  - poikiloderma on the trunk and limbs
  - Gottron papules on fingers
  - may have muscle weakness

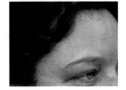

- **Flushing** – see www.dermnetnz.org/topics/flushing
  - intermittent redness, e.g. when hot, embarrassed or with certain foods
  - often lifelong tendency
  - systemically well
  - consider rosacea

- **Sunburn** – see www.dermnetnz.org/topics/sunburn
  - sun exposed site
  - spares eyelids, furrows, under chin

- **Systemic LE** – see Section 3.4
  - butterfly erythematous rash
  - systemic symptoms: tiredness, lethargy, arthralgia
  - check CBC, ANA, ENA

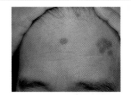
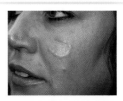
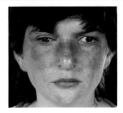

- **Telangiectasia** – see Section 5.13
    - ☐ may accompany flushing
    - ☐ vascular dilatation
    - ☐ various types

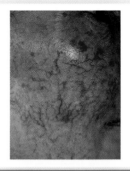

Face: brown macules/patches

Pigmentation is more pronounced in dark skin.

- **Erythema dyschromicum perstans** – see www.dermnetnz.org/topics/erythema-dyschromicum-perstans
    - ☐ grey–brown discoloration
    - ☐ any distribution
    - ☐ distinct border, sometimes red at first

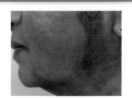

- **Melasma** – see Section 4.7
    - ☐ usually adult female
    - ☐ centrofacial, malar and mandibular patterns
    - ☐ spares eyelids, rare below jawline
    - ☐ symmetrical pigmentation with ragged border

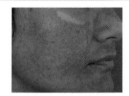

- **Post-inflammatory pigmentation** – see Section 4.9
    - ☐ preceding eczema, psoriasis, acne, etc.
    - ☐ distribution depends on cause

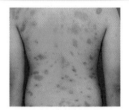

Face: pale or white macules/patches

- **Guttate hypomelanosis** – see Section 4.8
    - ☐ more commonly observed on limbs

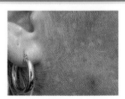

- **Pityriasis alba** – see Section 3.6.10
    - ☐ young child
    - ☐ cheeks, forehead
    - ☐ hypopigmentation, light scale

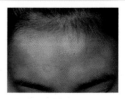

- **Post-inflammatory hypopigmentation** – see Section 4.8
  - ☐ preceding eczema, psoriasis, acne, etc.
  - ☐ distribution depends on cause

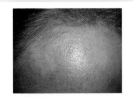

- **Vitiligo** – see Section 4.10
  - ☐ most often periocular, perioral
  - ☐ white, smooth surface

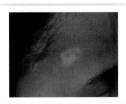

1.4.5 Flexures

Flexures: unilateral, asymmetrical rashes

- **Chronic dermatophyte infection** – see Section 2.2.3
  - ☐ athlete's foot (maceration between toes, left)
  - ☐ tinea cruris (groin, right)
  - ☐ mycology microscopy and culture positive

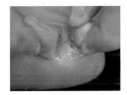
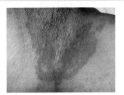

- **Candidiasis** – see Section 2.2.2
  - ☐ itchy moist peeling red and white skin
  - ☐ small superficial papules and pustules

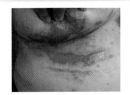

- **Erythrasma** – see www.dermnetnz.org/topics/erythrasma
  - ☐ irregular pigmented, dry plaque
  - ☐ positive Wood lamp examination
  - ☐ often asymptomatic

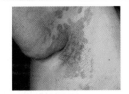

- **Folliculitis/furunculosis** – see Section 2.1.3
  - ☐ based on hair follicle
  - ☐ culture *Staph. aureus*

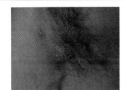

- **Impetigo** – see Section 2.1.4
  - ☐ irregular enlarging plaque
  - ☐ honey-coloured crusts
  - ☐ swabs: *Staph. aureus* +/– *Strep. pyogenes*

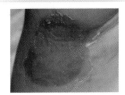

Flexures: bilateral, symmetrical rashes

- **Atopic dermatitis** – see Section 3.6.3
  - very itchy, scratched
  - acute flares are erythematous
  - chronic eczema is lichenified

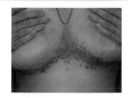

- **Benign familial pemphigus** (Hailey–Hailey disease) –
  see www.dermnetnz.org/topics/hailey-hailey-disease
  - genodermatosis
  - blisters and erosions

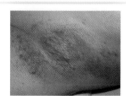

- **Contact allergic dermatitis** (reaction to clothing dye) – see Section 3.6.4
  - rash may also have asymmetrical distribution
  - itchy, may blister
  - positive patch tests
  - allergen may be:
    - fragrance, preservative or medicament
    - component of underwear, e.g. rubber in elastic, nickel in bra wire

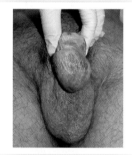

- **Irritant contact dermatitis** (due to postsurgical incontinence) –
  see Section 3.6.4
  - irritants: body fluids – sweat, urine, friction, soap, excessive washing
  - convexities > creases

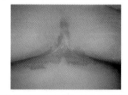

- **Flexural psoriasis** – see Section 3.19
  - chronic
  - circumscribed red shiny plaques

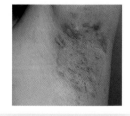

- **Hidradenitis suppurativa** – see Section 3.10
  - boil-like follicular papules and nodules
  - discharging sinuses and scars

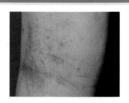

- **Scabies** – see Section 2.4.3
  - ☐ nodular form has papules in axillae, groin, and on buttocks
  - ☐ burrows between fingers, wrists
  - ☐ intense itch, especially at night
  - ☐ dermatoscopy of burrow reveals mite

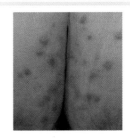

- **Seborrhoeic dermatitis** – see Section 3.6.12
  - ☐ patchy, salmon pink plaques
  - ☐ mild symptoms

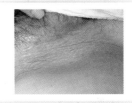

1.4.6 Genitalia

Anogenital region: itchy conditions

- **Allergic contact dermatitis** – see Section 3.6.4
  - ☐ positive patch tests
  - ☐ allergen may be:
    - ▪ fragrance, preservative or medicament
    - ▪ plant allergen transferred on fingers may cause penile oedema (figure)
    - ▪ component of underwear, e.g. rubber in elastic, nickel in bra wire

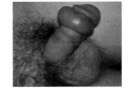

- **Irritant contact dermatitis** – see Section 3.6.4
  - ☐ irritants: body fluids – sweat, urine, friction, soap, excessive washing
  - ☐ convexities > creases

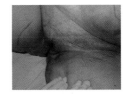

- **Lichen sclerosus** – see Section 3.12
  - ☐ mostly females >40 years
  - ☐ white thickened plaques on clitoral hood, labia minora, perineum (females) or glans penis (males)
  - ☐ petechiae, atrophy, scarring

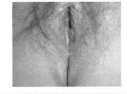

- **Lichen planus** (cutaneous, mucosal types) – see Section 3.11
  - ☐ violaceous, polymorphous or annular plaques on skin
  - ☐ lacy pattern on mucosa
  - ☐ similar to lichen sclerosus
  - ☐ also examine mouth

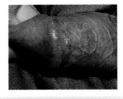

Lichen simplex – see Section 3.6.8

- ☐ unilateral > bilateral thickened plaque
- ☐ increased skin markings
- ☐ secondary to pruritus

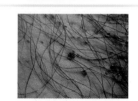

Psoriasis – see Section 3.19

- ☐ well-defined, erythematous, scaly thick plaques
- ☐ itch is variable

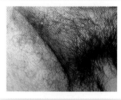

Pubic lice – see www.dermnetnz.org/topics/pubic-lice

- ☐ moving lice
- ☐ brown egg cases on hair shafts
- ☐ blood spots

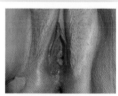

Tinea cruris – see Section 2.2.3

- ☐ slowly spreads over weeks to months
- ☐ irregular annular plaques
- ☐ peeling, scaling
- ☐ mycology positive

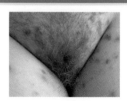

Vulvovaginitis or balanitis due to *Candida albicans* – see Section 2.2.2

- ☐ itchy moist peeling red and white skin
- ☐ small superficial papules and pustules

Anogenital region: painful conditions

Vulvitis, balanitis.

Bacterial infection (impetigo) – see Section 2.1.1

- ☐ boils
- ☐ impetigo
- ☐ folliculitis

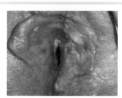

Erosive lichen planus – see Section 3.11

- ☐ very tender, red vaginal orifice
- ☐ may have other signs of lichen planus

Hidradenitis suppurativa – see Section 3.10
- boil-like follicular papules and nodules
- discharging sinuses and scars

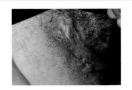

Non-infectious ulcer – see www.dermnetnz.org/topics/
non-sexually-acquired-genital-ulceration
- aphthous ulceration
- Behçet syndrome
- erythema multiforme
- fixed drug eruption

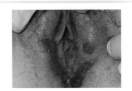

Scrotodynia or vulvodynia (pain without signs)
- provoked vestibulodynia – see www.dermnetnz.org/topics/vestibulodynia
- peno-scrotoynia – see www.dermnetnz.org/topics/scrotodynia
- dysaesthetic or neuropathic vulvodynia – see www.dermnetnz.org/topics/
  generalised-vulvodynia

Sexually transmitted infection – see www.dermnetnz.org/
topics/sexually-transmitted-infections
- primary syphilis
- lymphogranuloma venereum
- chancroid
- granuloma inguinale

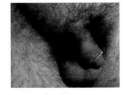

Viral infection – see Section 2.3
- herpes simplex (left)
- herpes zoster

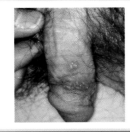
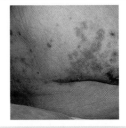

Anogenital region: variable symptoms

Atrophic vulvovaginitis – see www.dermnetnz.org/topics/atrophic-vulvovaginitis
- pale or patchy red vaginal orifice
- thin vaginal wall that bleeds easily

Extramammary Paget disease – see www.dermnetnz.org/topics/
extramammary-paget-disease
- unilateral or bilateral
- irregular slowly enlarging plaque
- red, white, pigmented

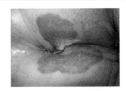

Molluscum contagiosum – see Section 2.3.7
- crop of umbilicated white papules

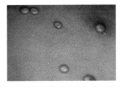

- **Squamous intraepithelial lesions** (vulval high-grade SIL) – see www.dermnetnz.org/topics/vulval-intraepithelial-neoplasia
  - ☐ unilateral or bilateral
  - ☐ irregular slowly enlarging plaque
  - ☐ red, white, pigmented

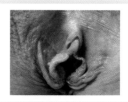

- **Viral warts** – see www.dermnetnz.org/topics/anogenital-warts
  - ☐ irregular crop of firm, soft, flattish and superficial papules

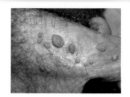

1.4.7 Hands and feet

Hands and feet: localised asymmetrical vesicles/pustules

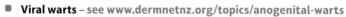

- **Acute dermatophyte infection** – see Section 2.2.3
  - ☐ tinea pedis: interdigital, sides of heel, instep
  - ☐ tinea manuum: inflammatory (zoophilic origin)
  - ☐ mycology microscopy and culture positive

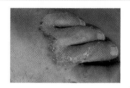

- **Herpes simplex** – see Section 2.3.4
  - ☐ often paronychia
  - ☐ painful crop of umbilicated vesicles, then crusts

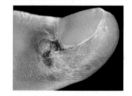

- **Impetigo** – see Section 2.1.4
  - ☐ often wound infection or scabies or paronychia
  - ☐ culture: *Staph. aureus* +/– *Strep. pyogenes*

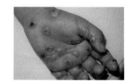

- **Neutrophilic dermatosis** – see www.dermnetnz.org/topics/acute-febrile-neutrophilic-dermatosis
  - ☐ dorsal hands (reaction to myeloid disease)
  - ☐ purplish plaques/nodules or bullae
  - ☐ pseudovesicular plaques

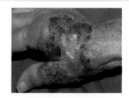

- **Orf** – see www.dermnetnz.org/topics/orf
  - ☐ single or several
  - ☐ flat-topped haemorrhagic nodule
  - ☐ appearance of pus but firm red tissue on incising
  - ☐ can be followed by erythema multiforme

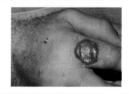

Hands and feet: diffuse, bilateral vesicles/pustules

- **Contact dermatitis** – see Section 3.6.4
  - ☐ mainly dorsal hand
  - ☐ affects sites in contact with irritant/allergen

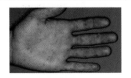

- **Enteroviral vesicular stomatitis** (HFM) – see Section 2.3.3
  - ☐ mild, febrile illness
  - ☐ mainly young children
  - ☐ vesicles are oval

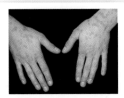

- **Erythema multiforme** – see Section 3.7
  - ☐ single episode or recurrent (herpes simplex)
  - ☐ fixed target lesions in acral sites

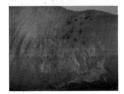

- **Palmoplantar pustulosis** – see www.dermnetnz.org/topics/palmoplantar-pustulosis
  - ☐ sterile tender, itchy, pustules
  - ☐ often based on erythematous plaques

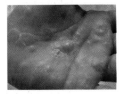

- **Pompholyx** – see Section 3.6.11
  - ☐ sides of fingers/toes, palms/soles
  - ☐ recurring crops of intensely itchy vesicles

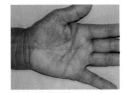

- **Scabies** – see Section 2.4.3
  - ☐ burrows: dermatoscopy finds mite at distal end
  - ☐ vesicles, pustules on palms, especially in infants
  - ☐ generalised itchy rash

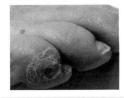

Hands and feet: localised dry/scaly rash

- **Corns and calluses** – see www.dermnetnz.org/topics/corns-and-calluses
  - ☐ pressure sites
  - ☐ tender on direct pressure

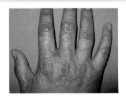

■ **Chronic dermatophyte infection** – see Section 2.2.3
  - ☐ tinea pedis

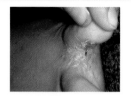

■ **Photosensitivity** – see Section 3.16
  - ☐ dorsal hand with sparing of the web spaces and body creases
  - ☐ sharp cut-off at sleeve cuff
  - ☐ various types

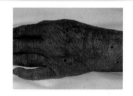

■ **Viral warts** – see Section 2.3.9
  - ☐ pressure sites and elsewhere
  - ☐ tender on lateral pressure

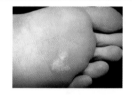

Hands and feet: diffuse dry/scaly rash

■ **Actinic keratoses** – see Section 5.2
  - ☐ persistent firm scaly papules
  - ☐ work or recreational exposure to sun

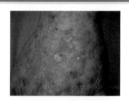

■ **Chronic dermatophyte infection** – see Section 2.2.3
  - ☐ moccasin pattern
  - ☐ tinea manuum: non-inflammatory scale '2 foot 1 hand syndrome'

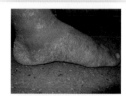

■ **Contact dermatitis** – see Section 3.6.4
  - ☐ mainly dorsal hand
  - ☐ affects sites in contact with irritant/allergen

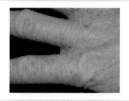

■ **Exfoliative keratolysis** – see www.dermnetnz.org/topics/exfoliative-keratolysis
  - ☐ palmar/plantar peeling
  - ☐ seasonally recurrent

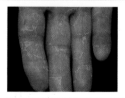

- **Keratoderma** – see www.dermnetnz.org/topics/
  palmoplantar-keratoderma
  - ☐ palms/soles hyperkeratotic/thickened
  - ☐ various types

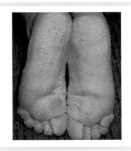

1.4.8 Legs

Legs: red papules/pustules

- **Insect bites** – see Section 2.4.1
  - ☐ lower legs, ankles
  - ☐ crops of grouped itchy papules
  - ☐ central punctum
  - ☐ may blister

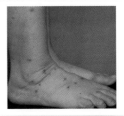

- **Lichen planus** – see Section 3.11
  - ☐ shins
  - ☐ firm, violaceous papules + white streaks
  - ☐ favour areas of earlier injury
  - ☐ Koebner phenomenon
  - ☐ also examine mouth

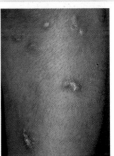

Legs: erosions/crusting

- **Herpes zoster** – see Section 2.3.5
  - ☐ dermatomal
  - ☐ painful
  - ☐ erythema may precede vesicles
  - ☐ culture/PCR: varicella-zoster virus

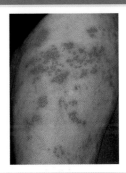

- **Impetigo** – see Section 2.1.4
  - ☐ irregular enlarging plaque
  - ☐ honey-coloured crusts
  - ☐ swabs: *Staph. aureus* +/– *Strep. pyogenes*

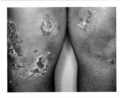

Legs: dry/scaly and very itchy

May also blister and swell.

- **Allergic contact dermatitis** – see Section 3.6.4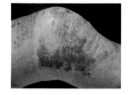
  - ☐ acute flares on any site
  - ☐ asymmetrical, odd-shaped patches/plaques
  - ☐ patch tests positive

- **Asteatotic dermatitis** – see Section 3.6.2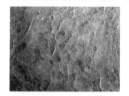
  - ☐ shins often elderly
  - ☐ reticulate pattern

- **Atopic dermatitis** – see Section 3.6.3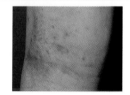
  - ☐ popliteal fossa, ankles
  - ☐ acute flares are erythematous plaques +/– mild vesicular plaques
  - ☐ chronic eczema is lichenified

- **Discoid eczema** – see Section 3.6.5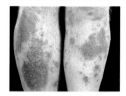
  - ☐ coin-shaped plaques
  - ☐ exudative and dry types

- **Stasis dermatitis** – see Section 3.6.13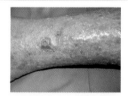
  - ☐ lower legs
  - ☐ associated lymphoedema, venous disease, lipodermatosclerosis, ulceration, obesity

Legs: scaly with minimal itch

- **Disseminated superficial actinic porokeratosis** (DSAP) – see www.dermnetnz.org/topics/disseminated-superficial-actinic-porokeratosis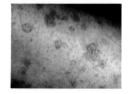
  - ☐ genodermatosis
  - ☐ multiple polycyclic plaques
  - ☐ each has rim of scale

- **Psoriasis** – see Section 3.19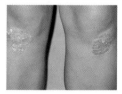
  - ☐ extensor knees, shins
  - ☐ roughly symmetrical distribution
  - ☐ well-circumscribed erythematous scaly plaques

Tinea corporis – see Section 2.5.5

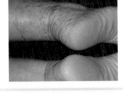

- ☐ asymmetrical annular or discoid plaques
- ☐ peripheral scale
- ☐ variable itch
- ☐ mycology microscopy and culture positive

Xerosis – see Section 4.2

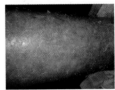

- ☐ dry skin

Legs: erythema without surface change

Erythema is less pronounced in dark skin.

Sunburn – see www.dermnetnz.org/topics/sunburn

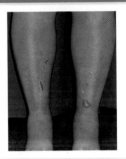

- ☐ sun-exposed site

Urticaria – see Section 3.22

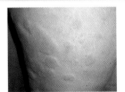

- ☐ weals can arise on any site
- ☐ spontaneous and induced types

Legs: multiple skin coloured papules

Granuloma annulare – see Section 3.9

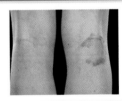

- ☐ over joints or buttocks
- ☐ arranged in rings

Legs: tender subcutaneous nodules

Erythema nodosum – see Section 3.14

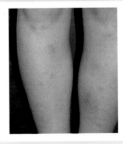

- ☐ mainly young women
- ☐ shins
- ☐ associated swelling of knees, ankles
- ☐ chest X-ray may show hilar lymphadenopathy if acute form of sarcoidosis

■ **Other forms of panniculitis** – see Section 3.14

   ☐ persistent

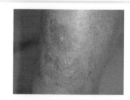

■ **Pretibial myxoedema** – see www.dermnetnz.org/topics/pretibial-myxoedema

   ☐ thickened, bumpy, tender plaques on shins
   ☐ thyrotoxicosis with diffuse goitre/Graves' disease

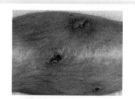

Legs: purple lesions

■ **Capillaritis** – see www.dermnetnz.org/topics/capillaritis

   ☐ various kinds
   ☐ 'cayenne pepper' macules

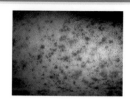

■ **Coagulopathy or bleeding**

   ☐ purpuric petechiae and ecchymoses
   ☐ if febrile/unwell, consider meningococcal disease –
      see www.dermnetnz.org/topics/meningococcal-disease

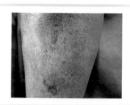

■ **Cryoglobulinaemia** – see www.dermnetnz.org/topics/cryoglobulinaemia

   ☐ essential or associated with hepatitis C or other systemic disease

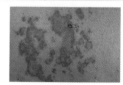

■ **Senile/solar purpura** – see www.dermnetnz.org/topics/senile-purpura

   ☐ sun damaged sites
   ☐ skin fragility
   ☐ often stellate ecchymotic macules

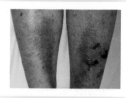

■ **Trauma**

   ☐ history of injury

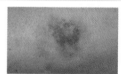

■ **Vasculitis** – see Section 3.23

   ☐ lower legs
   ☐ palpable purpura
   ☐ may ulcerate
   ☐ various kinds

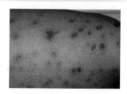

Legs: very painful ulcers

- **Arterial ulcer** – see www.dermnetnz.org/topics/arterial-ulcer
  - ☐ located on feet: heels or toes
  - ☐ painful, especially when legs elevated
  - ☐ punched out ulceration
  - ☐ lack of or reduced arterial pulse

- **Calciphylaxis** – see www.dermnetnz.org/topics/calciphylaxis
  - ☐ end stage renal disease + diabetes
  - ☐ stellate necrosis
  - ☐ retiform purpura

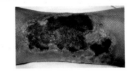

- **Infection** – see Section 2.1.4
  - ☐ superficial ulceration from impetigo
  - ☐ can be malodorous

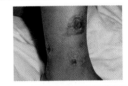

- **Pyoderma gangrenosum** – see www.dermnetnz.org/topics/pyoderma-gangrenosum
  - ☐ often associated with underlying inflammatory bowel disease, rheumatoid arthritis, myeloid blood dyscrasia
  - ☐ very painful autoinflammatory ulceration
  - ☐ irregular shape with overhanging purple edge

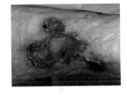

- **Trauma**
  - ☐ linear or triangular shape
  - ☐ bruising

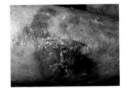

- **Vasculitis** – see Section 3.23
  - ☐ various kinds
  - ☐ often very painful
  - ☐ sharp margin

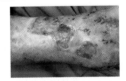

Legs: ulcers with minimal pain

- **Diabetic ulcer** – see www.dermnetnz.org/topics/diabetic-foot-ulcers
  - ☐ located on pressure points
  - ☐ callus around edge of ulcer

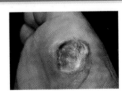

- **Infection** – see Section 2.1
  - ☐ deeper ulceration from cellulitis
  - ☐ necrosis associated with necrotising fasciitis
  - ☐ can be malodorous
  - ☐ infection is more often painful

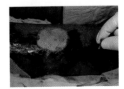

- **Malignant tumour: squamous cell carcinoma, basal cell carcinoma, lymphoma and others** – see www.dermnetnz.org/topics/skin-cancer
    - ☐ irregular shape
    - ☐ irregular structure and colour
    - ☐ infiltrated base

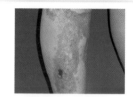

- **Necrobiosis lipoidica** – see www.dermnetnz.org/topics/necrobiosis-lipoidica
    - ☐ yellowish plaque, with telangiectasia
    - ☐ atrophic; can ulcerate
    - ☐ plaques mainly found on shins

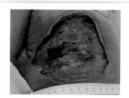

- **Trauma with neuropathy**
    - ☐ pressure sores – see www.dermnetnz.org/topics/bedsores
    - ☐ thermal burns – see www.dermnetnz.org/topics/thermal-burns

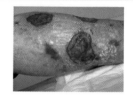

- **Venous ulcer** – see www.dermnetnz.org/topics/venous-leg-ulcers
    - ☐ located medial lower leg
    - ☐ not especially painful
    - ☐ associated mottled pigmentation, lipodermatosclerosis, oedema

1.4.9 Lips

Lips: asymptomatic lesions

- **Chronic granulomatous cheilitis** – see www.dermnetnz.org/topics/granulomatous-cheilitis
    - ☐ firm persistent swelling
    - ☐ associated Crohn disease, sarcoidosis

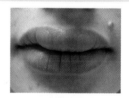

- **Exfoliative cheilitis** – see www.dermnetnz.org/topics/exfoliative-cheilitis
    - ☐ repetitive peeling

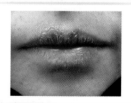

- **Glandular cheilitis** – see www.dermnetnz.org/topics/glandular-cheilitis
    - ☐ prominent salivary ducts

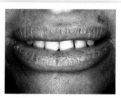

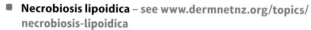

- **Mucous retention cyst** – see www.dermnetnz.org/topics/mucocoele-of-the-lip/
  - ☐ translucent papule

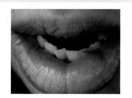

- **Venous lake** – see Section 5.13
  - ☐ bluish patch or papule

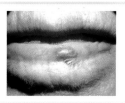

- **Vitiligo** – see Section 4.10
  - ☐ loss of normal pigment

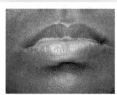

Lips: symptomatic lesions

- **Actinic cheilitis** – see Section 5.1
  - ☐ lower lip
  - ☐ diffuse or isolated
  - ☐ tender adherent scale

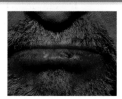

- **Angular cheilitis** – see www.dermnetnz.org/topics/angular-cheilitis/
  - ☐ red, dry or exudative
  - ☐ irritant contact dermatitis to saliva
  - ☐ most often culture *Candida albicans* (left)
  - ☐ impetigo: *Staph. aureus* (right)

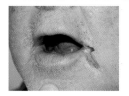 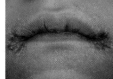

- **Cutaneous lupus erythematosus** – see Section 3.4
  - ☐ discoid LE, systemic LE
  - ☐ scaling, erosions, scarring

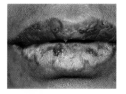

- **Drug-induced cheilitis** – see www.dermnetnz.org/topics/cheilitis
  - ☐ isotretinoin, acitretin
  - ☐ dryness, erosions, fissuring

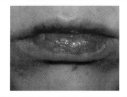

- **Eczematous cheilitis** – see www.dermnetnz.org/topics/
eczematous-cheilitis/
  - contact irritant (e.g. lip licker's dermatitis)
  - contact allergic
  - photosensitive, in actinic prurigo

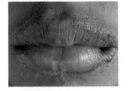

- **Fixed drug eruption** – see www.dermnetnz.org/topics/
fixed-drug-eruption/
  - central blister
  - hyperpigmentation
  - within 24 hours of exposure to drug

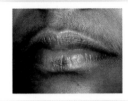

- **Herpes simplex** – see Section 2.3.4
  - recurrent groups of vesicles, erosions
  - positive swab: *Herpes simplex*

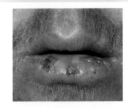

- **Lichen planus** – see Section 3.11
  - sometimes drug-induced
  - scaling, erosions, ulcers

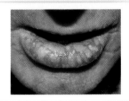

1.4.10 Nails

Examine the nails to determine whether any abnormality affects a single nail (infection, tumour) or multiple nails (inflammatory disorders). Evaluate the surface of the nail plate, its colour and shape, the cuticle and nail folds.

Nails: disorder affecting single or multiple nails

- **Acute bacterial paronychia** – see Section 2.2.6
  - tender, red pustule
  - swelling of nail fold
  - culture: *Staph. aureus*

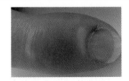

- **Chronic paronychia** – see Section 2.2.6
  - swelling of nail fold
  - sometimes pus expression
  - irregular ridging, discoloration of nail plate
  - culture: *Candida albicans*

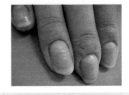

- **Discoloured nail plate –**
  see www.dermnetnz.org/topics/
  nail-terminology/
  - black: candidiasis
  - green, black: pseudomonas
  - purple: subungual haemorrhage
  - red/purple streak: splinter
    haemorrhage
  - white: trauma, superficial
    onychomycosis
  - yellow: psoriasis, dermatophyte
    infection
  - brown: melanonychia, fungal nail
    infection

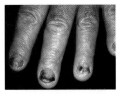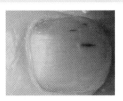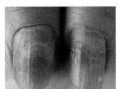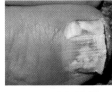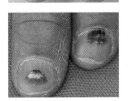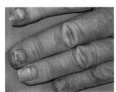

- **Fungal nail infection/onychomycosis/tinea unguium –**
  see Section 2.2.3
  - yellowish distal linear streaks
  - irregular ridging, discoloration of nail plate
  - onycholysis, subungual hyperkeratosis
  - mycology microscopy and culture *Trichophyton rubrum*,
    T. interdigitale

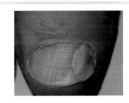

- **Glomus tumour – see Section 5.13**
  - red or blue, tender spot

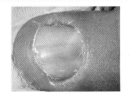

- **Herpetic whitlow – see Section 2.3.4**
  - tender, red, crop of vesicles
  - swelling of nail fold
  - culture/PCR: *Herpes simplex*

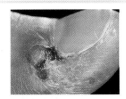

- **Median canaliform dystrophy –**
  see www.dermnetnz.org/topics/
  nail-terminology/
  - wide longitudinal furrow centre of
    both thumbnails
  - may have feathered edge
  - can be due to repeated habitual
    trauma to nail matrix (right)

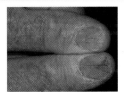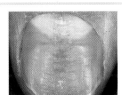

Melanonychia (brown longitudinal band) – see www.dermnetnz. org/topics/melanonychia/

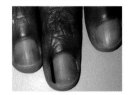

- ☐ stable: naevus, lentigo, rarely drug
- ☐ widening, irregular, loss of parallelism: melanoma

Malignant tumour (amelanotic melanoma) – see www.dermnetnz. org/topics/melanoma-of-nail-unit

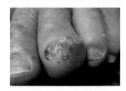

- ☐ tumour
- ☐ erosion, ulceration, loss of nail plate

Myxoid pseudocyst – see www.dermnetnz.org/topics/ digital-mucous-or-myxoid-cyst/

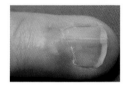

- ☐ translucent papule distal phalanx
- ☐ longitudinal furrow in nail plate

Onychocryptosis (ingrown nail) – see www.dermnetnz.org/topics/ ingrown-toenails/

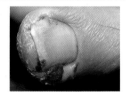

- ☐ paronychia or retronychia
- ☐ aggravated by oral retinoid

Onychopapilloma – see www.dermnetnz.org/topics/ onychopapilloma

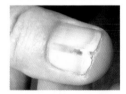

- ☐ erythronychia (longitudinal red band) + distal subungual hyperkeratosis

Subungual exostosis, fibroma, osteoma and other tumours – see www.dermnetnz.org/topics/subungual-exostosis/

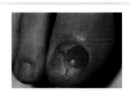

- ☐ diagnosed by X-ray and biopsy

Nails: disorder affecting multiple nails

Ageing – see www.dermnetnz.org/topics/nail-terminology/

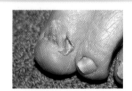

- ☐ slow growth
- ☐ increased longitudinal ridging
- ☐ increased curvature of nail plate
- ☐ various results: onychogryphosis, onychochauxis, pincer nail

Alopecia areata – see Section 4.1

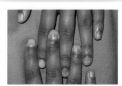

- ☐ regular pitting

- **Beau line** – see www.dermnetnz.org/topics/nail-terminology/
  - ☐ single or multiple transverse furrow
  - ☐ indicate previous illness

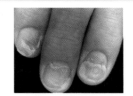

- **Clubbing** – see www.dermnetnz.org/topics/
  hypertrophic-osteoarthropathy-and-digital-clubbing/
  - ☐ longitudinal curvature
  - ☐ chronic pulmonary insufficiency or thyroid acropachy

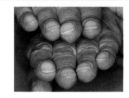

- **Connective tissue disease + vasculitis** – see www.dermnetnz.org/topics/connective-tissue-diseases/
  - ☐ ragged cuticles
  - ☐ nail fold capillary ectasia and loss
  - ☐ distal digital infarcts

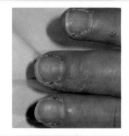

- **Crusted scabies** – see Section 2.4.3
  - ☐ subungual scaling

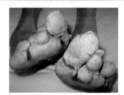

- **Darier disease** – see www.dermnetnz.org/topics/darier-disease/
  - ☐ split distal nail
  - ☐ erythronychia (red longitudinal band)

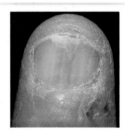

- **Discoloured nail plates** – see www.dermnetnz.org/topics/nail-terminology/
  - ☐ blue: minocycline
  - ☐ brown: hydroxyurea
  - ☐ white: low albumin, chronic kidney disease
  - ☐ yellow: psoriasis, dermatophyte infection

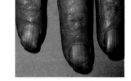

- **Hand dermatitis** – see www.dermnetnz.org/topics/hand-dermatitis/
  - ☐ irregular transverse ridges, furrows, pits

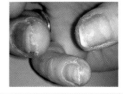

- **Koilonychia** – see www.dermnetnz.org/topics/nail-terminology/
  - ☐ genetic or due to iron deficiency or retinoid

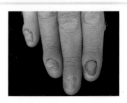

- **Lichen planus** – see Section 3.11
  - ☐ longitudinal ridging
  - ☐ angel-wing deformity
  - ☐ pterygium
  - ☐ rough nail plate (trachyonychia)
  - ☐ twenty nail dystrophy or loss of nails

- **Onycholysis** – see www.dermnetnz.org/topics/onycholysis/
  - ☐ multiple causes
  - ☐ photo-onycholysis drug-induced, e.g. doxycycline

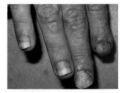

- **Psoriasis** – see Section 3.19
  - ☐ irregular transverse ridges, furrows, pits
  - ☐ onycholysis, subungual hyperkeratosis

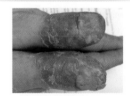

- **Pustulosis: Hallopeau acrodermatitis** – see Section 3.19
  - ☐ sterile periungual pustules
  - ☐ erythema, swelling

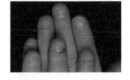

- **Trauma: picking, biting** – see nail biting (onychophagia) www.dermnetnz.org/topics/onychophagia
  - ☐ hang nail
  - ☐ nail plate irregularities

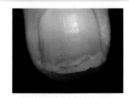

- **Water damage** – see www.dermnetnz.org/topics/nail-terminology/
  - ☐ longitudinal splitting (onychoschizia, shown)
  - ☐ brittle nails (onychorrhexis)

- **Yellow nail syndrome** – see www.dermnetnz.org/topics/yellow-nail-syndrome/
  - ☐ slow-growing, greenish yellow nails
  - ☐ increased curvature, irregular
  - ☐ lymphatic obstruction
  - ☐ cardiopulmonary disease

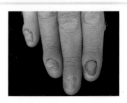

1.4.11 Oral mucosa

Oral mucosa: localised, asymmetrical blisters/pustules/ulcers

- **Aphthous ulcer/stomatitis** – see Section 3.13
  - minor: 2–3mm yellow ulcer with red halo
  - major: >5mm, slow to heal

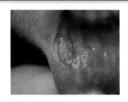

- **Behçet disease** – see www.dermnetnz.org/topics/behcet-disease/
  - recurrent oral and genital ulcers
  - ocular inflammation
  - skin lesions including pathergy
  - multisystem disease

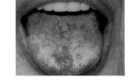

- **Complex aphthosis** – see Section 3.13
  - recurrent oral and genital ulcers

- **Contact stomatitis** – see www.dermnetnz.org/topics/contact-stomatitis
  - irritants such as nicotine
  - allergens such as rubber

- **Epstein–Barr virus or cytomegalovirus** – see www.dermnetnz.org/topics/infectious-mononucleosis/
  - acute solitary or few large ulcers
  - adolescent

- **Fixed drug eruption** – see www.dermnetnz.org/topics/fixed-drug-eruption/
  - recurring blister, ulcer

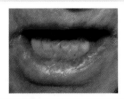

- **Herpes simplex** – see Section 2.3.4
  - primary or recurrent secondary disease
  - crops of tender vesicles, ulcers, swelling
  - may be within the distribution of a cutaneous nerve

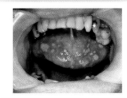

- **Herpes zoster** – see Section 2.3.5
  - unilateral vesicles
  - dermatomal

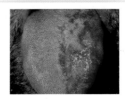

- **Trauma**

Oral mucosa: generalised blisters/pustules/ulcers

- **Candidiasis** – see Section 2.2.2
  - ☐ usually risk factors present
  - ☐ white, red, peeling, tender tongue, buccal mucosa
  - ☐ culture: *Candida albicans*

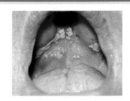

- **Drug-induced stomatitis** – see www.dermnetnz.org/topics/
  stomatitis/
  - ☐ new drug (fig. shows reaction to amoxicillin)

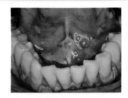

- **Enteroviral vesicular stomatitis (HFM)** – see Section 2.3.3
  - ☐ mild febrile illness
  - ☐ other sites affected

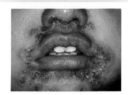

- **Erythema multiforme** – see Section 3.7
  - ☐ reaction to virus (e.g. *Herpes simplex*) > drug
  - ☐ ulcers in mouth, lips, sometimes genitals
  - ☐ acral rash, often targetoid, may blister

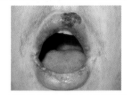

- **Gingivitis and periodontitis** – see www.dermnetnz.org/topics/
  gingivitis-and-periodontitis/
  - ☐ tender swollen inflamed gums that bleed easily
  - ☐ gums shrink and teeth may loosen
  - ☐ may be associated with lichen planus, pemphigus, etc.

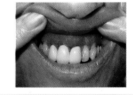

- **Herpangina** – see www.dermnetnz.org/topics/herpangina/
  - ☐ mild febrile illness
  - ☐ multiple 2mm ulcers on tongue, oropharynx

- **Immunobullous diseases** (pemphigus vulgaris) –
  see www.dermnetnz.org/topics/pemphigus-vulgaris/
  - ☐ fluid-filled blisters and/or erosions

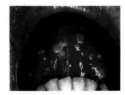

- **Lichen planus** – see Section 3.11
  - ☐ may affect skin and other mucous membranes
  - ☐ white lacy pattern in buccal mucosa typical
  - ☐ erosive lichen planus is painful variant

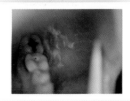

- **Orofacial granulomatosis** – see www.dermnetnz.org/topics/orofacial-granulomatosis/
  - ☐ swollen lips
  - ☐ facial palsy
  - ☐ sometimes associated with inflammatory bowel disease
  - ☐ variable ulceration

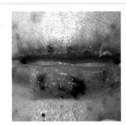

- **Secondary syphilis** – see www.dermnetnz.org/topics/syphilis/
  - ☐ snail track ulcers

- **Stevens–Johnson / toxic epidermal necrolysis** – see Section 3.5.4
  - ☐ severe adverse drug eruption
  - ☐ patient very unwell
  - ☐ extensive mucosal ulceration (eyes, mouth, genitals, anus)
  - ☐ painful erythema, morbilliform eruption or diffuse extensive painful red skin which soon evolves to blistering, loss of epidermis

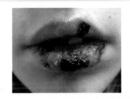

- **Systemic lupus erythematosus** – see Section 3.4
  - ☐ red patches and ulcers
  - ☐ may be painful or painless

1.4.12 Scalp

Patients may present with a skin problem that they believe to be confined to the scalp, but a full medical and focused cutaneous history should be followed by a brief examination of relevant sites.

Scalp: special tests

Hair pull test: pinch a group of hairs and tug them; evaluate scalp end for anagen or telogen hair shafts.
  Trichoscopy is dermatoscopy of the hair and scalp.

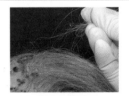

Scalp: scaly without hair loss

- **Atopic dermatitis** – see Section 3.6.3
  - ☐ ill-defined erythematous blistered or dry plaques
  - ☐ pruritic and very itchy
  - ☐ involves other body sites; check elbow flexures, popliteal fossae and eyelids

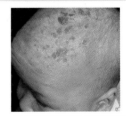

- **Head lice** – see Section 2.4.2
    - ☐ usually but not always young child
    - ☐ look for lice and egg cases close to scalp at nape of neck
    - ☐ blood spots behind ears

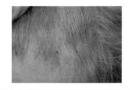

- **Pityriasis amiantacea** – see www.dermnetnz.org/topics/pityriasis-amiantacea
    - ☐ thick, perifollicular scale adherent to the hair shaft
    - ☐ scale is like asbestos

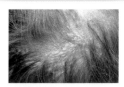

- **Psoriasis** – see Section 3.19
    - ☐ any age but mostly in those over 15 years
    - ☐ well defined, erythematous, thick plaques with white scale
    - ☐ may be localised or diffuse
    - ☐ resistant to anti-dandruff shampoo

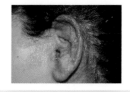

- **Seborrhoeic dermatitis** – see Section 3.6.12
    - ☐ infantile type (cradle cap)
    - ☐ adolescent/adult types
    - ☐ ill-defined, flaky, thin salmon-pink plaques
    - ☐ responds to anti-dandruff shampoo

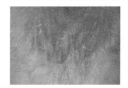

Scalp: scaly with hair loss

Hair loss from psoriasis, seborrhoeic dermatitis and atopic eczema is uncommon.

- **Actinic keratoses** – see Section 5.2
    - ☐ affect top of a bald scalp
    - ☐ tender, persistent erythematous plaques
    - ☐ adherent scale

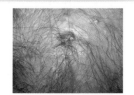

- **Discoid lupus erythematosus** – see Section 3.4
    - ☐ vertex and anterior scalp
    - ☐ localised irregular erythematous plaques
    - ☐ scarring alopecia
    - ☐ sometimes regrowth occurs
    - ☐ may involve other body sites; check nose, cheeks and ear concha

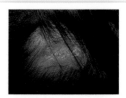

- **Head lice** – see Section 2.4.2
    - ☐ hair loss due to hair-pulling
    - ☐ look for lice and egg cases close to scalp at nape of neck
    - ☐ blood spots behind ears

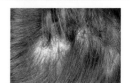

- **Frontal fibrosing alopecia** – see www.dermnetnz.org/topics/frontal-fibrosing-alopecia/
    - ☐ eyebrows to frontal hairline
    - ☐ perifollicular scale
    - ☐ scarring alopecia with shiny, hypopigmented skin

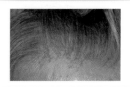

- **Lichen planopilaris** – see www.dermnetnz.org/topics/
  lichen-planopilaris/
  - ☐ any area of scalp
  - ☐ perifollicular scale
  - ☐ scarring alopecia

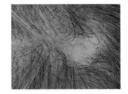

- **Pityriasis amiantacea** – see www.dermnetnz.org/topics/
  pityriasis-amiantacea
  - ☐ thick, perifollicular scale adherent to the hair shaft
  - ☐ hair comes out with the scale

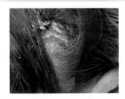

- **Tinea capitis** – see Section 2.2.3
  - ☐ young child
  - ☐ hair extracts easily
  - ☐ hair usually regrows after treatment
  - ☐ positive microscopy and fungal culture

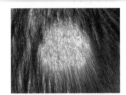

Scalp: pustules/erosions without hair loss

- **Dermatitis herpetiformis** (low-power histology) –
  see www.dermnetnz.org/topics/dermatitis-herpetiformis
  - ☐ intense itch means vesicles rarely observed
  - ☐ itchy spots elsewhere (variable)
  - ☐ biopsy confirmatory

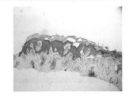

- **Folliculitis** – see Section 2.1.3
  - ☐ itchy or painful papules around the hair follicle
  - ☐ poor response to topical steroid
  - ☐ swabs: sterile or *Staph. aureus*

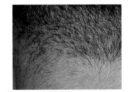

- **Impetigo** – see Section 2.1.4
  - ☐ associated with head lice in young children
  - ☐ secondary to inflammatory seborrhoeic dermatitis
  - ☐ swabs: *Staph. aureus* +/– *Strep. pyogenes*

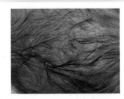

- **Herpes zoster** – see Section 2.3.5
  - ☐ acute dermatomal eruption
  - ☐ painful; pain may precede rash
  - ☐ erythema may precede vesicles
  - ☐ culture/PCR: varicella-zoster virus

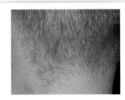

Scalp: pustules/erosions with hair loss

- **Erosive pustular dermatosis of the scalp** – see www.dermnetnz.org/topics/erosive-pustular-dermatosis/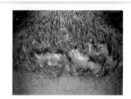
  - ☐ elderly
  - ☐ sun damaged scalp: actinic keratosis, squamous cell carcinoma
  - ☐ yellow–green hardened carapace overlies greenish pus
  - ☐ often several centimetres in diameter or multifocal

- **Folliculitis keloidalis** – see www.dermnetnz.org/topics/folliculitis-keloidalis/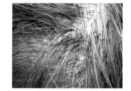
  - ☐ occipital scalp
  - ☐ follicular pustules + keloidal scars
  - ☐ alopecia between scars

- **Folliculitis decalvans** – see www.dermnetnz.org/topics/folliculitis-decalvans/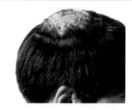
  - ☐ precipitated by scalp injury or infection
  - ☐ irregular bald areas
  - ☐ perifollicular pustules
  - ☐ multiple hairs in one follicle
  - ☐ biopsy confirmatory

- **Kerion** (inflammatory tinea capitis) – see www.dermnetnz.org/topics/kerion/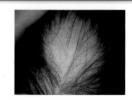
  - ☐ abscess
  - ☐ hair may be extracted easily
  - ☐ hair usually regrows after treatment
  - ☐ negative microscopy but positive fungal culture
  - ☐ mycology culture dermatophyte, usually zoophilic

Scalp: localised hair loss without scarring

- **Alopecia areata** – see Section 4.1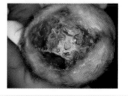
  - ☐ round bald patches
  - ☐ exclamation hairs
  - ☐ regrowing hair is often white
  - ☐ diffuse, totalis and universalis variants

- **Treated bacterial or fungal infection**

Scalp: localised hair loss with scarring

- **Aplasia cutis** – see www.dermnetnz.org/topics/aplasia-cutis/
  - ☐ eroded or thin skin at birth

- **Central centrifugal cicatricial alopecia** (CCCA, photo courtesy Dr Stavonnie Patterson) – see **www.dermnetnz.org/topics/central-centrifugal-cicatricial-alopecia/**
  - ☐ African ancestry
  - ☐ hair style that pulls on the hair

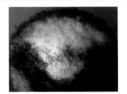

- **Ectodermal dysplasia** – see **www.dermnetnz.org/topics/ectodermal-dysplasia/**
  - ☐ various syndromes

- **Pseudopelade** (Brocq) – see **www.dermnetnz.org/topics/pseudopelade-of-brocq/**
  - ☐ 'footprints in the snow'

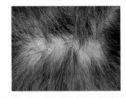

- **Sebaceous naevus** – see **www.dermnetnz.org/topics/sebaceous-naevus/**
  - ☐ yellowish–orange–pink plaque at birth
  - ☐ thickens at puberty

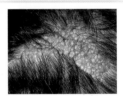
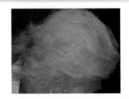

- **Trauma or surgery**

Scalp: diffuse hair loss without scarring

- **Ageing** – see Section 4.4

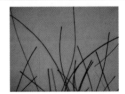

- **Alopecia areata** – see Section 4.1
  - ☐ alopecia totalis/universalis
  - ☐ hair pull reveals anagen hairs

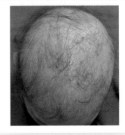

- **Drug-induced hair loss** – see **www.dermnetnz.org/topics/alopecia-from-drugs/**
  - ☐ chemotherapy, retinoids, warfarin, statins
  - ☐ diffuse hair loss

- **Pattern balding:** slow onset with reduced hair shaft diameter and minimal shedding – see Section 4.4
  - ☐ males: vertex, anterior scalp (left)
  - ☐ females: frontal scalp (right)

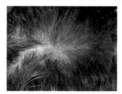
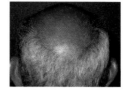

- **Systemic disease** – see Section 4.4
  - ☐ patchy hair thinning
  - ☐ moth-eaten appearance in systemic lupus erythematosus, syphilis
  - ☐ suggestive clinical features and investigations

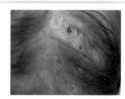

- **Telogen effluvium** – see Section 4.4
  - ☐ diffuse shedding
  - ☐ hair pull reveals telogen hairs
  - ☐ no bald areas

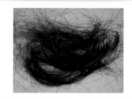

1.4.13 Trunk

Trunk: red papules/pustules

- **Acne vulgaris** – see Section 3.1
  - ☐ upper trunk
  - ☐ open and closed comedones
  - ☐ nodules + cysts if severe

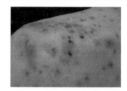

- **Hot tub folliculitis** – see Section 2.1.3
  - ☐ bathing costume distribution
  - ☐ exposed to hot tub
  - ☐ papulopustules
  - ☐ rarely, fever

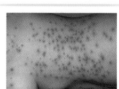

- **Lichen planus** – see Section 3.11
  - ☐ lower back
  - ☐ firm, violaceous papules + white streaks
  - ☐ favour areas of earlier injury
  - ☐ also examine mouth, distal limbs

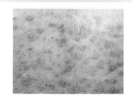

- **Malassezia folliculitis** – see Section 2.2.5
  - ☐ upper trunk
  - ☐ monomorphous superficial papulopustules

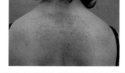

- **Miliaria** – see www.dermnetnz.org/topics/miliaria
  - ☐ mid trunk
  - ☐ acute non-follicular papulopustules
  - ☐ follows heat/sweating

- **Morbilliform drug or viral eruption** – see Section 3.5.3
  - ☐ entire trunk spreading to limbs
  - ☐ commenced new drug within 10 days
  - ☐ monomorphic macules and papules
  - ☐ variable itch

Trunk: erosions/crusting

- **Herpes zoster** (in this case there are 2 affected dermatomes, one on each side of the body)– see Section 2.3.5
  - ☐ dermatomal
  - ☐ painful
  - ☐ erythema may precede vesicles
  - ☐ culture/PCR: varicella-zoster virus

- **Impetigo** – see Section 2.1.4
  - ☐ irregular enlarging plaque
  - ☐ honey-coloured crusts
  - ☐ swabs: *Staph. aureus* +/– *Strep. pyogenes*

- **Scabies rash** – see Section 2.4.3
  - ☐ very itchy follicular and non-follicular papules on trunk
  - ☐ blisters and pustules, especially in children
  - ☐ look for burrows on hands and wrists

- **Transient acantholytic dermatosis** – see Section 3.21
  - ☐ acute or chronic
  - ☐ itchy or asymptomatic
  - ☐ elderly males
  - ☐ crusted papules

- **Varicella** (chickenpox) – see Section 2.3.3
  - ☐ febrile illness
  - ☐ also involves face, oral mucosa
  - ☐ monomorphic eruption
  - ☐ culture/PCR: varicella-zoster virus

Trunk: dry/scaly and very itchy

May also blister and swell.

- **Allergic contact dermatitis** – **see Section 3.6.4**
  - ☐ acute flares on any site
  - ☐ asymmetrical, odd-shaped patches/plaques, e.g. square corresponding to belt buckle
  - ☐ patch tests positive, e.g. nickel

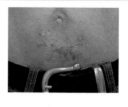

- **Atopic dermatitis** – **see Section 3.6.3**
  - ☐ patchy or diffuse
  - ☐ acute flares are erythematous
  - ☐ chronic eczema is lichenified

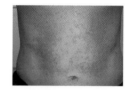

- **Discoid eczema/nummular dermatitis** – **see Section 3.6.5**
  - ☐ coin-shaped plaques
  - ☐ consider autoeczematisation from other site

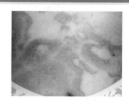

Trunk: dry/scaly with minimal itch

- **Annular erythema** – **see www.dermnetnz.org/topics/ erythema-annulare-centrifugum/**
  - ☐ mid or lower trunk
  - ☐ slowly enlarging rings
  - ☐ scale just inside periphery

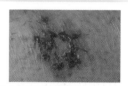

- **Pityriasis rosea** (herald patch – left and generalised rash – right) – **see Section 2.3.8**
  - ☐ larger herald patch appears several days before others (left)
  - ☐ distribution along Langers lines (fir tree pattern, right)
  - ☐ oval shaped plaques with scale just inside periphery
  - ☐ variable itch

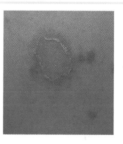 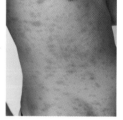

- **Pityriasis versicolor** – **see Section 2.2.5**
  - ☐ mid–upper back and mid chest
  - ☐ pale, pink or brown macules, patches
  - ☐ diffuse bran-like scale
  - ☐ mycology microscopy negative, culture positive

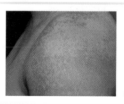 

- **Psoriasis** – **see Section 3.19**
  - ☐ roughly symmetrical distribution
  - ☐ well-circumscribed erythematous scaly plaques
  - ☐ variable itch

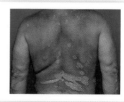

- **Seborrhoeic dermatitis** – see Section 3.6.12
  - ☐ mid–upper back and mid chest
  - ☐ erythema, flaking
  - ☐ skin feels rough on palpation
  - ☐ often, follicular prominence

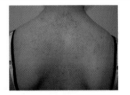

- **Secondary syphilis** – see www.dermnetnz.org/topics/syphilis/
  - ☐ rash involves palms, soles
  - ☐ condyloma lata umbilicus, mucosa
  - ☐ positive syphilis serology

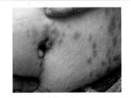

- **Subacute lupus erythematosus** – see Section 3.4
  - ☐ upper trunk
  - ☐ thin, annular erythematous plaques
  - ☐ peripheral scale
  - ☐ check CBC, ANA, ENA
  - ☐ biopsy confirmatory

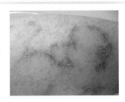

- **Tinea corporis** – see Section 2.2.3
  - ☐ asymmetrical annular or discoid plaques
  - ☐ peripheral scale
  - ☐ variable itch
  - ☐ mycology microscopy and culture positive

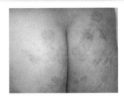

Trunk: erythema without surface change

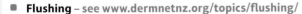

Erythema is less pronounced in dark skin.

- **Flushing** – see www.dermnetnz.org/topics/flushing/
  - ☐ intermittent redness, e.g. when hot, embarrassed or with certain foods
  - ☐ often lifelong tendency
  - ☐ systemically well
  - ☐ may precede/accompany inflammatory rosacea

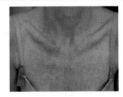

- **Urticaria** – see Section 3.22
  - ☐ Weals can arise on any site
  - ☐ Spontaneous and inducible types

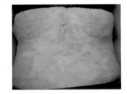

Trunk: multiple skin-coloured papules

- **Granuloma annulare** – see Section 3.9
  - ☐ Often arranged in rings
  - ☐ Plaques are more prevalent on limbs

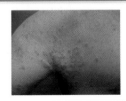

Chapter 2

Infections

2.1 Bacteria

2.1.1 Common bacterial skin infections

Introduction

Bacterial skin infections are primarily caused by *Staphylococcus aureus* and/or group A beta-haemolytic *Streptococcus pyogenes*, which originate from the environment.

Staphylococci colonise the nostrils, pharynx, axillae and perineum of about 20% of healthy individuals permanently and more transiently. *Strep. pyogenes* colonises the oropharynx of about 10% of individuals.

Under some circumstances, these bacteria can cause skin infection, including:
- Impetigo and ecthyma (see *Section 2.1.4*).
- Folliculitis and furunculosis (see *Section 2.1.3*).
- Erysipelas, cellulitis and necrotising fasciitis (see *Section 2.1.2*).

They can also rarely give rise to toxic reactions:
- Staphylococcal scalded skin syndrome.
- Scarlet fever.
- Erythema marginatum.

What are the predisposing factors?

Skin infections are seen worldwide. Predisposing factors include:
- Warm temperature.
- High humidity.
- Poor hygiene.
- Underlying skin disease.
- Malnutrition, diabetes, renal insufficiency or other debility.

How are bacterial skin infections diagnosed?

Bacterial skin infections cause typical symptoms and signs. It can be useful to confirm the diagnosis by swabs for microscopy (Gram stain) and culture. In a sick patient, blood culture may be necessary. Skin biopsy may be added to exclude an inflammatory disease.

How are bacterial skin infections treated?

Local care of a skin infection depends on presentation. Topical, oral and intravenous antibiotics are also used, the choice depending on the extent and severity of the infection.

TOPICAL ANTIBIOTIC FOR LOCALISED INFECTION
- Mupirocin ointment.
- Fusidic acid cream or ointment.
- Retapamulin ointment.

ORAL ANTIBIOTIC FOR SEVERE OR WIDESPREAD INFECTION

Prevalence and pattern of community acquired or nosocomial methicillin resistant *Staph. aureus* (MRSA) vary and account for regional choices of first-line and second-line antibiotics:
- Flucloxacillin.
- Beta-lactamase resistant penicillin.
- Erythromycin.
- Azithromycin.
- Cephalexin.
- Trimethoprim/sulfamethoxazole.
- Clindamycin.
- Rifampicin.
- Doxycycline.

INTRAVENOUS ANTIBIOTICS IF ORAL ANTIBIOTICS FAIL OR IMMUNOCOMPROMISED HOST
- Ceftriaxone.
- Cefuroxime.
- Vancomycin.
- Clindamycin.
- Other.

PREVENTION OF BACTERIAL SKIN INFECTION

Chronic *Staph. aureus* carriage in nostrils, axillae/groin and/or submammary area can be treated with 5–7 day courses of:
- Antiseptic cleansers containing chlorhexidine or triclosan.
- Topical antibiotic applied 3 times daily to the nose; this can be repeated from time to time if infections recur.

Other cutaneous bacterial infections

Skin signs are sometimes due to infection with other bacteria:
- Erythrasma, due to *Corynebacterium minutissimum*.
- Spa pool folliculitis, due to *Pseudomonas aeruginosa*.

For information about other less common bacterial infections giving rise to cutaneous signs, see DermNetNZ.org.

2.1.2 Erysipelas and cellulitis

Erysipelas and cellulitis are common acute skin infections characterised by localised and spreading redness, swelling, heat, pain and fever.

What is erysipelas?

Erysipelas involves the superficial dermis and epidermis, often resulting in superficial blistering. Lymphangitis is common.

What is cellulitis?

Cellulitis involves the deep dermis and subcutaneous tissue.

What causes erysipelas and cellulitis?

Erysipelas and cellulitis are usually caused by group A beta-haemolytic streptococcus (*Strep. pyogenes*). Group B, C, D and G streptococci, *Staph. aureus,* and rarely other bacteria may also cause erysipelas and cellulitis. *Haemophilus influenzae* is an occasional cause in non-vaccinated children. Cellulitis around ulcers may be due to mixed infection.

Who gets erysipelas and cellulitis?

Erysipelas and cellulitis can occur in children and adults. Erysipelas most often affects adult women aged 40–60 years. Infection can be due to a break in the skin barrier or, in the case of cellulitis in immune suppressed individuals, blood borne.

Predisposing factors include:
- Previous episode of erysipelas or cellulitis causing lymphatic damage.
- Venous insufficiency, lymphoedema, vascular disease and obesity.
- Diabetes, alcoholism and immune compromise.
- Wound from fungal infection, trauma or surgery.

Despite being frequently blamed, there is little evidence that cellulitis is caused by spider bite.

What are the clinical features of erysipelas and cellulitis?

Erysipelas and cellulitis have an abrupt onset. They are preceded by fever, rigors, malaise and nausea. Skin infection may be accompanied by tender lymphadenopathy, often with a red streak leading from the primary site of infection to the regional lymph node (lymphangitis).

Mixed superficial (erysipelas) and deep (cellulitis) infections may occur.

ERYSIPELAS

The most common sites for erysipelas are lower legs and mid face (*Fig. 2.1*).
- Single circumscribed hot red indurated plaque.
- Advancing border.
- Skin surface develops translucent or haemorrhagic flaccid bullae and pustules.
- Tender lymphadenopathy, often with red streak from plaque to lymph node (lymphangitis, *Fig. 2.2*).
- Resolves with desquamation and post-inflammatory dyspigmentation.

CELLULITIS

The most common sites for cellulitis are lower legs of adults (*Fig. 2.3*) and face of children.

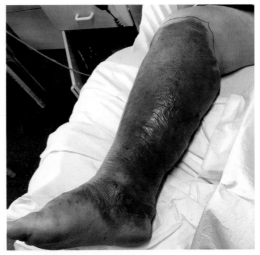

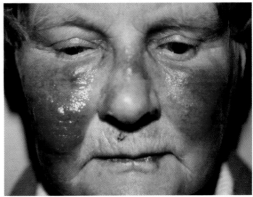

Figure 2.1. Erysipelas of the lower leg and face.

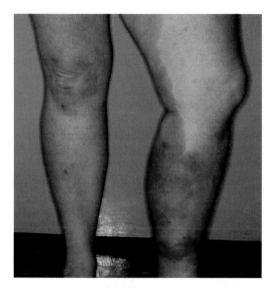

Figure 2.2. Erysipelas with lymphangitis.

Upper limbs are also commonly involved, particularly in IV drug users.

- Ill-defined hot, red, painful swelling (see *Fig. 2.3*).
- Advancing border.
- Slow resolution of swelling once redness and tenderness has settled.

Complications of erysipelas and cellulitis

Complications of erysipelas and cellulitis may include:

- Necrotising fasciitis (*Fig. 2.4*): sick patient with rapidly progressing and life-threatening necrosis of subcutaneous fat and fascia.
- Post-streptococcal acute glomerulonephritis.
- Subacute bacterial endocarditis.
- Recurrent infection at the same site.

Erysipelas and cellulitis of the lower limb may lead to:

- Leg ulceration (*Fig. 2.4*).
- Persistent oedema.

How are erysipelas and cellulitis diagnosed?

Erysipelas and cellulitis are clinical diagnoses.

- Blood count may be normal or reveal neutrophil leucocytosis.
- Skin swabs, needle aspiration and blood cultures may reveal causative organism.
- Rising streptococcal anti-DNase B and ASO titres are confirmatory.

Skin biopsy is rarely necessary. Histological features may include:

- Dermal-epidermal separation in erysipelas.
- Dermal oedema, spreading in cellulitis to involve subcutis.
- Lymphatic and vascular dilatation.
- Suppurative necrosis.
- Streptococci may be seen using direct immunofluorescence and latex agglutination tests.

What is the treatment for erysipelas and cellulitis?

- Rest.
- Wet dressings if blistered or oozing.
- Immobilise and elevate affected limb.
- Avoid non-steroidal anti-inflammatories in cellulitis.
- Hospitalise if facial infection, systemic features of concern, or failure of oral antibiotics.

As it is nearly always streptococcal in origin, erysipelas usually responds to oral or intravenous penicillin or amoxicillin. However, when treating

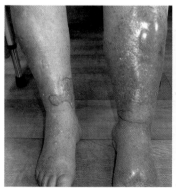
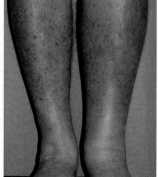
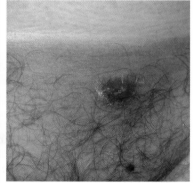

Figure 2.3. Cellulitis of lower leg and around a boil.

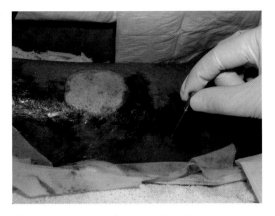 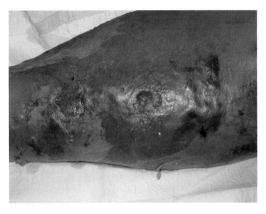

Figure 2.4. Necrotising fasciitis (left) and leg ulceration (right) as a complication of erysipelas and cellulitis.

cellulitis, include anti-staphylococcal cover, and if it is a complication of a chronic ulcer, use broad-spectrum antibiotics.

Long-term therapy after erysipelas and/or cellulitis

Long-term therapy should consider:
- Low-dose penicillin to prevent recurrence.
- Management of venous disease and lymphoedema.

2.1.3 Folliculitis and furunculosis – bacterial

What is folliculitis?

Folliculitis is inflammation of the hair follicle due to infection, chemical irritation or physical injury. Bacterial folliculitis is the most common form of infectious folliculitis.

What causes bacterial folliculitis?

Bacterial folliculitis is usually due to *Staph. aureus*. Less often, coagulase-negative staphylococci and gram-negative organisms are responsible, including anaerobes.

Who gets bacterial folliculitis?

Bacterial folliculitis affects children and adults, with adolescents and young adult males most often infected. It is prevalent worldwide.

The following factors predispose to bacterial folliculitis:
- Maceration and occlusion (clothing, dressings, ointments).
- Frequent shaving, waxing or other forms of depilation.
- Friction from tight clothing.

- Atopic dermatitis.
- Use of topical corticosteroids.
- Anaemia, obesity, diabetes.
- Previous long-term use of antibiotics.

Bathing in an inadequately cleansed spa pool or hot tub can lead to folliculitis caused by *Pseudomonas*.

What are the clinical features of bacterial folliculitis?

Bacterial folliculitis may be superficial or involve the whole hair follicle (a boil). It may arise on any body site, but is most often diagnosed on the scalp, beard area, axilla, buttocks and extremities. Systemic symptoms are uncommon.

SUPERFICIAL FOLLICULITIS

Superficial folliculitis presents with one or more follicular pustules. They may be itchy or mildly sore. Superficial folliculitis heals without scarring (see *Fig. 2.5*).

A hordeolum or stye is bacterial folliculitis affecting an eyelash.

FURUNCULOSIS/BOILS

Furunculosis or boils presents as one or more painful, hot, firm or fluctuant, red nodules (*Fig. 2.6*) or walled-off abscesses (collections of pus). A carbuncle (*Fig. 2.6*) is the name used when a focus of infection involves several follicles and has multiple draining sinuses. Recovery leaves a scar.

Complications of bacterial folliculitis

SOFT TISSUE INFECTION

Bacterial folliculitis can lead to cellulitis (see *Fig. 2.4*) and lymphangitis; subsequent

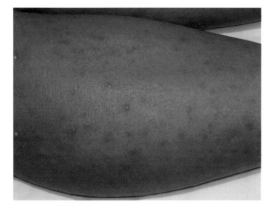

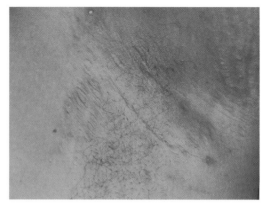

Figure 2.5. Superficial folliculitis on leg and in armpit.

bacteraemia might result in osteomyelitis, septic arthritis or pneumonia.

How is bacterial folliculitis diagnosed?

Bacterial folliculitis is usually diagnosed clinically but can be confirmed by bacterial swabs sent for microscopy (Gram-positive cocci), culture and sensitivity.

Blood count may reveal neutrophil leucocytosis when folliculitis is widespread.

Skin biopsy is rarely necessary. Histology shows dense neutrophilic infiltrate in subcutaneous tissue and foreign body reaction around a hair shaft.

What is the treatment for bacterial folliculitis?

- Avoid shaving and/or waxing.
- Warm compresses.
- Incise and drain fluctuant lesions and abscesses.

- Antiseptic cleansers (e.g. hydrogen peroxide, chlorhexidine, triclosan).
- Topical, oral or intravenous antibiotic depending on extent and severity.

2.1.4 Impetigo

What is impetigo?

Impetigo is a common acute superficial bacterial skin infection (pyoderma). It is characterised by pustules and honey-coloured crusted erosions (*Fig. 2.7*) ('school sores').

The term *impetiginisation* is used for superficial secondary infection of a wound or other skin condition. Ulcerated impetigo is called *ecthyma*.

What causes impetigo?

Impetigo is most often caused by *Staph. aureus*. Non-bullous impetigo can also be caused by group A beta-haemolytic *Streptococcus* (*Strep. pyogenes*).

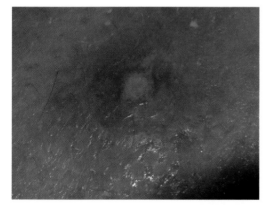

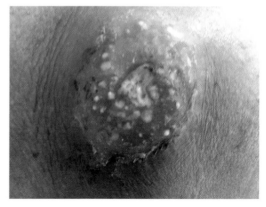

Figure 2.6. Furunculosis (left) and a carbuncle (right).

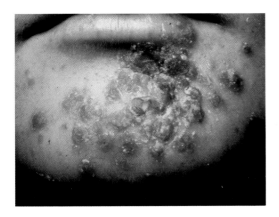

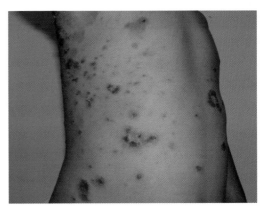

Figure 2.7. Impetigo on face and trunk.

NON-BULLOUS IMPETIGO
In non-bullous impetigo, staphylococci and/or streptococci invade a site of minor trauma where exposed proteins allow the bacteria to adhere.

ECTHYMA
Ecthyma is usually due to *Strep. pyogenes*, but co-infection with *Staph. aureus* may occur.

BULLOUS IMPETIGO
Bullous impetigo is due to staphylococcal exfoliative toxins (exfoliatin A–D), which target desmoglein 1 (a desmosomal adhesion glycoprotein), and cleave off the superficial epidermis through the granular layer. No trauma is required, because the bacteria can infect intact skin.

Who gets impetigo?
Impetigo is most common in children (especially boys), but may also affect adults if they have low immunity to the bacteria. It is prevalent worldwide. Peak onset is during summer and it is more prevalent in developing countries.

The following factors predispose to impetigo:
- Atopic eczema.
- Scabies.
- Skin trauma: chickenpox, insect bite, abrasion, laceration, thermal burn, dermatitis, surgical wound.

What are the clinical features of impetigo?
Primary impetigo mainly affects exposed areas such as the face and hands, but may also affect trunk, perineum and other body sites (see *Fig. 2.8*). It presents with single or multiple, irregular crops of irritable superficial plaques. These extend as they heal, forming annular or arcuate lesions.

Although many children are otherwise well, lymphadenopathy, mild fever and malaise may occur.

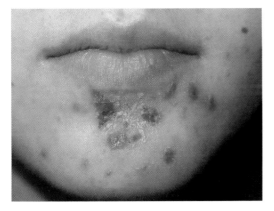

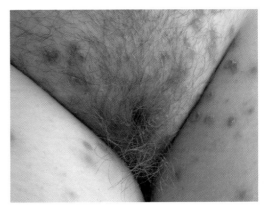

Figure 2.8. Impetigo of face and groin.

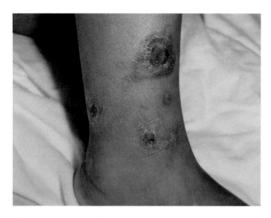

Figure 2.9. Non-bullous impetigo and ecthyma.

NON-BULLOUS IMPETIGO
Non-bullous impetigo starts as a pink macule that evolves into a vesicle or pustule and then into crusted erosions. Untreated impetigo usually resolves within 2–4 weeks without scarring (*Fig. 2.8*).

ECTHYMA
Ecthyma starts as non-bullous impetigo but develops into a punched-out necrotic ulcer (*Figs 2.9* and *2.10*). This heals slowly, leaving a scar.

BULLOUS IMPETIGO
Bullous impetigo presents with small vesicles that evolve into flaccid transparent bullae (*Fig. 2.11*). It heals without scarring.

Complications from impetigo

SOFT TISSUE INFECTION
The bacteria causing impetigo can become invasive, leading to cellulitis and lymphangitis; subsequent bacteraemia might result in osteomyelitis, septic arthritis or pneumonia.

STAPHYLOCOCCAL SCALDED SKIN SYNDROME
In infants under 6 years of age or adults with renal insufficiency, localised bullous impetigo due to certain staphylococcal serotypes can lead to a sick child with generalised staphylococcal scalded skin syndrome (SSSS). Superficial crusting then tender cutaneous denudation on face, in flexures, and elsewhere is due to circulating exfoliatin/epidermolysin, rather than direct skin infection (*Fig. 2.12*). It does not scar.

TOXIC SHOCK SYNDROME
Toxic shock syndrome is rare and rarely preceded by impetigo. It causes fever, diffuse erythematous then desquamating rash, hypotension and involvement of other organs.

POST-STREPTOCOCCAL GLOMERULONEPHRITIS
Group A streptococcal infection may rarely lead to acute post-streptococcal glomerulonephritis 3–6 weeks after the skin infection. It is associated with anti-DNase B and antistreptolysin O (ASO) antibodies.

RHEUMATIC FEVER
Group A streptococcal skin infections have rarely been linked to cases of rheumatic fever and rheumatic heart disease. It is thought that this occurs because strains of group A streptococci usually found on the skin have moved to the throat.

How is impetigo diagnosed?
Impetigo is usually diagnosed clinically but can be confirmed by bacterial swabs sent for

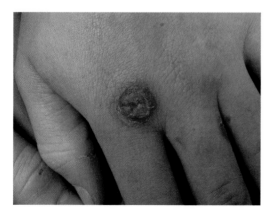

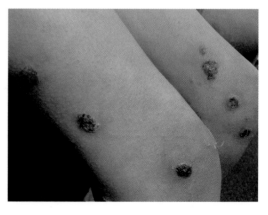

Figure 2.10. Ecthyma.

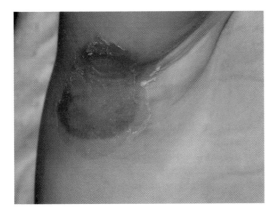

Figure 2.11. Bullous impetigo.

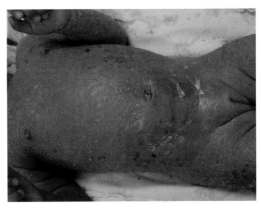

Figure 2.12. Staphylococcal scalded skin syndrome.

microscopy (Gram-positive cocci are observed), culture and sensitivity.

Blood count may reveal neutrophil leucocytosis when impetigo is widespread.

Skin biopsy is rarely necessary. Histological features are characteristic.

Non-bullous impetigo
- Gram-positive cocci.
- Intra-epidermal neutrophilic pustules.
- Dense inflammatory infiltrate in upper dermis.

Bullous impetigo
- Split through granular layer of epidermis without inflammation or bacteria.
- Acantholytic cells.
- Minimal inflammatory infiltrate in upper dermis.
- Resembles pemphigus foliaceus.

Ecthyma
- Full thickness skin ulceration.
- Gram stain shows cocci within dermis.

What is the treatment for impetigo?

The following steps are used to treat impetigo:
- Cleanse the wound.
- Remove the crusts.
- Apply wet dressings.
- Cover affected areas and avoid direct contact with others.
- Recommend antiseptic cleansers (e.g. hydrogen peroxide, chlorhexidine, triclosan, bleach baths).
- Topical, oral or intravenous antibiotic depending on extent and severity of the infection.

2.2 Fungi

2.2.1 Fungal infections

Introduction

Fungal infection commonly causes chronic superficial mycoses that result in minor symptoms. Refer to other resources for information about deep dermal, subcutaneous or systemic mycoses.

What causes fungal skin infections?

Common superficial fungal skin infections are due to dermatophytes (fungi that cause tinea, see *Section 2.2.3*) and yeasts (candida, see *Section 2.2.2*, and malassezia, see *Section 2.2.5*).

Deeper fungal skin infections are rarely seen outside of the tropics in healthy individuals, but may be a cause of an unusual crusted swelling or ulcer in an immune compromised individual.

How are fungal infections diagnosed?

Fungal infections are diagnosed clinically and by mycology: microscopy and culture of skin, hair or nails. Biopsy is occasionally necessary, particularly when a deep fungal infection is possible.

How are fungal infections treated?

Topical antifungal agents are available in various vehicles and can be purchased over the counter in pharmacies with or without prescription. They are suitable for minor or localised infections with responsive organisms.

Oral antifungal agents should be considered for extensive, severe, recurrent infections. These medications have potential side-effects and may interact with other drugs. The choice of oral antifungal agent depends on whether it is a yeast, when an azole should be prescribed, or a dermatophyte, which can be treated with an azole, terbinafine or, if available, griseofulvin.

2.2.2 Candida infections

What is candida?

Candida is the name for a group of yeasts that normally live in the human digestive tract. Infections of mucous membranes and skin are dominated by *Candida albicans*, but at times non-albicans species are cultured, usually *C. tropicalis*, *C. parasilosis*, *C. glabrata*, *C. guilliermondii*.

What are candida infections?

Candida is an opportunistic pathogen and infects mucosa, skin or both when host defences are lowered; the fungus appears to undergo rapid genetic and epigenetic changes in response to environmental cues. Common acute and chronic presentations include:
- Oral candidiasis (*Fig. 2.15*).
- Candida napkin dermatitis (*Fig. 2.16*).
- Vulvovaginal candidiasis (*Fig. 2.17*).
- Candida balanitis (*Fig. 2.18*).
- Candida intertrigo (*Fig. 2.19*).

Systemic infection in immune suppressed individuals is rare.

Candida is also often cultured from chronic paronychia in wet workers with hand dermatitis (*Fig. 2.13*). It is unclear whether it is a primary pathogen or acting as an allergen, because it is often associated with an eczematous dermatitis. It may also be present in some dystrophic fingernails and toenails (see *Fig. 2.14*), often primarily affected by trauma or an inflammatory skin disease such as psoriasis (see *Sections 1.4.10* and *3.19.2*).

Who gets candida infections?

There are usually predisposing factors for active candida infections:
- Infancy or old age.
- Tropical climate with hyperhidrosis.
- Occlusion.
- Use of broad-spectrum antibiotics.
- Pregnancy or high-oestrogen oral contraceptive.
- Smoking.

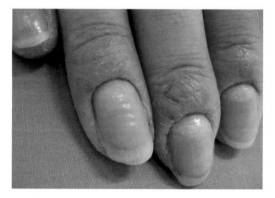

Figure 2.13. Chronic paronychia caused by hand dermatitis and candida infection.

- Topical or systemic steroids or chemotherapy.
- Underlying diabetes mellitus, iron deficiency, Cushing syndrome, malnutrition, cancer, immune deficiency.
- Skin disease, particularly psoriasis.

What are the clinical features of candida disease?

ORAL CANDIDIASIS

An acute presentation is usual (*Fig. 2.15*), but candida may cause chronic disease in the mouth of patients with underlying mucosal disease (such as lichen planus), in those using inhaled steroids, or with chronic illness. Clinical variations include angular cheilitis (red fissured moist furrows in the skin at the corners of the lips), pseudomembranous (peeling white patches), atrophic (sore, red, shiny patches), and hyperplastic (chronic red and white plaques) variants.

CANDIDA NAPKIN DERMATITIS

Candida colonises wet skin and complicates irritant contact dermatitis due to urine and faeces in contact with

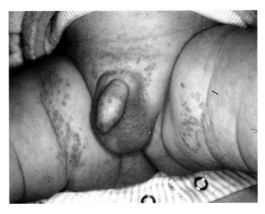

Figure 2.16. Candida napkin dermatitis.

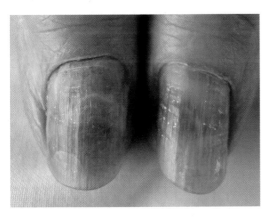

Figure 2.14. Onycholysis and greenish discoloration of nail plates caused by candida infection.

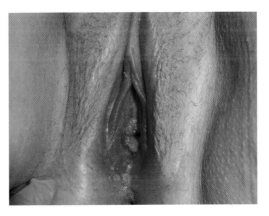

Figure 2.17. Acute vulvovaginitis as a result of candida infection.

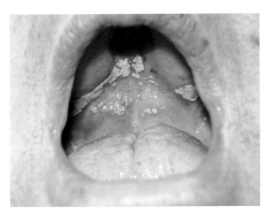

Figure 2.15. Oral thrush as a result of candida infection.

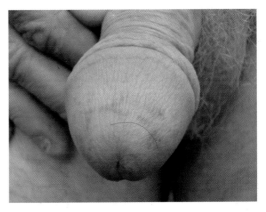

Figure 2.18. Candida ballanitis.

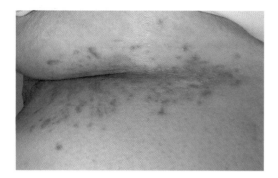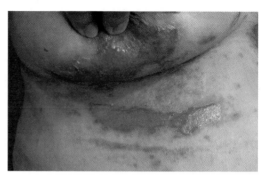

Figure 2.19. Candida intertrigo; erosive form on the right.

the skin. It has an acute presentation with erythematous papules and plaques with small satellite spots or superficial pustules that rapidly peel (*Fig. 2.16*).

VULVOVAGINAL CANDIDIASIS
Candida albicans thrives on glycogen, present within the normal vagina in women aged 15–55 or that are using topical or systemic hormone replacement. Overgrowth of candida leads to a white curd-like vaginal discharge, a burning sensation in the vagina and vulva and sometimes a bright red, itchy secondary dermatitis on vulva and surrounding skin (*Fig. 2.17*). Symptoms tend to be worse premenstrually and after intercourse.

CANDIDA BALANITIS
Balanitis is an inflammation of the glans penis and mainly affects uncircumcised men. *Candida albicans* can cause spotty or diffuse redness (*Fig. 2.18*), swelling, itch, tenderness and discharge. Most often balanitis is a non-specific dermatitis, with multiple organisms cultured.

CANDIDA INTERTRIGO
Intertrigo is a rash in skin folds (see *Section 1.4.5; flexures*). Candida can cause an acute flare with erythema, fissuring, peeling and satellite pustules (*Fig. 2.19*), or be a component of chronic non-specific intertrigo.

How is candida diagnosed?
Candida infection is generally diagnosed clinically because of its typical location and appearance. Microscopy and culture of skin swabs and scrapings may support the diagnosis;

note that candida may be found in up to 50% of normal mouths and about 20% of normal vaginas.

What is the treatment for candida?
Minimise predisposing factors where possible. Acute candidal skin infections are usually treated with topical imidazoles or nystatin.
Vaginal candidiasis is treated with antifungal pessaries or cream inserted high into the vagina, usually clotrimazole or miconazole for 1–7 days.
Eczematous nail-fold infections, intertrigo and vulvovaginitis may also require topical corticosteroid, e.g. hydrocortisone cream or combination hydrocortisone/miconazole cream.
Refractory or recurrent candidiasis can be treated with oral fluconazole or itraconazole.

2.2.3 Dermatophyte skin infections: tinea

What are dermatophytes?
Dermatophytes are common fungal pathogens that infect keratin in skin, hair and nails. Clinical infection is known as tinea. Dermatophytes almost never cause invasive or disseminated infection.

What organisms cause tinea?
The dermatophytes include three genera of moulds in the class Euascomycetes: *Trichophyton*, *Microsporum*, and *Epidermophyton*.
Human-associated dermatophytes are classified as anthropophilic dermatophytes and are the most common causes of tinea. Zoophilic (animal-associated) and geophilic (soil-dwelling) dermatophytes can also sometimes infect human skin.

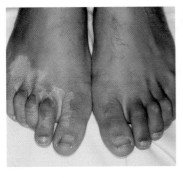
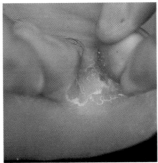
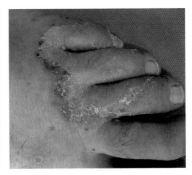

Figure 2.20. Tinea pedis.

Who gets dermatophyte infections?

Predisposing causes of dermatophyte infections include:

- Tropical climate.
- Overcrowding.
- Occlusive footwear and clothing.
- Community showers.
- Participation in sports.

What are the clinical features of dermatophyte infections?

ANTHROPOPHILIC DERMATOPHYTES

Anthropophilic dermatophytes, particularly *Trichophyton rubrum*, cause chronic persistent skin disease with mild inflammation. Itch tends to be mild.

- **Tinea pedis** (foot) is a common cause of athlete's foot (interdigital maceration), which can also be due to bacteria or yeast infection and/or a skin disease, particularly psoriasis and eczema. Tinea pedis may also cause dryness, peeling and/or irregular clusters of pustules on one or both soles (*Fig. 2.20*).
- **Tinea unguium** (nail) is the most common cause of onychomycosis, which can also be due to yeast and mould infections. Tinea unguium most often affects the great toenail. It presents with one or more discoloured, thickened, ridged or crumbling nail plates. Differential diagnosis of nail dystrophy includes trauma, psoriasis, lichen planus and other skin diseases (*Fig. 2.21*).
- **Tinea cruris** (groin) is one cause of intertrigo. Others are irritant dermatitis due to moisture and occlusion, *Candida albicans* infection, and skin diseases such as psoriasis and seborrhoeic dermatitis. Tinea cruris presents with unilateral or bilateral plaques spreading from the inguinal or crural folds and with a prominent erythematous, scaly border (*Fig. 2.22*).
- **Tinea corporis** (trunk, limbs) due to *T. rubrum* is most often seen in diabetics, patients using steroids or other immune suppressives, or the elderly. It causes unilateral or bilateral irregular annular scaly plaques (*Fig. 2.23*).

ZOOPHILIC OR GEOPHILIC ORGANISMS

Zoophilic or geophilic organisms present with acute inflammation and can be self-healing. In developed countries, *Microsporum canis*

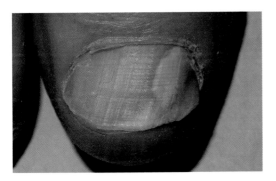
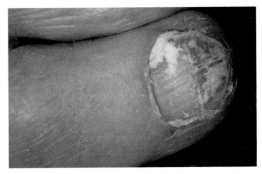

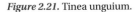
Figure 2.21. Tinea unguium.

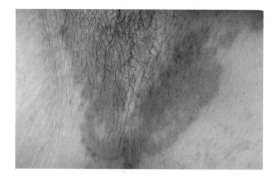
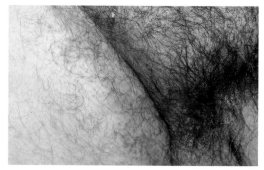

Figure 2.22. Tinea cruris.

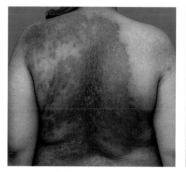
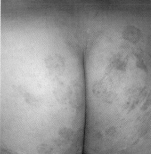
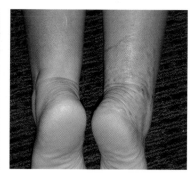

Figure 2.23. Tinea corporis.

is most often cultured, and is usually due to contact with an infected kitten.

- **Tinea capitis** (scalp) usually affects preschool children, who have one or more hairless scaly plaques on the scalp (*Fig. 2.24*). Strands of hair can be readily extracted from affected sites.
- **Tinea corporis** (body) is classic ringworm: multiple irregularly distributed and itchy, annular plaques on sites exposed to a pet or other animal (*Fig. 2.25*).
- **Kerion** is a fungal abscess. As there is a vigorous immune reaction, it may be difficult to ascertain the causative organism (*Fig. 2.26*).

How are dermatophyte infections diagnosed?

The diagnosis of fungal infection may be suspected by the presence of irregular plaques with superficial scaling. It should be confirmed by taking skin scrapings for mycology. Put samples in a clean, dry container and send to the laboratory.

- Use a dull blade to scrape off surface scale and loose hair.
- Scrape debris underneath infected nails and add nail clippings.

- An interim microscopy report may reveal mycelia and arthrospores in scrapings stained with potassium hydroxide (KOH).
- The final report of culture of the causative fungus may take several weeks.

What is the treatment for dermatophyte infections?

Topical therapy using one of a variety of antifungal agents is appropriate for localised skin infections of limited extent. Continue for

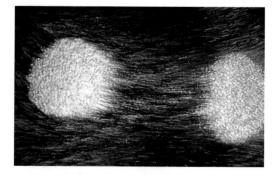

Figure 2.24. Tinea capitis on scalp.

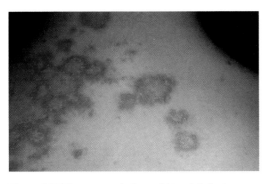

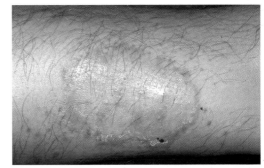

Figure 2.25. Tinea corporis due to *M. canis* infection.

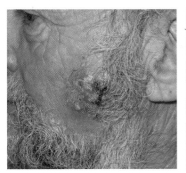

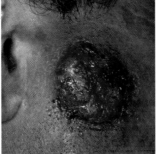

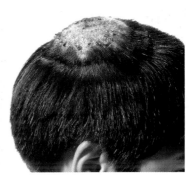

Figure 2.26. Kerion.

several days after apparent resolution of infection.

Oral therapy with terbinafine or an azole antifungal is usual for the following mycologically confirmed infections:

- Extensive skin involvement.
- Tinea capitis.
- Symptomatic confirmed nail plate infections.

2.2.4 Fungal nail infections

What is fungal nail infection?

Fungal nail infection starts in one nail and, over time, may involve others. The great toenail is affected most commonly.

Fungal nail infection is also called onychomycosis. When due to a dermatophyte fungus, it is called tinea unguium (see *Fig. 2.21*).

Who gets fungal nail infection?

Uncommon in children, prevalence of fungal nail infection increases with age. It is more common and severe in patients with diabetes or immune deficiencies or immune suppression. Spores are long-lived, and healthy family members may present with similar infections due to sharing bathing facilities.

What causes fungal nail infection?

Fungal nail infection often follows trauma and can co-exist with another disease of the nails. It spreads from local tinea pedis of the hyponychium. Culture may reveal:

- Dermatophyte fungus: 90% of cases are either due to *T. rubrum* (*Fig. 2.27*), *T. interdigitale* (*Fig. 2.28*), or *Epidermophyton floccosum*.
- *Candida albicans:* associated with paronychia (*Fig. 2.29*) or underlying psoriatic nail dystrophy.
- Moulds: scytalidinum, scopulariopsis (*Fig. 2.30*), fusarium and others.
- Mixed.

What are the clinical features of fungal nail infection?

Fungal nail infection can cause:

- Nail plate dystrophy: irregular ridging, thickening, brittle nails.
- Discoloration in longitudinal streaks, blotches or of entire nail plate: yellow, brown, green, black.

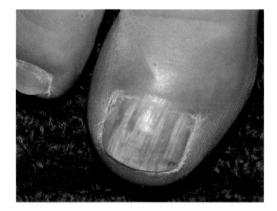

Figure 2.27. Fungal nail infection caused by *T. rubrum*.

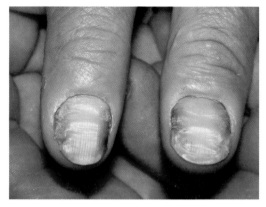

Figure 2.29. Fungal nail infection caused by *C. albicans*.

Typical patterns include:
- Lateral onychomycosis: a white or yellow opaque streak appears at one side of the nail (see *Fig. 2.27*).
- Subungual hyperkeratosis: scaling occurs under the nail (*Fig. 2.31*).
- Distal onycholysis: the end of the nail lifts up and the free edge often crumbles (see *Fig. 2.30*).
- Superficial white onychomycosis: flaky white patches and pits appear on the top of the nail plate (see *Fig. 2.28*).
- Proximal onychomycosis: yellow or white spots appear in the half-moon (lunula, *Fig. 2.32*).
- Onychoma or dermatophytoma. This is a thick localised area of infection in the nail plate (*Fig. 2.33*).
- Complete destruction of the nail (see *Fig. 2.31*).

Complications of fungal nail infection

Fungal nail infection is unsightly. It can also give rise to:
- Lack of dexterity (fingernails).
- Pain or discomfort.
- A reservoir of dermatophytes.

How is fungal nail infection diagnosed?

Clinical examination alone can be unreliable, so confirmation prior to treatment is recommended. Distal nail clippings, scrapings of the surface of the nail plate, and scrapings of subungual debris are taken. Microscopy may show mycelia and arthrospores. Cultures are reported at 4–6 weeks.

What is the treatment for fungal nail infections?

Mild distal nail infection is treated with topical lacquers or solutions. Efficacy is poor. Systemic

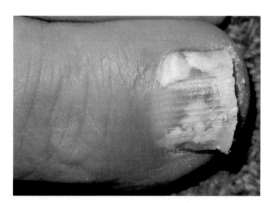

Figure 2.28. Fungal nail infection caused by *T. interdigitale*.

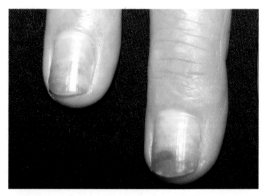

Figure 2.30. Fungal nail infection caused by the scopulariopsis mould.

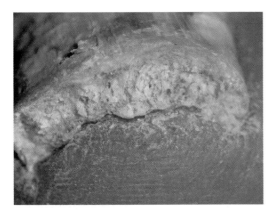

Figure 2.31. Subungal hyperkeratosis.

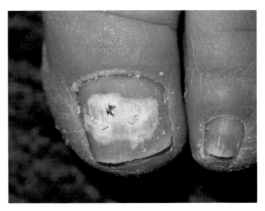

Figure 2.33. Onychoma or dermatophytoma.

therapy has higher cure rates but may fail to clear severe infections or disease in the elderly. Failure can also be due to concominant underlying nail disease, usually due to repetitive trauma or psoriasis.

- Dermatophytes are treated with oral terbinafine for 3–6 months.
- Yeasts are treated with oral azoles, in 7-day pulses each month or continuously.
- Moulds and mixed infections are treated with both.

Physical nail removal, chemical nail removal (e.g. using urea paste) and laser treatment may be of limited benefit.

How can fungal nail infections be prevented?

Regular foot inspections are recommended. Athlete's foot and other forms of tinea pedis should be promptly treated with topical antifungal cream.

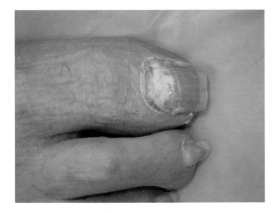

Figure 2.32. Proximal onychomycosis.

Bathrooms and pool surrounds should receive regular treatment with hypochlorite solution to reduce transmission of infection.

What is the outlook for fungal nail infections?

Fungal nail infections rarely clear spontaneously. Mild to moderate dermatophyte infections usually clear with oral therapy in young to middle-aged adults. Treatment of confirmed fungal infection may be unhelpful if the dystrophy is mainly due to another cause.

2.2.5 Malassezia infections

What are malassezia?

Malassezia are yeasts that are part of the normal cutaneous flora of the scalp, face and upper trunk from the neonatal period. There are up to 14 subspecies. They are dependent on host lipids and secrete lipase and phospholipases. Under some circumstances malassezia may cause:

- Infantile and adult seborrhoeic dermatitis (*Fig. 2.34*).
- Pityriasis versicolor (*Fig. 2.35*).
- Malassezia folliculitis (*Fig. 2.36*).
- Atopic eczema (*Fig. 2.37*).
- Systemic infections in immunocompromised hosts.

Who gets malassezia infections?

Predisposing causes of chronic malassezia infections include:

- Hyperhidrosis associated with tropical and subtropical climates and occlusive clothing.
- Oily skin—hence prevalence in young adults, especially those using oily emollient creams.

- Corticosteroid therapy, malnutrition and immune suppression.

What are the clinical features of malassezia disease?

- Seborrhoeic dermatitis causes flaking and inflammation in sites normally colonised by malassezia, especially scalp and face. The eczematous reaction is most prominent within the skin folds (*Fig. 2.34*).
- Pityriasis versicolor is also flaky, but not inflamed, and affects the trunk with multiple thin, hypopigmented, pink or brown plaques (*Fig. 2.35*).
- Malassezia folliculitis is a monomorphic superficial follicular papulopustular eruption of the upper trunk, notably itchy (*Fig. 2.36*).
- Malassezia plays a role in some patients with atopic eczema (*Fig. 2.37*), leading to flaky eczematous dermatitis on scalp, face and neck.

How is malassezia diagnosed?

The diagnosis of malassezia may be suspected by the presence of flaky skin. It fluoresces yellow under a Wood lamp. Potassium hydroxide wet mount of a scraping of scale or pustule shows hyphae and bunches of spores. Culture is usually negative. On skin biopsy, spores and hyphae may be noted within the stratum corneum and dilated ostia of hair follicles.

What is the treatment for malassezia?

Topical therapy using one of a variety of antifungal agents is appropriate for localised skin infections of limited extent. Continue for several days after apparent resolution of infection. Ketoconazole and ciclopirox are particularly effective.

Intermittent use of low potency topical corticosteroid creams is also necessary for seborrhoeic dermatitis and atopic eczema flares.

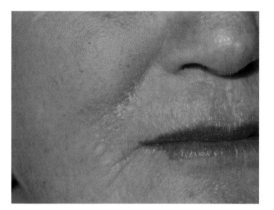

Figure 2.34. Seborrhoeic dermatitis.

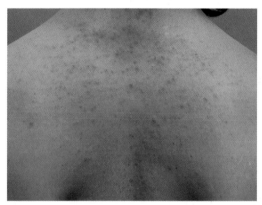

Figure 2.36. Malassezia folliculitis.

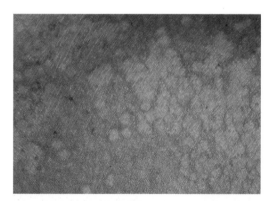

Figure 2.35. Pityriasis versicolor.

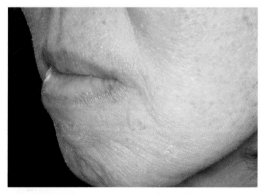

Figure 2.37. Atopic eczema with flaking due to malasezzia.

Oral therapy with an azole antifungal agent is usual for the following:

- Extensive skin involvement.
- Lack of response to topical therapy.

2.2.6 Paronychia

What is paronychia?

Paronychia is inflammation of the skin around a finger or toenail. It can be acute or chronic; both are common conditions. Paronychia is also called whitlow. It may be associated with felon (infection of the pulp of the fingertip).

Who gets paronychia?

Acute paronychia can affect anyone. However, it is more likely to follow a break in the skin, especially between the proximal nail fold/cuticle and the nail plate. For example:

- If the nail is bitten or the nail fold is habitually picked.
- In infants that suck their fingers or thumbs.
- Following manicuring.
- Ingrown toenails.
- On application of sculptured or artificial fingernails.
- Treatment with systemic retinoid that dries the skin (acitretin, isotretinoin).
- Other drugs, including epidermal growth factor receptor and *BRAF* inhibitors.

Chronic paronychia mainly occurs in people with hand dermatitis, or who have constantly cold and wet hands, such as:

- Dairy farmers.
- Fishermen.
- Bar tenders.
- Cleaners.
- Housewives.
- People with poor circulation.

Acute and chronic skin infections tend to be more frequent and aggressive in patients with diabetes or chronic debility, or that are immune suppressed.

What causes paronychia?

Acute paronychia is usually due to bacterial infection with *Staph. aureus*, or other bacterial pathogens less frequently. It can also be due to the cold sore virus, *Herpes simplex* (see *Section 2.3.4*).

The cause or causes of chronic paronychia are not fully understood. In many cases, it is due to dermatitis of the nail fold. Often several different micro-organisms can be cultured, particularly *C. albicans* (see *Section 2.2.2*) and Gram-negative bacilli.

What are the clinical features of paronychia?

Acute paronychia develops rapidly over a few hours, and usually affects a single nail fold (*Fig. 2.38*). This becomes painful, red and swollen. If herpes simplex is the cause, multiple tender vesicles may be observed (*Fig. 2.39*). Sometimes yellow pus appears under the cuticle and can evolve into an abscess. The nail plate may lift up. Acute paronychia due to *Strep. pyogenes* may be accompanied by fever, lymphangitis and tender lymphadenopathy.

Chronic paronychia (*Fig. 2.40*) is a gradual process. It may start in one nail fold but often spreads to several others. Each affected nail

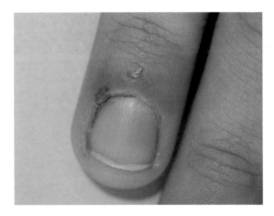

Figure 2.38. Bacterial paronychia.

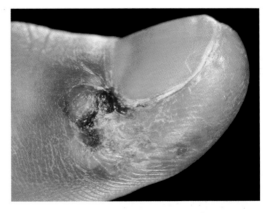

Figure 2.39. Paronychia due to herpes simplex.

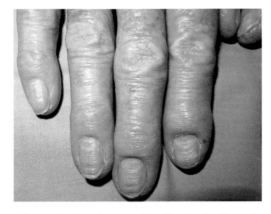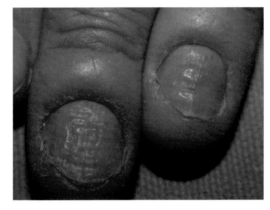

Figure 2.40. Chronic paronychia, also showing dystrophy of nails.

fold is swollen and lifted off the nail plate. The affected skin may be red and tender from time to time, and sometimes a little pus (white, yellow or green) can be expressed from under the cuticle.

What are the complications of paronychia?

Acute paronychia can spread to cause a serious hand infection (cellulitis, see *Section 2.1.2*) and may involve underlying tendons (infectious tendonitis).

The main complication of chronic paronychia is nail dystrophy. It is often associated with distorted, ridged nail plates (*Fig. 2.40*). They may become yellow or green/black and brittle. After recovery, it takes up to a year for the nails to grow back to normal.

How is paronychia diagnosed?

Paronychia is a clinical diagnosis, often supported by culture of bacterial and viral swabs and/or nail clippings for mycology.

What is the treatment for paronychia?

ACUTE PARONYCHIA
- Soak affected digit in warm water, several times daily.
- Topical antiseptic may be prescribed for localised, minor infection.
- Oral antibiotics may be necessary for severe or prolonged bacterial infection.
- Consider aciclovir or valaciclovir in case of severe herpes simplex infection.

- Surgical incision and drainage may be required for abscess followed by irrigation and packing with gauze.
- Rarely, the nail must be removed to allow pus to drain.

CHRONIC PARONYCHIA
Attend to predisposing factors.
- Keep the hands dry and warm.
- Avoid wet work, or use totally waterproof gloves.
- Keep fingernails scrupulously clean.
- Wash after dirty work with soap and water, rinse off and dry carefully.
- Apply emollient hand cream frequently – dimeticone barrier creams may help.

Treatment should focus on the dermatitis and any microbes grown on culture.
- Topical corticosteroid ointment for 2–4 weeks and for flares.
- Antiseptics or antifungal lotions or solutions for several months.
- Oral antifungal agent (itraconazole or fluconazole) if *C. albicans* confirmed.

What is the outlook for paronychia?

Acute paronychia usually clears completely in a few days, and rarely recurs in healthy individuals.

Chronic paronychia may persist for months or longer, and can recur in predisposed individuals.

2.3 Viruses

2.3.1 General viral infections

Introduction

Numerous viral infections cause specific and non-specific widespread exanthems (rashes) and some also cause enanthems (mucositis). These are often experienced during childhood and can last anything from a few hours to several weeks.

Specific exanthems (see *Section 2.3.3*) are:
- Measles (morbilli, *Fig. 2.41*).
- Rubella (German measles).
- Varicella (chickenpox, *Fig. 2.42*).
- Erythema infectiosum (fifth disease, *Fig. 2.43*).
- Roseola (exanthem subitum).
- Enteroviral vesicular stomatitis (HFM, *Fig. 2.44*).

Other viral syndromes include:
- Pityriasis rosea (see *Section 2.3.8* and *Fig. 2.45*).

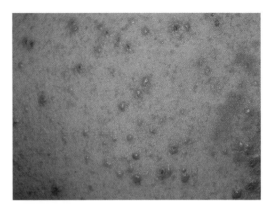

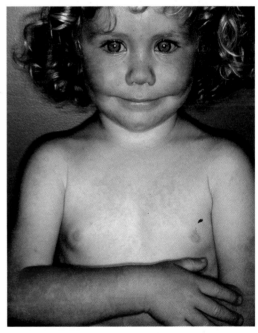

Figure 2.42. Chickenpox.

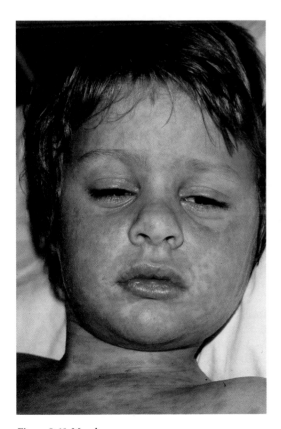

Figure 2.41. Measles.

Figure 2.43. Erythema infectiosum.

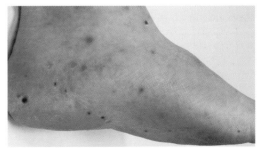

Figure 2.44. Enteroviral vesicular stomatitis (HFM).

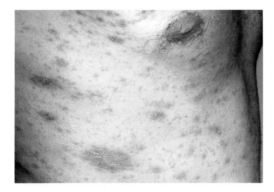

Figure 2.45. Pityriasis rosea.

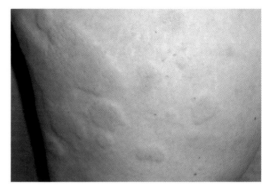

Figure 2.48. Acute urticaria.

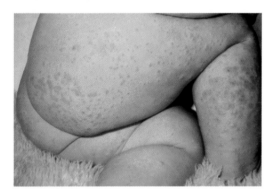

Figure 2.46. Infantile papular acrodermatitis.

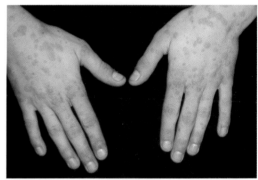

Figure 2.49. Erythema multifome.

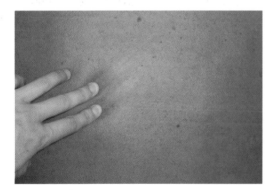

Figure 2.47. Erythema.

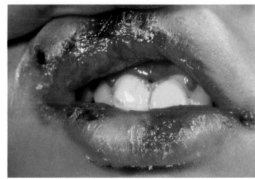

Figure 2.50. Herpes simplex infection.

- Infantile papular acrodermatitis (see *Section 2.3.6* and *Fig. 2.46*).

Non-specific reactions to viral infection can include:
- Erythema (*Fig. 2.47*).
- Acute urticaria (see *Section 3.22* and *Fig. 2.48*).
- Erythema multiforme (see *Section 3.7* and *Fig. 2.49*).

Localised viral infections are most frequently due to:
- Herpes simplex (see *Section 2.3.4* and *Fig. 2.50*).
- Herpes zoster (see *Section 2.3.5* and *Fig. 2.51*).
- Molluscum contagiosum (see *Section 2.3.7* and *Fig. 2.52*).
- Viral warts, including anogenital warts (see *Sections 2.3.9* and *2.3.2*, and *Fig. 2.53*).

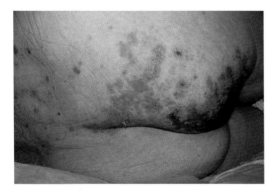

Figure 2.51. Herpes zoster infection.

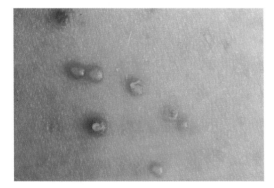

Figure 2.52. Molluscum contagiosum.

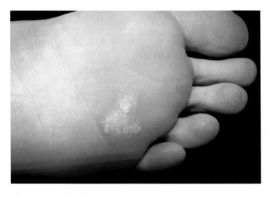

Figure 2.53. Viral warts.

How are viral skin infections diagnosed?

Diagnosis is often made by the clinical appearance. Tests depend on the suspected infection, and may include:

- Viral swab for viral culture, immunofluorescence and PCR.
- Blood tests for serology, PCR, RNA/DNA.
- Genotyping.

How are viral skin infections prevented and treated?

Prevention requires vaccination. Vaccines are available to measles, rubella, varicella and anogenital warts.

Treatment of viral infection is most often supportive, because there is no specific treatment for the majority of viral infections.

- Aciclovir, most often taken orally, is effective for herpes virus infections. Alternatives are valaciclovir and famciclovir.
- Antiretroviral treatment controls human immunodeficiency virus.
- Viral warts and molluscum can be locally destroyed.

For information about other viral infections giving rise to cutaneous signs, see DermNetNZ.org

2.3.2 Anogenital warts

What are anogenital warts?

Anogenital warts are common superficial skin lesions in the anogenital area that are caused by human papillomavirus. They are also called condyloma acuminata, genital warts, venereal warts and squamous cell papilloma.

What is the human papillomavirus?

The human papillomavirus (HPV) is actually a group of viruses.

- There are at least 100 different types of HPV; at least 40 can infect the anogenital area. Many others cause warts on other areas of skin.
- At least 75% of sexually active adults have been infected with at least one type of anogenital HPV at some time in their life.
- HPV is incorporated into skin cells and stimulates them to proliferate, causing a visible wart.
- Visible anogenital warts are often easy to diagnose by their typical appearance. They are usually due to HPV types 6 and 11.
- Most do not develop visible warts. However, the infection may show up on a cervical smear. This is known as subclinical infection.
- Some strains of HPV cause anogenital cancer. These oncogenic strains may not cause visible warts but they remain contagious.

Who gets anogenital warts?

As anogenital warts are sexually acquired during close skin contact, they are most commonly observed in young adults between the ages of

15 and 30 years. They are highly contagious, and occur in equal numbers in unvaccinated males and females. However, they are rare in people that have been vaccinated against HPV in childhood before beginning sexual activity.

What do anogenital warts look like?

Anogenital warts are flesh coloured papules a few millimetres in diameter that may join together to form warty plaques several centimetres across. They may occur in the following sites:

- Vulva (*Fig. 2.54*).
- Vagina.
- Cervix.
- Urethra.
- Penis (*Fig. 2.55*).
- Scrotum.
- Anus (*Fig. 2.56*).

Warts due to the same types of HPV can also arise on the lips or within the oral mucosa.

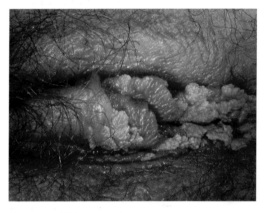

Figure 2.54. Vulval warts.

Normal anatomical structures may be confused with warts. These include:

- Pearly papules (these are in a ring around the glans of the penis).
- Sebaceous glands on the labia (known as 'Fordyce spots').
- Vestibular papillae (the fronds found in the opening to the vagina).

How is HPV transmitted?

Visible genital warts and subclinical HPV infection nearly always arise from direct skin-to-skin contact.

- Sexual contact – this is the most common method of transmission amongst adults.
- Transmission is more likely from visible warts than from subclinical HPV infection.
- Oral sex – HPV is relatively more common in the genital area than the mouth, however.
- Vertical (mother to baby) transmission through the birth canal.
- Auto-inoculation from one site to another.
- Fomites (i.e. from objects like bath towels) – it remains very controversial whether warts can spread this way.
- Often, warts will appear 3–6 months after infection, but they may appear months or even years later.

How can transmission of warts be reduced?

Transmission of warts to a new sexual partner can be reduced but not completely prevented by using condoms. Condoms do not prevent all genital skin-to-skin contact, but they also protect against other STDs.

Successful treatment of the warts decreases the chance of passing on the infection.

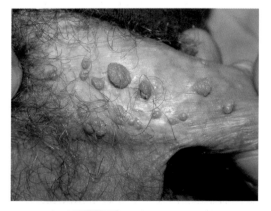

Figure 2.55. Penile warts.

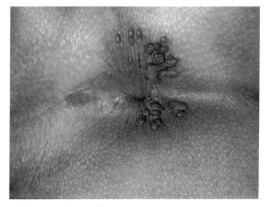

Figure 2.56. Anal warts.

What is the treatment for genital warts?

The primary goal of treatment is to eliminate warts that cause physical or psychological symptoms such as:

- Pain.
- Bleeding.
- Itch.
- Embarrassment.

Options include:

- No treatment.
- Self-applied treatments at home.
- Treatment at a doctor's surgery or medical clinic.

The underlying viral infection may persist after the visible warts have cleared. Warts sometimes re-emerge years later because the immune system has weakened.

SELF-APPLIED TREATMENTS

To be successful the patient must identify and reach the warts, and follow the application instructions carefully. Available treatments include:

- Podophyllotoxin.
- Imiquimod.
- Sinecatechins.

TREATMENT AT THE CLINIC

Options include:

- Cryotherapy.
- Podophyllin resin.
- Trichloroacetic acid applications.
- Electrosurgery.
- Curettage and scissor or scalpel excision.
- Laser ablation.
- Fluorouracil cream.

Genital warts and cancer

The HPV types that cause external visible warts (HPV types 6 and 11) rarely cause cancer. Other HPV types (most often types 16, 18, 31, 33 and 35) are less common in visible warts but are strongly associated with anogenital cancer (*Fig. 2.57*), including:

- Intraepithelial neoplasia of penile, vulval and anal skin.
- Invasive squamous cell carcinoma (SCC) of cervix, penis, vulva and anus.

HPV also causes some cases of oral and nasopharyngeal cancers.

Only a small percentage of infected people develop genital cancer. This is because HPV

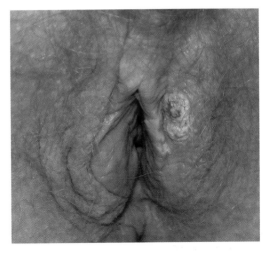

Figure 2.57. Warts evolving into carcinoma.

infection is only one factor in the process; cigarette smoking and the immune system are also important.

Cervical smears, as recommended in National Cervical Screening guidelines, detect early abnormalities of the cervix, which can then be treated. If these abnormalities were ignored over a long period, they could progress to cancer.

Human papillomavirus vaccine

Two vaccines are available to prevent HPV infection, Gardasil and Cervarix. More are under development.

- Gardasil is effective against HPV types 6, 11, 16 and 18. In the UK, Gardasil is offered to all girls aged 12–13y at school and a catch-up programme for girls aged 14–17y is now complete. In New Zealand, Gardasil 9 (against HPV types 6, 11, 16, 18, 31, 33, 45, 52 and 58) is funded and recommended for males and females up to the age of 26y. It can also be prescribed for older individuals but this is unfunded.
- Cervarix is effective against HPV types 16 and 18. Available in many countries for prevention of cervical cancer, it is not subsidised in New Zealand, but was the original vaccination in the UK prior to the change to Gardasil in 2012.

HPV vaccination is most effective when offered at a young age, before the onset of sexual activity. However, girls that are already sexually active may not have been infected with the types of HPV covered by the vaccine and may still benefit from vaccination. Women that receive an HPV vaccine should continue to participate in cervical screening programmes, because the vaccine will not prevent all cervical cancers.

HPV vaccines are also effective in boys. Vaccination of boys is recommended to reduce transmission of HPV to unvaccinated females. It also reduces the incidence of cancers related to HPV infection. However, at present there is no vaccination HPV programme for boys in the UK, though this is being reviewed.

There has been interest in developing therapeutic HPV vaccines for the treatment of genital warts and cervical cancer in those already infected.

2.3.3 Exanthems

What is an exanthem?

Exanthem is the medical name given to a widespread rash that is usually accompanied by systemic symptoms such as fever, malaise and headache. It is usually caused by an infectious condition such as a primary infection with a contagious virus, or bacterial toxin, and represents either a reaction to a toxin produced by the organism, damage to the skin by the organism, or an immune response. Exanthems may also be due to a drug (especially antibiotics and non-steroidal anti-inflammatory drugs).

What causes exanthems?

Viral acute exanthems generally occur during childhood.
- Enteroviral vesicular stomatitis (HFM, *Fig. 2.58*).
- Erythema infectiosum (fifth disease, *Fig. 2.59*).

- Measles (morbilli, *Fig. 2.60*).
- Roseola (erythema subitum).
- Rubella (German measles, *Fig. 2.61*).
- Varicella (chickenpox, *Fig. 2.62*).

What are the signs and symptoms of exanthems?

In most cases, prior to the rash appearing, patients may have systemic symptoms indicative of infection:
- Fever.
- Malaise.
- Headache.
- Loss of appetite, nausea.
- Abdominal pain, vomiting, diarrhoea.
- Muscular aches and pains.

ENTEROVIRAL VESICULAR STOMATITIS
- Also called hand, foot and mouth disease (see *Fig. 2.58*).
- Most frequently due to Coxsackie A viruses.
- Spreads via respiratory secretions, the oral–faecal route, or by direct contact with vesicles.
- Incubation period is 3–5 days.
- Contagious until blisters have gone.
- Oral papules evolve into vesicles as similar lesions occur on hands and feet and sometimes elsewhere.
- Blisters peel within 7 days.
- Fingernails may be shed a few weeks later.

ERYTHEMA INFECTIOSUM
- Also called fifth disease (see *Fig. 2.59*).
- Due to erythrovirus, parvovirus B19.
- Spreads via respiratory secretions.
- Incubation period is 7–10 days to viral symptoms and another 7 days to the rash.

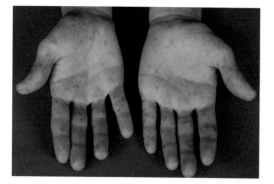
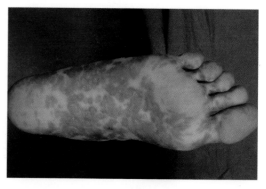

Figure 2.58. Hand, foot and mouth (enteroviral vesicular stomatitis).

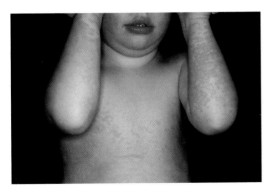

Figure 2.59. Fifth disease (erythema infectiosum).

- Contagious from onset of viral symptoms until rash appears.
- Swelling and redness of cheeks for 2–4 days (slapped cheek appearance).
- Diffuse erythema followed by lace-like reticular pattern on limbs that fades and recurs over several weeks when warm.
- Rarely, in adults can cause papular purpuric gloves-and-socks syndrome.
- Complications may occur in adults, the immune compromised and those with haemolytic anaemia or haemoglobinopathies: polyarthropathy, aplastic anaemia and other syndromes.
- *In utero* vertical infection in early pregnancy (10% maternal infections) leads to hydrops fetalis and fetal death.

MEASLES (MORBILLIVIRUS)
- Due to morbillivirus (see *Fig. 2.60*).
- Spreads via respiratory droplets or direct contact.
- Incubation period is 7–14 days.
- Contagious from 2 days before symptoms to 5 days after onset of the rash.
- Cough, conjunctivitis and oral blue–white Koplik spots occur early.
- Asymptomatic maculopapular rash appears on face within 3–5 days.
- Rash spreads to trunk and limbs at a peak with high point of fever then fades through purplish copper colour with fine scaling.
- Complications more common in malnourished children: diarrhoea, otitis media and deafness, pneumonia, corneal ulceration and blindness, renal disease.
- Prevented by 2-dose vaccination, usually MMR (with mumps, rubella).
- Aciclovir is prescribed for adults and immune-suppressed children.

ROSEOLA
- Also known as exanthem subitum.
- Due to type 6 and 7 herpes virus infection (HHV6, HHV7).
- Spreads via respiratory droplets or direct contact with saliva.
- Incubation period is 9–10 days.
- Contagious during febrile period.
- Rash appears as high fever experienced in previous 3–5 days subsides.
- Pale pink macules on trunk spreading to face, neck and limbs.
- Similar spots occur on soft palate and uvula (Nagayama spots).
- Rash fades within hours or up to 2 days.
- Complications include febrile convulsions.
- Reactivation of HHV6 and HHV7 can lead to pityriasis rosea (see *Section 2.3.8*).
- Drug hypersensitivity syndrome is associated with reactivation of HHV6 (see *Section 3.5.2*).

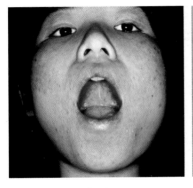
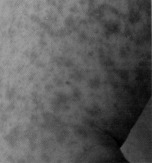
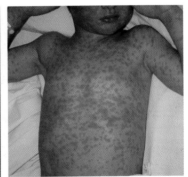

Figure 2.60. Measles.

Figure 2.61. German measles (rubella).

Rubella

- Also known as German measles (see *Fig. 2.61*).
- Due to rubella virus infection.
- Spreads via direct contact with nasal or throat secretions.
- Incubation period is 12–23 days.
- Contagious 7 days before rash until 7 days after rash clears.
- Lymphadenopathy is often prominent behind ears and back of neck.
- Pale pink macules on face, neck, trunk and limbs.
- Rash fades within 5 days.
- If infected in first trimester, fetus has 50% chance of congenital rubella syndrome.
- Prevented by vaccination (MMR with mumps, measles) but remains common in developing countries.

Varicella

- Chickenpox is due to a herpes virus, varicella-zoster (see *Fig. 2.62*).
- Spreads via respiratory droplets or direct contact with blister fluid.

- Incubation period is up to 21 days.
- Contagious from 2 days before rash to when all lesions have crusted over.
- Itchy papules that evolve to vesicles then crust.
- Located on scalp, face, inside mouth, trunk with fewer lesions on limbs.
- Complications more common in adults and immune-suppressed children: viral pneumonia, CNS infection, thrombocytopenia and purpura, secondary streptococcal skin infection. Rarely, may be fatal in the immune suppressed, who can develop recurrent primary infection.
- Most cases can be prevented by vaccination.
- Treatment is supportive. Healthy children do not require antiviral therapy.
- High-dose aciclovir or valaciclovir is prescribed for adults and immune-suppressed children.
- Varicella-zoster immunoglobulin may be administered in immune suppression, pregnancy and neonates and for prophylaxis in such patients. Refer to local guidelines.
- Reactivation of varicella-zoster virus causes herpes zoster (see *Section 2.3.5*).

Specific bacterial exanthems are less common and include:
- Scarlet fever (scarlatina, *Fig. 2.63*).
- Staphylococcal scalded skin syndrome (*Fig. 2.64*).
- Toxic shock syndrome (staphylococcal, streptococcal).

Scarlet fever

- Also called scarlatina (see *Fig. 2.63*).
- Due to a toxin-producing strain of Group A beta-haemolytic streptococci.
- Mostly affects school-aged children.
- Incubation period is 12 hours to 7 days.

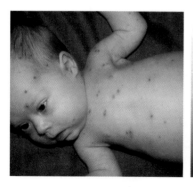
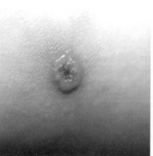
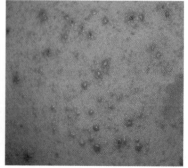

Figure 2.62. Chickenpox (varicella).

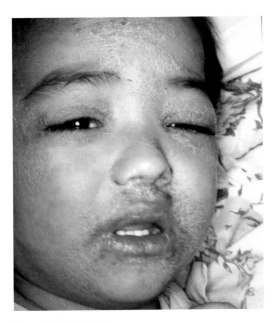

Figure 2.63. Scarlet fever.

- Contagious during the acute illness.
- Associated with acute exudative pharyngitis, or less often wound infection or other streptococcal disease.
- Diffusely punctate rash spreads from neck to trunk and limbs, variable redness with linear arrays of petechiae.
- Affected skin feels dry 'like sandpaper'.
- Flushed face with circumoral pallor.
- Red papules on mucous membranes, white then red, strawberry tongue.
- Fine desquamation after 7–10 days, especially face, palms and soles.
- Treatment requires antibiotics.
- Can lead to post-streptococcal disease, e.g. rheumatic fever, and other complications.

STAPHYLOCOCCAL SCALDED SKIN SYNDROME
- Due to a toxin-producing strain of *Staph. aureus* (see *Fig. 2.64*).
- Affects infants, and rarely adults that are immune compromised or have renal impairment.
- Starts as localised focus of bullous impetigo around the mouth or in armpit or groin.
- Rash spreads to other sites of body.
- Skin peels like tissue paper, leaving moist red and tender areas.
- Children usually recover rapidly without scarring.
- Treatment requires antibiotics.

Non-specific exanthems may also be caused by other infections, including:
- Infectious mononucleosis (*Fig. 2.65*).
- Viral hepatitis.
- Mycoplasma (*Fig. 2.66*).
- Rickettsial diseases, dengue, chikungunya and zika infections (*Fig. 2.67*) associated with arthropod bites.

TOXIC SHOCK SYNDROME
- Due to a toxin-producing strain of *Staph. aureus*.
- Toxin-producing strain of *Strep. pyogenes* causes toxic shock-like syndrome with similar symptoms and signs.
- Associated with localised focus or systemic infection at any age.
- Cytokine release causes fever, hypotension, multiorgan disease.
- Skin becomes diffusely red.
- Skin peels after 1–2 weeks, especially palms and soles.

Non-specific exanthems are usually widespread and may be more extensive on the trunk and

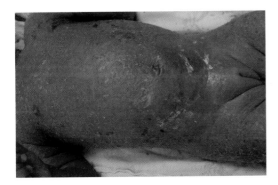

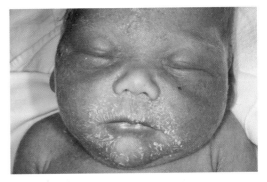

Figure 2.64. Staphylococcal scalded skin syndrome.

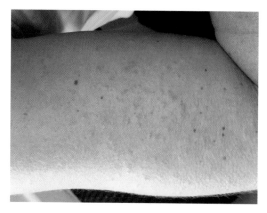

Figure 2.65. Infectious mononucleosis.

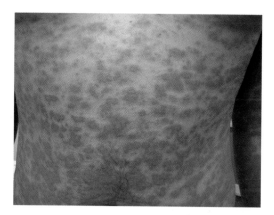

Figure 2.66. Mycoplasma.

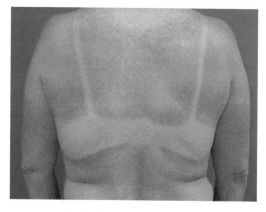

Figure 2.67. Zika infection.

extremities. Viral exanthems often occur in small epidemics so there may be other children affected at the same time.

For descriptions of drug eruptions, see *Section 3.5*.

Diagnosis of exanthems

The exanthems described above have distinct patterns of rashes and prodromal (pre-rash) symptoms allowing clinical diagnosis.

Consult local laboratory resources to determine the most suitable tests in case of doubt, particularly in a very sick patient or if the exanthem arises during pregnancy.

What is the treatment for exanthems?

Treatment of specific exanthems will depend on the cause.

Symptomatic treatment may include:
- Paracetamol to reduce fever.
- Moisturising emollients to reduce itch.

2.3.4 Herpes simplex

What is herpes simplex?

Herpes simplex is a common viral infection that presents with localised blistering. It affects most people on one or more occasions during their lives.

Herpes simplex is commonly referred to as cold sores or fever blisters, because recurrences are often triggered by a febrile illness, such as a cold.

What causes herpes simplex?

Herpes simplex is caused by one of two types of herpes simplex virus (HSV), members of the *Herpesvirales* family of double-stranded DNA viruses.
- Type 1 is mainly associated with oral and facial infections (*Fig. 2.68*).
- Type 2 is mainly associated with genital and rectal infections (anogenital herpes, *Fig. 2.69*).

However, either virus can affect almost any area of skin or mucous membrane.

After the primary episode of infection, HSV resides in a latent state in spinal dorsal root nerves that supply sensation to the skin. During a recurrence, the virus follows the nerves onto the skin or mucous membranes, where it multiplies, causing the clinical lesion. After each attack and lifelong, it enters the resting state.

During an attack, the virus can be inoculated into new sites of skin, which can then develop blisters as well as the original site of infection.

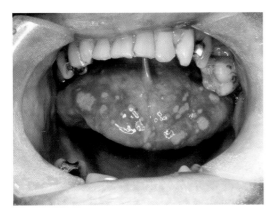

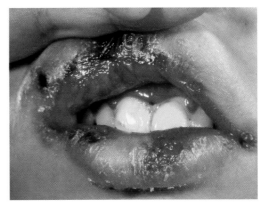

Figure 2.68. Herpes simplex type 1.

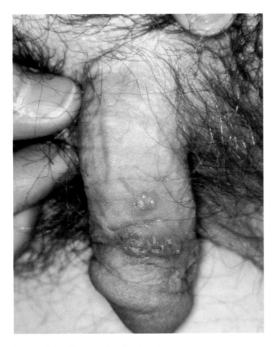

Figure 2.69. Herpes simplex type 2.

Who gets herpes simplex?

Primary attacks of type 1 HSV infections occur mainly in infants and young children. In crowded, underdeveloped areas of the world, nearly all children have been infected by the age of 5. In less crowded places, the incidence is lower, for example, less than half of university entrants in the UK have been infected. Type 2 HSV infections occur mainly after puberty, and are often transmitted sexually.

HSV is transmitted by direct or indirect contact with someone with active herpes simplex, which is infectious for 7–12 days.

Asymptomatic shedding of the virus in saliva or genital secretions can also lead to transmission of HSV, but this is infrequent, because the amount shed from inactive lesions is 100 to 1000 times less than when it is active. The incubation period is 2–12 days.

Minor injury helps inoculate HSV into the skin. For example:
- A thumb sucker may transmit the virus from their mouth to their thumb.
- A healthcare worker may develop herpetic whitlow (see *Section 2.2.6, Fig. 2.70*).
- A rugby player may get a cluster of blisters on one cheek ('scrum pox').

What are the clinical features of herpes simplex?

PRIMARY HERPES SIMPLEX
Primary infection with HSV can be mild or subclinical, but symptomatic infection tends to be more severe than recurrences. Type 2 HSV is more often symptomatic than type 1 HSV.

Primary type 1 HSV most often presents as gingivostomatitis in children between 1 and 5 years of age. Symptoms include fever, which may be high, restlessness and excessive dribbling. Drinking and eating are painful and the breath is foul. The gums are swollen and red and bleed easily. Whitish vesicles evolve to yellowish ulcers on the tongue, throat, palate and inside the cheeks. Local lymph glands are enlarged and tender.

The fever subsides after 3–5 days and recovery is usually complete within 2 weeks.

Primary type 2 HSV usually presents as genital herpes after the onset of sexual activity. Painful vesicles, ulcers, redness and swelling

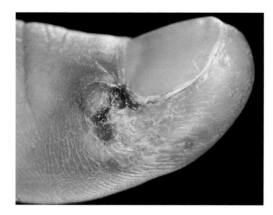

Figure 2.70. Herpetic whitlow.

last for 2–3 weeks, if untreated, and are often accompanied by fever and tender inguinal lymphadenopathy.

In males, herpes most often affects the glans, foreskin and shaft of the penis. Anal herpes is more common in males who have sex with men than with heterosexual partners.

In females, herpes most often arises on the vulva and in the vagina. Dysuria is common. Infection of the cervix may progress to severe ulceration.

RECURRENT HERPES SIMPLEX

After the initial infection, whether symptomatic or not, there may be no further clinical manifestations throughout life. Where viral immunity is insufficient, recurrent infections are common, particularly with type 2 genital herpes.

Recurrences can be triggered by:
- Minor trauma, surgery or procedures to the affected area.
- Upper respiratory tract infections.
- Sun exposure.
- Hormonal factors (in women, flares are not uncommon prior to menstruation).
- Emotional stress.

In many cases, no reason for the eruption is evident.

The vesicles tend to be smaller and more closely grouped in recurrent herpes, compared to primary herpes. They usually return to roughly the same site as the primary infection.
- Recurrent type 1 HSV can occur on any site, most frequently the face, particularly the lips (herpes simplex labialis).

- Recurrent type 2 HSV may also occur on any site, but most often affects the genitals or buttocks.

Itching or burning is followed an hour or two later by an irregular cluster of small, closely grouped, often umbilicated vesicles on a red base. They normally heal in 7–10 days without scarring. The affected person may feel well or suffer from fever, pain and have enlarged local lymph nodes.

Herpetic vesicles are sometimes arranged in a line rather like shingles, and are said to have a zosteriform distribution, particularly when affecting the lower chest or lumbar region.

White patches or scars may occur at the site of recurrent HSV attacks, and these are more obvious in those with skin of colour.

How is herpes simplex diagnosed?

If there is clinical doubt, HSV can be confirmed by culture or PCR of a viral swab taken from fresh vesicles. HSV serology is not very informative, because it is positive in most individuals and thus not specific for the lesion with which they present.

What are the complications of herpes simplex?

EYE INFECTION

Herpes simplex may cause swollen eyelids and conjunctivitis with opacity and superficial ulceration of the cornea (dendritic ulcer).

THROAT INFECTION

Throat infections may be very painful and interfere with swallowing.

ECZEMA HERPETICUM

In patients with a history of atopic dermatitis or Darier disease, HSV may result in severe and widespread infection, known as eczema herpeticum. The skin disease can be active or historical. Numerous blisters erupt on the face or elsewhere, associated with swollen lymph glands and fever (*Fig. 2.71*).

ERYTHEMA MULTIFORME

Recurrent erythema multiforme (see *Section 3.7*) is an uncommon reaction to herpes simplex. The rash of erythema multiforme appears as symmetrical plaques on hands, forearms, feet and lower legs. It is characterised

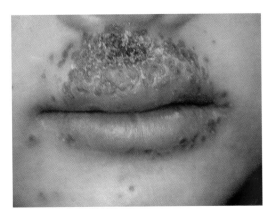

Figure 2.71. Eczema herpeticum.

by target lesions, which sometimes have central blisters.

NERVOUS SYSTEM

Cranial/facial nerves may be infected by HSV, producing temporary paralysis of the affected muscles. Rarely, neuralgic pain may precede each recurrence of herpes by 1 or 2 days (Maurice's syndrome). Meningitis is rare.

WIDESPREAD INFECTION

Disseminated and/or persistent ulceration due to HSV can be serious in debilitated or immune deficient patients, e.g. people with human immunodeficiency virus (HIV) infection.

What is the treatment for herpes simplex?

Mild uncomplicated eruptions of herpes simplex require no treatment. Blisters may be covered if desired, e.g. with a hydrocolloid patch. Severe infection may require treatment with an antiviral agent.

Antiviral drugs used for herpes simplex and their usual doses are:

- Aciclovir – 200 mg 5 times daily for 5 days.
- Valaciclovir – 1 g 3 times daily for 7 days.
- Famciclovir – as a single dose of 3 × 500 mg (New Zealand) or 500 mg twice daily for 7d (UK).

Higher doses are used for eczema herpeticum or for disseminated herpes simplex.

Topical aciclovir or penciclovir may shorten attacks of recurrent herpes simplex, provided the cream is started early enough.

Can herpes simplex be prevented?

As sun exposure often triggers facial herpes simplex, sun protection using high protection factor sunscreens and other measures are important.

Antiviral drugs will stop HSV multiplying once it reaches the skin or mucous membranes but cannot eradicate the virus from its resting stage within the nerve cells. They can therefore shorten and prevent attacks but a single course cannot prevent future attacks. Repeated courses may be prescribed or the medication may be taken continuously to prevent frequent attacks.

Topical aciclovir or penciclovir cream may shorten attacks of recurrent herpes simplex, provided it is started early enough, e.g. within a few hours of a prodromal tingling sensation.

2.3.5 Herpes zoster

What is herpes zoster?

Herpes zoster is a localised, blistering and painful rash caused by reactivation of varicella-zoster virus (VZV). It is characterised by dermatomal distribution, i.e. the blisters are confined to the cutaneous distribution of one or two adjacent sensory nerves (*Fig. 2.72*).

Herpes zoster is also called shingles. VZV is also called herpesvirus 3, and is a member of the *Herpesvirales* order of double-stranded DNA viruses.

Who gets herpes zoster?

Anyone who has previously had varicella (chickenpox) may subsequently develop zoster. This can occur in childhood (*Fig. 2.73*) but is much more common in adults, especially the elderly. People who have had zoster rarely get it again; the risk of getting a second episode is about 1%.

Herpes zoster often affects people with poor immunity.

What causes herpes zoster?

After primary infection – varicella – VZV remains dormant in dorsal root ganglia nerve cells for years before it is reactivated and migrates down sensory nerves to the skin to cause herpes zoster.

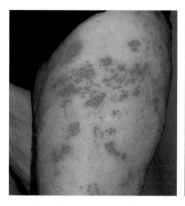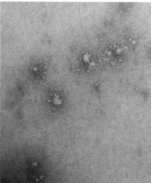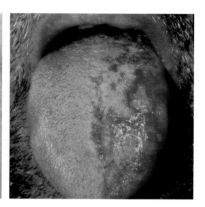

Figure 2.72. Herpes zoster infection.

It is not clear why herpes zoster affects a particular nerve fibre. Triggering factors are sometimes recognised, such as:

- Pressure on the nerve roots.
- Radiotherapy at the level of the affected nerve root.
- Spinal surgery.
- An infection.
- An injury (not necessarily to the spine).
- Contact with someone with varicella or herpes zoster.

What are the clinical features of herpes zoster?

The clinical presentation of herpes zoster depends on the age and health of the patient and which dermatome is affected.

The first sign of herpes zoster is usually pain, which may be severe, relating to one or more sensory nerves. The pain may be just in one spot or it may spread out. The patient usually

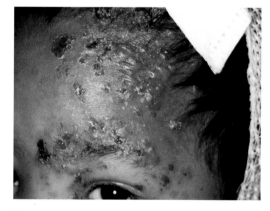

Figure 2.73. Herpes zoster in a child.

feels quite unwell with fever and headache. The lymph nodes draining the affected area are often enlarged and tender.

Within 1 to 3 days of the onset of pain, a blistering rash appears in the painful area of skin. It starts as a crop of red papules. New lesions continue to appear for several days within the distribution of the affected nerve, each blistering or becoming pustular then crusting over.

The chest (thoracic), neck (cervical), forehead (ophthalmic) and lumbar/sacral sensory nerve supply regions are most commonly affected at all ages. Frequency of ophthalmic herpes zoster increases with age. Herpes zoster occasionally causes blisters inside the mouth or ears, and can also affect the genital area. Occasionally there is pain without rash – herpes zoster 'sine eruptione' – or rash without pain, most often in children.

Pain and general symptoms subside gradually as the eruption disappears. In uncomplicated cases, recovery is complete within 2–3 weeks in children and young adults, and within 3–4 weeks in older patients.

What are the complications of herpes zoster?

Herpes zoster may cause:

- Blisters to erupt over several dermatomes or bilateral eruptions (*Fig. 2.74*).
- Deep blisters that destroy the skin, taking weeks to heal (*Fig. 2.75*) followed by scarring (*Fig. 2.76*).
- Muscle weakness in about 1 in 20 patients. Facial nerve palsy is the most common result. There is a 50% chance of complete recovery

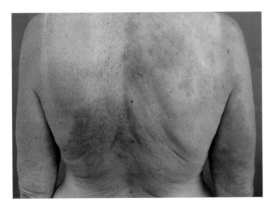

Figure 2.74. Bilateral eruptions in herpes zoster infection.

but some improvement can be expected in nearly all cases.
- Infection of internal organs, including the gastrointestinal tract, lungs and brain (encephalitis).

Herpes zoster in the early months of pregnancy can harm the fetus, but luckily this is rare. The fetus may be infected by chickenpox in later pregnancy, and then develop herpes zoster as an infant.

Post-herpetic neuralgia

Post-herpetic neuralgia is defined as persistence or recurrence of pain in the same area more than a month after the onset of herpes zoster. It becomes increasingly common with age, affecting about one-third of patients over the age of 40. It is particularly likely if there is facial infection. Post-herpetic neuralgia may be a continuous burning sensation with increased sensitivity in the affected areas or a spasmodic shooting pain. The overlying skin is often numb or exquisitely sensitive to touch. Sometimes, instead of pain, the neuralgia results in a persistent itch (neuropathic pruritus).

Treatment of herpes zoster

Antiviral treatment can reduce pain and the duration of symptoms if started within 1–3 days after the onset of herpes zoster. Aciclovir 800 mg 5 times daily for 7 days is prescribed most often. Valaciclovir and famciclovir are also effective. The efficacy of prescribing systemic steroids is unproven.

Note that herpes zoster is infectious to people who have not previously had chickenpox.

Management of acute herpes zoster may include:
- Rest and pain relief.
- Protective ointment applied to the rash, such as petroleum jelly.
- Oral antibiotics for secondary infection.

Post-herpetic neuralgia may be difficult to treat successfully. It may respond to any of the following:
- Local anaesthetic applications.
- Topical capsaicin.
- Tricyclic antidepressant medications.
- Anti-epileptic medications gabapentin and pregabalin.
- Transcutaneous electrical nerve stimulation or acupuncture.
- Botulinum toxin injections into the affected area.

Non-steroidal anti-inflammatories and opioids are generally unhelpful.

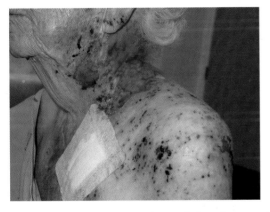

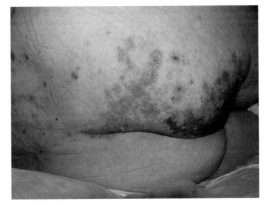

Figure 2.75. Deep necrosis, erosions and ulceration caused by herpes zoster.

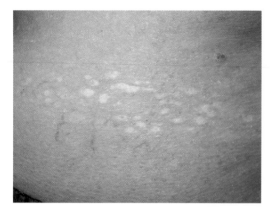

Figure 2.76. Scarring following herpes zoster infection.

Prevention of herpes zoster

Because the risk of severe complications from herpes zoster is more likely in older people, those aged over 60 years might consider zoster vaccine, which can reduce the incidence of herpes zoster by half. In people who do get herpes zoster despite being vaccinated, the symptoms are usually less severe and post-herpetic neuralgia is less likely to develop.

2.3.6 Infantile papular acrodermatitis

What is infantile papular acrodermatitis?

Infantile papular acrodermatitis is a characteristic response of the skin to viral infection in which there is a papular rash that lasts for several weeks.

Other names sometimes used for this skin condition include Gianotti–Crosti syndrome, papulovesicular acrodermatitis of childhood, papular acrodermatitis of childhood and acrodermatitis papulosa infantum.

Who gets infantile papular acrodermatitis?

As the name suggests, infantile papular acrodermatitis mainly affects children between the ages of 6 months and 12 years. However, it has rarely been described in adults.

A clustering of cases is often observed, and a preceding upper respiratory infection is common.

What causes infantile papular acrodermatitis?

The specific viruses causing infantile papular acrodermatitis include:
- Hepatitis B infection.
- Epstein–Barr virus (the cause of glandular fever).
- Enterovirus infections.
- Echo viruses.
- Respiratory syncytial virus.

Vaccination has also occasionally been associated with the onset of infantile papular acrodermatitis.

What are the clinical features of infantile papular acrodermatitis?

Infantile papular acrodermatitis presents over the course of 3 or 4 days. A profuse eruption of dull red spots develops first on the thighs and buttocks, then on the outer aspects of the arms, and finally on the face (*Fig. 2.77*). The rash is often asymmetrical.

The individual spots are 5–10 mm in diameter and are a deep red colour. Later they often look purple, especially on the legs, due to leakage of

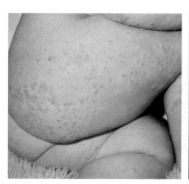
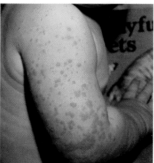
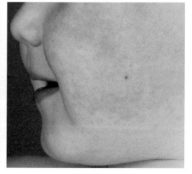

Figure 2.77. Infantile papular acrodermatitis showing progression from thighs and buttocks, to arms and then face.

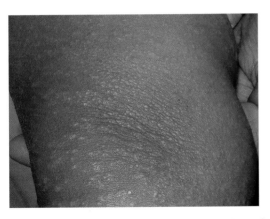

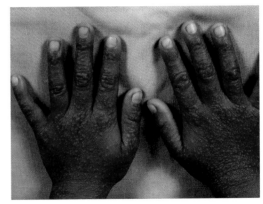

Figure 2.78. Infantile papular acrodermatitis: papules and vesicles.

blood from the capillaries (*Fig. 2.78*). They may develop vesicles.

Infantile papular acrodermatitis is not usually itchy.

A child with infantile papular acrodermatitis may feel quite well or have a mild temperature. Mildly enlarged lymph nodes in the armpits and groins may persist for months.

How is infantile papular acrodermatitis diagnosed?

The clinical appearance is quite characteristic, and many children do not require any specific tests. However, blood tests may include:

- Blood count.
- Liver function.
- Viral serology or PCR.

What is the treatment for infantile papular acrodermatitis?

There is no specific treatment for infantile papular acrodermatitis. A mild topical steroid cream or emollient may be prescribed for itch.

What is the outlook for infantile papular acrodermatitis?

Infantile papular acrodermatitis fades in 2–8 weeks with mild scaling. Recurrence is unlikely but has been reported.

If hepatitis B is present, the liver takes between 6 months and 4 years to fully recover. Sometimes there is persistent hepatitis and long-term viral carriage.

2.3.7 Molluscum contagiosum

What is molluscum contagiosum?

Molluscum contagiosum is a common viral skin infection of childhood that causes localised clusters of epidermal papules called mollusca.

Who gets molluscum contagiosum?

Molluscum contagiosum mainly affects infants and young children under the age of 10 years. It is more prevalent in warm climates than cool ones, and in overcrowded environments. Adolescents and adults are less often infected.

Mollusca tend to be more numerous and last longer in children who also have atopic eczema, due to deficiencies in the skin barrier. It can be very extensive and troublesome in patients with HIV infection or that have other reasons for poor immune function.

What causes molluscum contagiosum?

Molluscum contagiosum is caused by a poxvirus, the molluscum contagiosum virus. There are at least four viral subtypes.

There are several ways it can spread:

- Direct skin-to-skin contact.
- Indirect contact via shared towels or other items.
- Auto-inoculation into another site by scratching or shaving.
- Sexual transmission in adults.

Transmission of mollusca appears to be more likely in wet conditions, such as when children bathe or swim together. The incubation period is usually about 2 weeks but can be as long as 6 months.

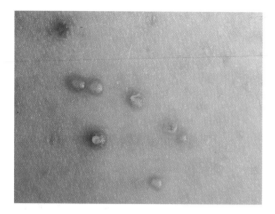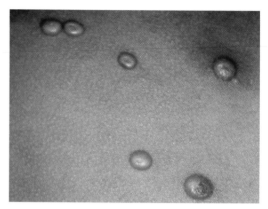

Figure 2.79. Typical umbilicated papules of molluscum contagiosum.

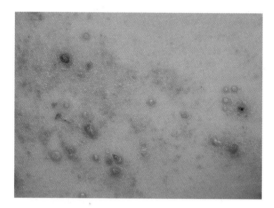

Figure 2.80. Eczematous reaction surrounding molluscum contagiosum papules.

What are the clinical features of molluscum contagiosum?

Molluscum contagiosum presents as clusters of small round papules. The papules range in size from 1 to 6 mm, and may be white, pink or brown. They often have a waxy, shiny look with a small central pit (this appearance is sometimes described as umbilicated). Each papule contains white cheesy material (*Fig. 2.79*).

There may be few or hundreds of papules on one individual. They mostly arise in warm moist places, such as the armpit, behind the knees, groin or genital areas. They can arise on the lips or rarely inside the mouth. They do not occur on palms or soles.

When mollusca are auto-inoculated by scratching, the papules often form a row.

Mollusca frequently induce dermatitis around them, which becomes pink, dry and itchy. As the papules resolve, they may become inflamed, crusted or scabby for a week or two (*Fig. 2.80*).

Complications of molluscum contagiosum

Complications of molluscum contagiosum can include:

- Secondary bacterial infection from scratching.
- Conjunctivitis when eyelid is infected.
- Dermatitis on distant sites; this represents an immunological reaction or 'id' to the virus.
- Numerous, widespread or giant mollusca in immune deficiency, e.g. uncontrolled HIV infection or on immune suppressing drugs.
- Scarring due to surgical treatment.

How is molluscum contagiosum diagnosed?

Molluscum contagiosum is usually recognised by its characteristic clinical appearance or on dermatoscopy. White molluscum bodies can often be expressed from the centre of the papules.

Sometimes, the diagnosis is made on skin biopsy. Histopathology shows characteristic intracytoplasmic inclusion bodies.

What is the treatment for molluscum contagiosum?

There is no single perfect treatment for molluscum contagiosum since we are currently unable to kill the virus. In many cases no specific treatment is necessary.

Physical treatments include:

- Picking out the soft white core (note, this could lead to auto-inoculation).

- Cryotherapy (can leave white marks).
- Gentle curettage or electrodessication (can scar).
- Laser ablation (can scar).

Medical treatments include:
- Antiseptics such as 1% hydrogen peroxide cream or 10% povidone iodine solution.
- Podophyllotoxin cream.
- Wart paints containing salicylic acid.
- Cantharidine solution.

Imiquimod cream and sinecatechins are sometimes used but are unproven.

Secondary dermatitis may be treated symptomatically with a mild topical corticosteroid such as hydrocortisone cream. It is unlikely to fully resolve until the molluscum infection has cleared up.

How can molluscum contagiosum be prevented?

Molluscum contagiosum is infectious while active. However, affected children and adults should continue to attend day care, school and work.

To reduce spread:
- Keep hands clean.
- Avoid scratching or shaving.
- Cover all visible lesions with clothing or watertight bandages.
- Dispose of all used bandages.
- Do not share towels, clothing or other personal effects.
- Adults should practice safe sex or abstinence.

What is the outlook for molluscum contagiosum?

In immune competent hosts, molluscum contagiosum is relatively harmless. The papules may persist for up to 2 years or longer. In children, about half of cases have cleared by 12 months, and two-thirds by 18 months, with or without treatment. Contact with another infected individual later on can lead to a new crop of mollusca.

Tiny pit-like scars may be left behind after the molluscum contagiosum clears up. The appearance improves over time.

2.3.8 Pityriasis rosea

What is pityriasis rosea?

Pityriasis rosea is a papulosquamous rash that lasts about 6–12 weeks. It is characterised by a herald patch followed by similar, smaller oval red patches that are located mainly on the chest and back.

Who gets pityriasis rosea?

Pityriasis rosea most often affects teenagers and young adults. However, it can affect males and females of any age.

What are the clinical features of pityriasis rosea?

SYSTEMIC SYMPTOMS

Many people with pityriasis rosea have no other symptoms, but the rash sometimes follows a few days after an upper respiratory viral infection (cough, cold, sore throat or similar).

THE HERALD PATCH

The herald patch is a single plaque that appears 1–20 days before the generalised rash of pityriasis rosea. It is an oval pink or red plaque 2–5 cm in diameter, with a scale trailing just inside the edge of the lesion like a collaret (*Fig. 2.81*).

SECONDARY RASH

A few days after the appearance of the herald patch, more scaly patches or plaques appear on the chest and back (*Fig. 2.82*). A few plaques may also appear on the thighs, upper arms and neck but are uncommon on the face or scalp. These secondary lesions of pityriasis rosea tend to be smaller than the herald patch. They are also oval in shape with a dry surface. Like the herald patch, they may have an inner collaret of scaling. Some plaques may be annular (ring-shaped).

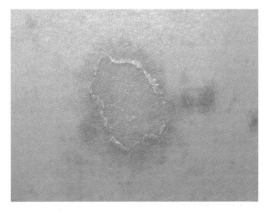

Figure 2.81. The herald patch preceding pityriasis rosea.

NSAIDs, Atypical antipsychotics, imatinib

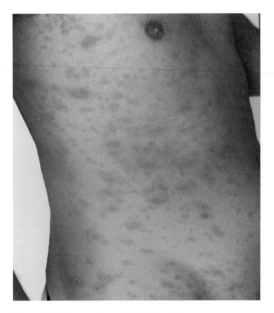

Figure 2.82. Secondary rash of pityriasis rosea.

Pityriasis rosea plaques usually follow the relaxed skin tension or cleavage lines (Langers lines) on both sides of the upper trunk. The rash has been described as looking like a fir tree. It does not involve the face, scalp, palms or soles.

Pityriasis rosea may be very itchy, but in most cases it doesn't itch at all.

ATYPICAL PITYRIASIS ROSEA

Pityriasis rosea is said to be atypical when diagnosis has been difficult. Atypical pityriasis rosea may be diagnosed when the rash has features such as:

- Atypical morphology, e.g. papules, vesicles, urticated plaques, purpura or target lesions.
- Large sized or confluent plaques.
- Unusual distribution of skin lesions, e.g. inverse pattern, with prominent involvement of the skin folds, or greater involvement of limbs than the trunk.
- Involvement of mucosal sites.
- Solitary herald patch without generalised rash.
- Multiple herald patches.
- Absence of herald patch.
- Severe itch.
- Prolonged course of disease.
- Multiple recurrences.

What causes pityriasis rosea?

Pityriasis rosea is associated with reactivation of herpes viruses 6 and 7, which cause the primary rash roseola in infants. Influenza viruses and vaccines have triggered pityriasis rosea in some cases.

Pityriasis rosea or atypical pityriasis rosea-like rashes can rarely arise as an adverse reaction to a medicine. Reactivation of herpes 6/7 is reported in some but not all cases of drug-induced pityriasis rosea. Pityriasis rosea-like drug eruptions have been caused by angiotensin-converting enzyme inhibitors, non-steroidal anti-inflammatory drugs, hydrochlorothiazide, imatinib, clozapine, metronidazole, terbinafine, gold and atypical antipsychotics.

How long does pityriasis rosea last?

Pityriasis rosea clears up in about 6–12 weeks. Post-inflammatory dyspigmentation may persist for a few months in darker skinned people, but eventually the skin returns to its normal appearance.

Second attacks of pityriasis rosea are uncommon (1–3%), but another viral infection may trigger recurrence years later.

Does pityriasis rosea cause any complications?

Pityriasis rosea during early pregnancy has been reported to cause miscarriage in 8 of 61 women studied. Premature delivery and other perinatal problems also occurred in some women.

Atypical pityriasis rosea due to reactivation of herpes 6/7 in association with a drug can also lead to the severe cutaneous adverse reaction, drug hypersensitivity syndrome.

How is pityriasis rosea diagnosed?

The diagnosis of pityriasis rosea is usually made clinically.

Subacute dermatitis is noted on histopathology of a skin biopsy. Eosinophils are typical of drug-induced pityriasis rosea.

Blood testing for HHV6 (IgG or PCR) is not indicated because nearly 100% of individuals have been infected with the virus in childhood and existing commercial tests do not measure HHV6 activity.

Treatment of pityriasis rosea

GENERAL ADVICE
- Bathe or shower with plain water and soap substitute.
- Apply moisturising creams to dry skin.
- Expose skin to sunlight cautiously (without burning).

PRESCRIPTION TREATMENTS
- Topical steroid cream or ointment may reduce the itch while waiting for the rash to resolve.

The following medicines have been reported to speed up clearance of pityriasis rosea but are unproven:
- A 7-day course of high-dose aciclovir.
- A 2-week course of oral erythromycin.

PHOTOTHERAPY
Extensive or persistent cases can be treated by ultraviolet-B phototherapy.

2.3.9 Viral warts

What are viral warts?
Warts are very common non-cancerous growths of the skin caused by infection with human papillomavirus (HPV). More than 100 HPV subtypes are known, giving rise to a variety of presentations.

A viral wart on the sole of the foot is also called a verruca, and warty lesions are often described as verrucous.

Who gets viral warts?
Warts are particularly common in school-aged children, but they may arise at any age. They are more persistent and numerous in people that are immune suppressed (see *Fig. 2.83*) with medications such as azathioprine or ciclosporin, or with HIV infection. In these patients, the warts almost never disappear despite treatment.

What causes viral warts?
HPV is spread by direct skin-to-skin contact or auto-inoculation. This means that if a wart is scratched or picked, the viral particles may be spread to another area of skin. The incubation period can be as long as 12 months.

What are the clinical features of viral warts?
Warts have a hard surface. A tiny black dot may be observed in the middle of each scaly spot, due to a thrombosed capillary blood vessel.

COMMON WARTS
Common warts (*Fig. 2.84*) arise most often on the backs of fingers or toes, around the nails – where they can distort nail growth – and on the knees. Sometimes they resemble a cauliflower; these are known as butcher's warts.

PLANTAR AND PALMAR WARTS
Plantar (verrucas, *Fig. 2.85*) and palmar (*Fig. 2.86*) warts include tender inwardly growing and painful 'myrmecia' on the sole of the foot, and clusters of less painful mosaic warts.

PLANE WARTS
Plane warts have a flat surface. They are often numerous and may be inoculated by shaving or scratching, so that they appear in a line (*Fig. 2.87*).

FILIFORM WARTS
Filiform warts are on a long stalk like a thread. They commonly appear on the face.

MUCOSAL WARTS
Oral warts can affect the lips, nose (see *Fig. 2.88*) and even inside the cheeks, where they may be called squamous cell papillomas.

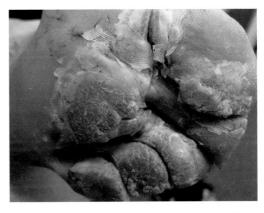

Figure 2.83. Giant warts in an immune suppressed patient.

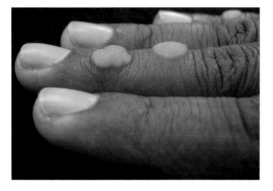
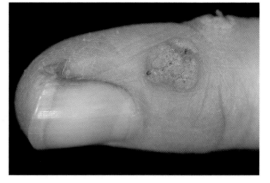

Figure 2.84. Typical common warts.

Complications of viral warts

Viral warts are very widespread in people with the rare inherited disorder epidermodysplasia verruciformis (*Fig. 2.89*).

Malignant change is rare in common warts, and causes verrucous carcinoma.

Oncogenic strains of HPV, the cause of some anogenital warts and warts arising in the oropharynx, are responsible for mucosal intraepithelial neoplastic lesions (see *www.dermnetnz.org/topics/squamous-intraepithelial-lesion*).

How are viral warts diagnosed?

Tests are rarely needed to diagnosis viral warts, because they are so common and have a characteristic appearance. Dermatoscopic examination is sometimes helpful to distinguish viral warts from other verrucous lesions such as seborrhoeic keratosis and skin cancers.

Sometimes, viral warts are diagnosed on skin biopsy because the histopathological features of common warts differ from those of plane warts.

What is the treatment for viral warts?

Many people don't bother to treat viral warts because treatment can be more uncomfortable and troublesome than the warts – they are hardly ever a serious problem. However, warts may be painful, and they often look ugly so cause embarrassment.

To get rid of them, we have to stimulate the body's own immune system to attack the wart virus. Persistence with the treatment and patience is essential!

TOPICAL TREATMENT

Topical treatment includes wart paints containing salicylic acid or similar compounds, which work by removing the dead surface skin cells. Podophyllin is a cytotoxic agent used in some products, and must not be used in pregnancy or in women considering pregnancy.

The paint is normally applied once daily. Treatment with wart paint usually makes the wart smaller and less uncomfortable;

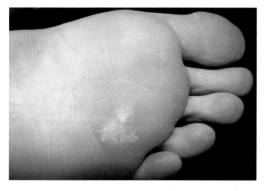
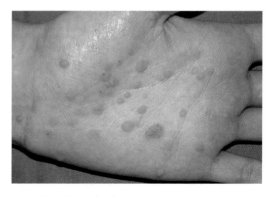

Figure 2.85. Typical plantar wart.

Figure 2.86. Typical palmar warts.

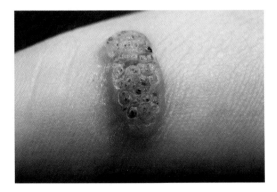

Figure 2.87. Linear arrangement of plane warts.

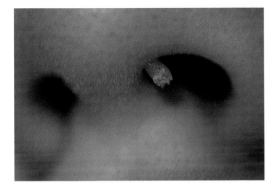

Figure 2.88. Mucosal wart in nose.

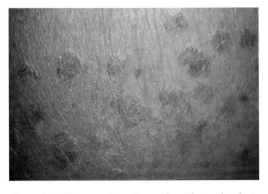

Figure 2.89. Flat warts in patient with epidermodysplasia verruciformis.

70% of warts resolve within 12 weeks of daily applications.
- Soften the wart by soaking in a bath or bowl of hot soapy water.
- Rub the wart surface with a piece of pumice stone or emery board.
- Apply wart paint or gel accurately, allowing it to dry.
- Cover with plaster or duct tape.

If the wart paint makes the skin sore, stop treatment until the discomfort has settled, then recommence as above. Take care to keep the chemical off normal skin.

CRYOTHERAPY
Cryotherapy is normally repeated at 1–3 week intervals. It is uncomfortable and may result in blistering for several days or weeks. Success is in the order of 70% after 3–4 months of regular freezing.

A hard freeze using liquid nitrogen might cause a permanent white mark or scar. It can also cause temporary numbness.

An aerosol spray with a mixture of dimethyl ether and propane (DMEP) can be purchased over the counter to freeze common and plantar warts. It is important to read and follow the instructions carefully.

ELECTROSURGERY
Electrosurgery (curettage and electrocautery) is used for large warts. Under local anaesthetic, the growth is pared away and the base burned. The wound heals in 2 weeks or longer; even then 20% of warts can be expected to recur within a few months. This treatment leaves a permanent scar.

OTHER TREATMENTS
Other experimental treatments for warts include:
- Topical retinoids, such as tretinoin cream or adapalene gel.
- Fluorouracil cream.
- Bleomycin injections.
- Photodynamic treatment.
- Laser vaporization.
- Pulse dye laser destruction of feeding blood vessels.
- The immune modulator imiquimod cream.
- Immune stimulation using diphencyprone or squaric acid.
- Systemic retinoids.

How can viral warts be prevented?
HPV vaccines are available to prevent genital warts. Anecdotally, these have been reported to result in clearance of non-genital warts in some people.

What is the outlook for viral warts?
No treatment is universally effective at eradicating viral warts. In children, even without treatment, 50% of warts disappear within 6 months, and 90% are gone in 2 years. They are more persistent in adults but they clear up eventually.

2.4 Arthropods

2.4.1 Arthropod bites and stings

What are arthropods?

Arthropods include insects, spiders (arachnids), mites and ticks.

- Arthropods can infest human skin, especially scabies (see *Section 2.4.3*) and head lice (see *Section 2.4.2*).
- They can inflict bites and stings.
- They can carry diseases such as malaria, yellow fever and filariasis.
- They can give rise to allergic conditions such as hay fever, asthma and eczema.

What causes arthropod bites and stings?

Insect bites and stings can be divided into two groups: venomous and non-venomous. A small number of spiders are also venomous.

VENOMOUS INSECTS (STINGERS)

A sting is usually an attack by a venomous insect, which injects toxic and painful venom through its stinger as a defence mechanism, e.g.

- Bees.
- Wasps.
- Hornets.
- Yellow jackets.
- Fire ants.

VENOMOUS SPIDERS

Venomous spider bites (see *Fig. 2.90*) are rare but have potentially serious systemic neurotoxicity (e.g. *Lactrodectus* species), or usually local, cytotoxic effects (e.g. *Loxosceles* species).

The majority of household spiders are harmless. Identification of the offending spider is essential to determine management including antivenin.

NON-VENOMOUS INSECT BITES

Non-venomous insects pierce the skin to feed on blood. This usually results in intense itching.

- Mosquitoes.
- Fleas.
- Ticks.
- Bed bugs.
- Lice.
- Sarcoptes scabiei (mite which causes scabies).
- Calyptra moths.

CATERPILLARS AND MOTHS

Some caterpillars and moths have irritating hairs and sharp spines, causing stinging, short-lasting papular urticaria, dermatitis and allergic reactions (*Fig. 2.91*).

Who gets arthropod bites and stings?

Anyone exposed to arthropods can be bitten or stung. Arthropod habitat is variable and individual risks depend largely on geographic and climatic factors. Time of day may be important, for example, some mosquitoes bite at night and others during daytime. Factors to consider include:

- Less clothing is worn in tropical areas or in summer elsewhere.
- There is increased exposure to insects in the garden or forest.
- Overcrowding, travel and poor hygiene.
- Current or previous pets.

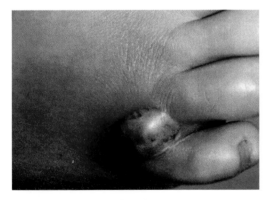

Figure 2.90. Katipo spider bite.

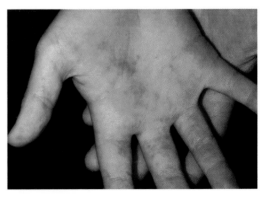

Figure 2.91. Response to hairs on a caterpillar. Photo courtesy of Prof Raimo Suhonen.

Mosquitoes are attracted to body heat, carbon dioxide in exhaled air, human sweat, and human microflora.

What are the clinical features of arthropod bites and stings?

The reaction to an encounter with an arthropod depends on the species involved, whether it carries disease, and individual factors such as host immunity.

A venomous sting from a bee or wasp (see *Fig. 2.92*) usually causes a stinging sensation or pain with redness and swelling of the area. Sensitisation to the venom affects response.

- A large localised reaction causes swelling to spread more widely over several hours.
- An anaphylactic systemic reaction results in immediate angioedema, urticaria and bronchospasm and can be life-threatening.

An insect bite presents as one or more intensely itchy papules on a body site exposed to the insect (*Fig. 2.93*).

- Insect bites often arise in crops.
- The papule usually subsides within a few hours.
- It may have a central clear or haemorrhagic blister, and persists for several days.
- Scratching results in an open sore.

Complications of arthropod bites and stings

Complications of insect bites include:

- Secondary infection with staphylococci and/or streptococci (impetigo, cellulitis).
- Papular urticaria.

- Persistent insect bite reaction.
- Arthropod-borne infection.

PAPULAR URTICARIA

Papular urticaria (*Fig. 2.94*) is a hypersensitivity reaction, most often in a young child due to fleabites and/or mosquito bites. New bites are accompanied by reactivation of old ones and present as symmetrical crops of itchy urticated papules. Papular urticaria resolves with the development of immunological tolerance.

PERSISTENT INSECT BITE REACTION

Solitary persistent insect bite reactions can be urticarial, bullous, vasculitic or granulomatous (*Fig. 2.95*).

ARTHROPOD-BORNE INFECTIONS

Diseases in which arthropods are the vector occur worldwide but are particularly prevalent in tropical and developing regions. They include:

- Parasites: malaria, leishmaniasis, trypanosomiasis.
- Bacteria: Lyme disease, plague, bacillary angiomatosis, relapsing fever, tularaemia, babesiosis.
- Viral disease: dengue fever, chikungunya fever, zika fever.
- Rickettsial disease: typhus.

How are arthropod bites and stings diagnosed?

Generally people are aware of bites, especially if they have observed the arthropod, but occasionally they are not.

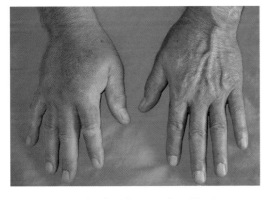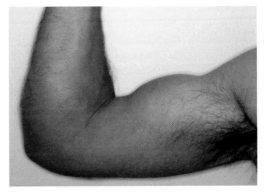

Figure 2.92. Localised erythema and swelling in response to (on the left) a bee sting (in the right hand) and (on the right) a wasp sting in the same individual.

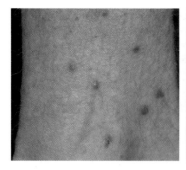
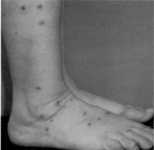
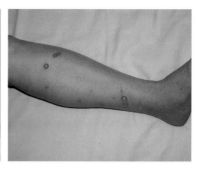

Figure 2.93. Itchy papules and vesicles following insect bites.

Skin biopsy can be suggestive if it shows central punctum, eosinophilic spongiosis, and a wedge-shaped mixed dermal infiltrate distributed around the sweat ducts/glands.

What is the treatment for arthropod bites and stings?

STINGS

If the reaction is mild, insect stings should be treated by first removing the stinger. This is necessary because the stinger continues to pump venom from its sack until it is empty or removed.

- Place a firm edge such as a knife or credit card against the skin next to the embedded stinger.
- Apply constant firm pressure and scrape across the skin surface to remove the stinger. This is preferred to using tweezers or fingers, which can accidentally squeeze more venom into the patient.
- Clean the site with disinfectant.

- Apply ice or a cold pack to reduce pain and swelling. Topical steroid cream or calamine lotion may be applied several times a day until symptoms subside. If necessary, oral antihistamines can also be taken.

If an insect sting causes a severe reaction or anaphylaxis, urgent medical attention should be sought. If a patient is known to have an allergy to insect stings they may carry with them an allergy kit containing adrenaline (epinephrine).

INSECT BITES

The main treatment aim for insect bites is to prevent itching.

- Cool the affected area.
- Apply topical calamine lotion or local anaesthetic agent.
- Oral antihistamine reduces itch and weal.
- Use moderate potency topical steroids for papular urticaria or persistent reactions.

Bites from insects carrying disease require specific antimicrobial therapy to treat the disease.

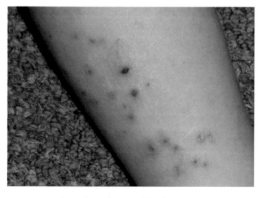

Figure 2.94. Papular urticaria in response to bites.

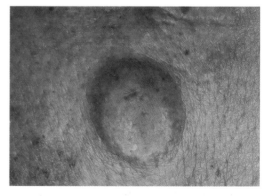

Figure 2.95. Persistent granulomatous reaction to an insect bite.

How can arthropod bites and stings be prevented?

The following measures can prevent or reduce insect stings and bites:

- Wear fully covering clothing.
- Keep windows and doors closed at night.
- Avoid perfume and bright-coloured clothing to reduce the risk of bee stings.
- Control odours at picnics and garbage areas that can attract insects.
- Destroy or relocate hives or nests away from the home.
- Drain pools of stagnating water that attract mosquitoes.
- Use electrical insect repelling devices and lit coils.
- De-flea cats, dogs and other household pets regularly.
- Apply insect repellents containing DEET (diethyltoluamide) to exposed skin.
- Apply permethrin to clothing for 2 week protection, through two washings. It can also be applied directly to exposed skin keeping the insects away for a few days.
- Thiamine (vitamin B1) can be used as a systemic insect repellent (the skin has a characteristic smell).

2.4.2 Head lice

What are head lice?

Head lice are small, wingless insects that infest the human scalp. They are the most common of the three human lice species. Infestation with head lice is also called pediculosis capitis.

Who gets head lice?

Head lice affect people of all ages and walks of life, all over the world. They are a very common problem in children aged 4–14 years of age.

Risk factors for infestation include:

- Female gender.
- Greater number of children in a family.
- Sharing beds, clothing and hair brushes.

Head lice can't jump or fly but spread by crawling along hair shafts by head to head contact.

What causes head lice?

The head louse, *Pediculus humanus capitis*, is an ectoparasite that feeds on human blood. It is 2–3 mm in length (*Fig. 2.96*) and has a flattened, elongated, grey-coloured body that becomes reddish after feeding. The louse clings to the hair shaft using its 6 claws and rapidly moves from hair to hair.

Lice inject anticoagulant saliva into a person's scalp to suck up the blood up to five times a day. They die within 1–2 days away from the scalp if they are unable to feed.

After mating, the female louse attaches her eggs to the hair shaft close to the scalp in cool climates, and further down the shaft in warmer climates. The female louse can lay 50–100 eggs at a rate of 3–6 per day. The new egg cases are brown and hard to see. They are carried away from the scalp as the hair grows.

The eggs hatch after about 8 days. The empty egg case then appears white and is more easily seen – the nit.

The louse nymph reaches full maturity around 10 days after hatching and the cycle begins again. An adult louse survives on the scalp for about 1 month, and off the scalp for up to 48 hours.

What are the clinical features of head lice?

Head lice usually cause an itch and irritation in the scalp. This can take several weeks to develop after the initial infestation.

- Lice favour the nape of the neck and the skin behind the ears.
- Nits are generally easy to see after the eggs have hatched, as adherent white grains on the hair shaft.
- Red–brown spots on the skin are due to excreted digested blood.

Occasionally the eyelashes can become infested, although this is more frequently due to a different insect, the pubic louse.

Scratching can cause crusting and scaling on the scalp. Hair pulling can lead to small areas of hair loss.

Complications of head lice

The head lice do not carry any other infectious disease. Heavy infestation can lead to:

- Dermatitis: red scaly itchy plaques.
- Secondary bacterial infection: crusted sores.
- Tender swollen lymph nodes.

How are head lice diagnosed?

It is important to identify the lice (or nits) to make a correct diagnosis. The lice can be hard to

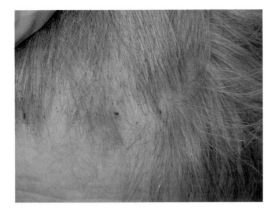
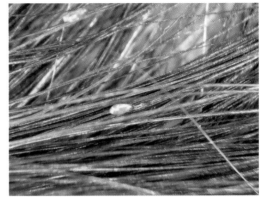

Figure 2.96. Head lice on the scalp and egg cases on the hair shaft.

detect, and there are usually only 10–20 adult lice in each colony.

- Look for lice and nits behind and above the ears and on the back of the neck.
- They may be observed scurrying to hide from the light to dwell in dark shadows.
- Unhatched eggs are mostly within a few millimetres of the scalp and have a dark area within the shell.
- Hatched eggs are transparent or whitish. These may persist after successful treatment unless physically removed. They are not infectious.
- White scale encircling the base of the hair shaft at the scalp surface is not due to head lice.

It is easier to identify (and remove) live lice by wet combing using a lice comb, compared to visual inspection alone.

What is the treatment for head lice?

Treatment of head lice usually consists of at least two applications of chemical insecticide and/or physical or other methods. Note:

- Treat all members of the family at the same time. Inform the day care or school.
- A second application of insecticide is required 7–10 days after the first one because the eggs may survive, allowing new louse nymphs to hatch out.
- Physical methods are required to remove the nits – simple washing is not effective.

CHEMICAL TREATMENT

The most commonly used topical insecticide for head lice has been permethrin, but it is no longer recommended in the UK because of resistance. Other options include:

- Malathion.
- Phenothrin.
- Spinosad.
- Ivermectin.

Lotions, liquids or cream are preferred to shampoo (which is too weak to be reliable). They are applied directly to the scalp. It is important to follow the manufacturer's advice on how long to use it and how often to repeat it due to potential toxicity.

PHYSICAL METHODS

Physical methods of removing nits and lice are used in conjunction with insecticide treatments and may be required daily for several weeks.

- Nit combs used in wet hair are the most effective way of physically removing the lice and nits. Metal combs are best for thick hair, and plastic combs are kinder on fine or long hair. Apply a conditioner to the hair.
- Work through the scalp in sections.
- Comb down the hair shaft towards the scalp.

Expect nit removal to take at least half an hour. Repeat daily until no lice are found on three consecutive occasions.

Electrical combs designed to 'zap' lice on the hair shaft are probably not effective.

OTHER METHODS

The effectiveness of these treatments has not been extensively studied.

- Suffocating agents such as dimeticone, petroleum jelly or benzyl alcohol are applied to dry hair from the scalp to the ends, covered with a shower cap for 20 minutes, and then washed out. Treatment is repeated once weekly until clear.

- Shaving the head or cutting the hair very short is effective, but rarely necessary.
- Daily 30 minute exposure to a hot air dryer over a period of 1 month destroys live eggs.
- Treatments using natural oils may be as effective as the chemical treatments that have been approved for use in head lice.
- Oral ivermectin 400 mcg/kg (off label) is no more effective than topical ivermectin.
- Oral sulfamethoxazole/trimethoprim) intended to kill the bacteria in the gut of the lice, which are essential for the digestion of nutrients, so they starve to death. It should be reserved as second-line treatment because co-trimoxazole may sometimes cause rare serious adverse reactions.

Why does head lice treatment fail?

Failure to eradicate lice is a common and frustrating problem. It can be due to:
- Inactive infestation (white nits do not contain live eggs).
- Reinfestation from another person.
- Less likely, reinfestation from contaminated clothes, hats, etc.
- Improperly applied treatment.
- Resistance of lice to insecticides.
- Misdiagnosis.

How do you prevent head lice spreading?

It is difficult to prevent head lice infestation in children. Discourage children from sharing or using another child's hat, comb, or brush.

Community-wide or school-based education programmes informing parents of methods to eradicate lice, and community health teams in schools, are the most effective ways in keeping infestation rates down.

2.4.3 Scabies

What is scabies?

Scabies is a very itchy rash caused by a parasitic mite that burrows in the skin surface. The human scabies mite's correct name is *Sarcoptes scabiei* var. *hominis*.

Who gets scabies?

Scabies affects families and communities worldwide. It is most common in children, young adults and the elderly. Factors leading to spread of scabies include:

- Poverty and overcrowding.
- Institutional care, such as rest homes, hospitals, prisons.
- Refugee camps.
- Individuals with immune deficiency or that are immune suppressed.
- Low rates of identification and proper treatment of the disease.

What causes scabies?

Scabies is nearly always acquired by skin-to-skin contact with someone else with scabies.
- The contact may be quite brief such as holding hands with an infested child.
- It is sometimes sexually transmitted.
- Occasionally scabies is acquired via bedding or furnishings.

Typically, several scabies mites infest an affected host. After mating, the male mite dies. The female scabies mite burrows into the outside layers of the skin, where she lays up to three eggs each day for her lifetime of 1–2 months. The development from egg to adult scabies mite takes 10–14 days.

What are the clinical features of scabies?

Scabies causes a very itchy rash. It's important to search for burrows carefully in a patient with severe itch, especially if the rash is mild. Contacts should be examined for burrows, whether or not they are itchy.

ITCH
- If it is the first episode, itch arises 4–6 weeks after transmission of a mite.
- It may occur within a few hours of subsequent infestation.
- Itch is characteristically more severe at night, disturbing sleep.
- It affects the trunk and limbs, sparing the scalp (except in infants and in crusted scabies).
- Itch is mild or absent in some patients with crusted scabies.
- Itch can persist for several weeks after successful treatment to kill the mites.

BURROWS
Scabies burrows appear as 0.5–1.5 cm grey irregular tracks in the web spaces between the fingers, on the palms and wrists (*Fig. 2.97*). They may also be found on or in elbows, nipples, armpits, buttocks, penis, insteps and heels.

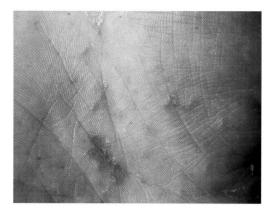

Figure 2.97. Scabies burrows on a palm.

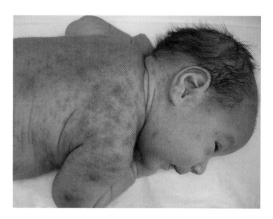

Figure 2.98. Vesicular scabies lesions in a baby.

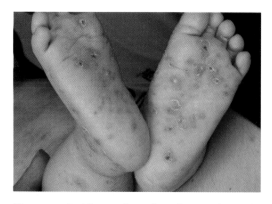

Figure 2.99. Scabies papules and vesicles on palms and soles.

Dermatoscopic or microscopic examination (see *Fig. 2.103*) of the contents of a burrow may reveal mites, eggs or mite faeces (scybala).

GENERALISED RASH

Scabies rash is a hypersensitivity reaction that arises several days to weeks after initial infestation. It has a varied appearance.

- Erythematous papules on the trunk and limbs, often follicular.
- In babies, lesions may be vesicular (*Fig. 2.98*).
- Diffuse or nummular dermatitis.
- Urticated erythema.
- Papules and vesicles on palms and soles (*Fig. 2.99*).
- Acropustulosis (sterile pustules on palms and soles) in infants.
- Papules or nodules in the armpits, groins, buttocks, scrotum and along the shaft of the penis (*Fig. 2.100*).
- Rare involvement of face and scalp.

Complications of scabies

SECONDARY INFECTION

Secondary infection is due to scratching.

- Staphylococcal or streptococcal infection results in crusted plaques and pustules (impetigo).
- Streptococcal cellulitis results in painful swelling and redness, and fever.
- Systemic sepsis with staphylococci and/or streptococci is potentially very serious.
- Scabies outbreaks may lead to cases of post-streptococcal glomerulonephritis and rheumatic fever.

CRUSTED SCABIES

Crusted scabies is a very contagious variant of scabies in which an individual is infested by thousands or millions of mites living in the surface of the skin.

- The patient presents with a generalised scaly rash. This is often misdiagnosed as psoriasis or seborrhoeic dermatitis (*Fig. 2.101*).
- Scale is often prominent in the finger webs, on wrists, elbows, breasts and scrotum, but in severe and prolonged infestations may spread more widely (see *Fig. 2.102*).
- Numerous burrows are present on palms and elsewhere.
- Itch may be absent or minimal.
- Crusted scabies may affect the scalp.

Risk factors for crusted scabies include:

- Very old age.

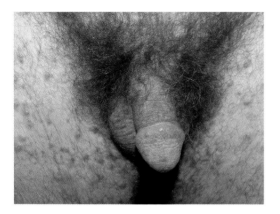

Figure 2.100. Scabies papules in groin and on penis.

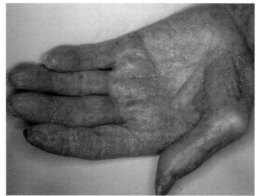

Figure 2.101. The scaly rash of crusted scabies.

- Malnutrition.
- Immune deficiency.
- Intellectual deficit.
- Neurological disease.
- Specific inherited immune defect in some otherwise healthy people.

A case of crusted scabies is the usual reason for an outbreak of scabies in an institution. Patients and staff in the institution may present with:
- Usual scabies.
- Crusted scabies.
- Hypersensitivity reaction but no burrows, i.e. not infested.

How is scabies diagnosed?

The clinical suspicion of scabies in a patient with an itchy rash, especially when reporting itchy household members, can be confirmed by:
- Dermatoscopy: the mite at the end of a burrow has characteristic jet-plane or hang-glider appearance (*Fig. 2.103*).
- Microscopic examination of the contents of a burrow.
- Skin biopsy, but this is often negative, e.g. if taken from the inflammatory rash rather than the surface of a burrow.

Crusted scabies reveals numerous mites on dermatoscopy or microscopy, raised immunoglobulin E (IgE) and eosinophilia.
    Differential diagnosis of scabies includes insect bites, skin infections, dermatitis and bullous pemphigoid.

What is the treatment for scabies?

Treatment involves identification and treatment of the disease and household contacts. Oral antibiotics are required for secondary infection.

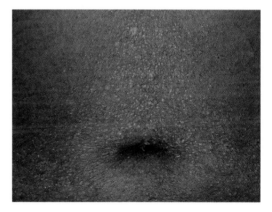

Figure 2.102. Scaly papules are seen here on the abdomen.

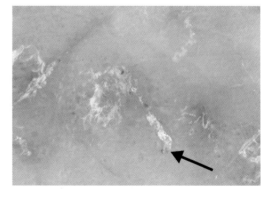

Figure 2.103. Dermatoscopic examination of scabies mite (arrowed) and burrow.

    Careful attention to instructions is essential if scabies is to be cured.
    Scabicides are chemical insecticides used to treat scabies. The scabicide is applied to the

whole body from the scalp to soles. The usual topical treatment is 5% permethrin cream, left on the entire skin for 8–14 hours. It should be applied under fingernails using a soft brush.

Oral ivermectin 200 mcg/kg is convenient, but more expensive than topical permethrin. It may be slightly less effective. It is mainly used for mass treatments in institutions, or in patients unable to use topical therapy.

Other treatments include:

- 0.5% aqueous malathion lotion, left on for 24 hours.
- 25% benzyl benzoate (black ▼ in UK) lotion, applied daily for 3 days. This is irritant and should not be used in children.
- 2–10% precipitated sulphur ointment.

Treatment should be repeated 8–10 days after the first application to catch mites that have newly hatched. Crotamiton cream can be used to reduce itch; it is a weak scabicide.

Patients with crusted scabies may need repeated oral and topical treatments over several weeks or longer; seek specialist advice.

ADDITIONAL MANAGEMENT

Contacts must be identified and treated. In addition:

- Bed linen, towels and clothing should be laundered after treatment.
- Non-washable items should be sealed in a plastic bag and stored for one week.
- Rooms should be thoroughly cleaned with normal household products. Fumigation or specialised cleaning is not required.
- Carpeted floors and upholstered furniture should be vacuumed.

What is the outlook for scabies?

Scabies itch and rash are expected to improve within a few days of successful treatment and to completely clear within a month.

A rash may persist after scabies treatment. Reasons for this include:

- Persistent infestation due to incorrectly applied treatment, treatment resistance, or re-infestation due to an untreated contact.
- The hypersensitivity reaction can be slow to settle, despite complete cure of parasitic infestation.
- On-going dermatitis can be due to the mite, the scratching, the treatment or other factors. Persistently itchy papules, nodules and eczematous plaques should be treated with frequent applications of emollients and mild topical steroids once or twice daily.
- Incorrect diagnosis.

Chapter 3

Inflammatory rashes

3.1 Acne

What is acne?

Acne is a common chronic pilosebaceous disorder in which there is follicular occlusion and inflammation.

Who gets acne?

Acne affects males and females of all races and ethnicities. It is prevalent in adolescents and young adults, with 85% of 16–18-year-olds affected. However, it may sometimes occur in children and adults of all ages.

What causes acne?

The pathogenesis of acne is multifactorial:
- familial tendency.
- endogenous and exogenous androgenic hormones.
- acne bacteria *Proprionibacterium acnes*.
- innate immune activation with inflammatory mediators.
- distension and occlusion of the hair follicles.

Acne flares can be provoked by:
- polycystic ovarian disease.
- drugs – steroids, hormones, anticonvulsants, epidermal growth factor receptor inhibitors and others.
- application of occlusive cosmetics.
- high environmental humidity.
- diet high in dairy products and high glycaemic foods.

What are the clinical features of acne?

Acne is often confined to the face but it may involve neck, chest and back. It is characterised by:
- uninflamed open and closed comedones (blackheads and whiteheads), see *Fig. 3.1*.
- inflamed papules and pustules, see *Fig. 3.2*.
- in severe acne, nodules and pseudocysts, see *Figs 3.3* and *3.4*.
- post-inflammatory erythematous or pigmented macules and scars, see *Figs 3.5* and *3.6*.
- adverse social and psychological effects.

How is acne diagnosed?

Acne is differentiated from other folliculocentric disorders by the presence of comedones. It is classified according to the proportion of specific lesion types (see *Figs 3.1–3.3*).

Severity is classified as mild, moderate or severe:
- mild acne: total lesion count <30.
- moderate acne: total lesion count 30–125.
- severe acne: total lesion count >125 (see *Fig. 3.4*).

What tests are necessary in acne?

In most cases, tests are unnecessary. If features are atypical consider:
- skin swabs for microscopy and culture.
- hormonal tests in females.

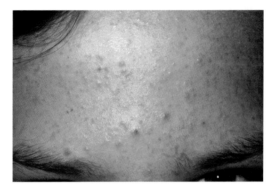

Figure 3.1. Comedonal acne.

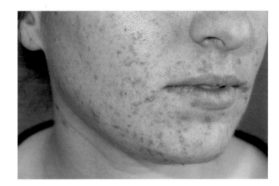

Figure 3.2. Papulopustular acne.

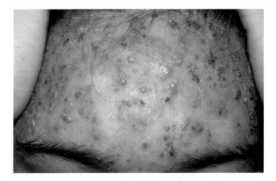

Figure 3.3. Severe acne fulminans. Patient had systemic symptoms.

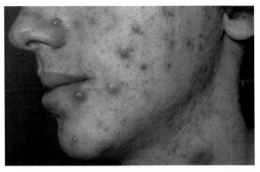

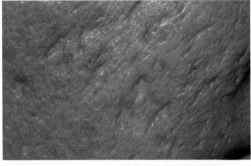

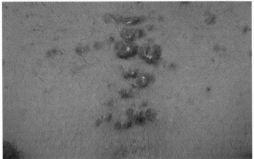

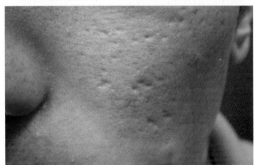

Figure 3.4. Nodulocystic acne (top) and keloid acne scars (bottom).

Figure 3.6. Typical ice-pick acne scarring (top) and scarring following infantile acne (bottom).

- Topical benzoyl peroxide and/or topical tretinoin or adapalene gel.
- Low-dose combined oral contraceptive.
- Antiseptic or keratolytic washes containing salicylic acid.
- Light/laser therapy.

MODERATE ACNE

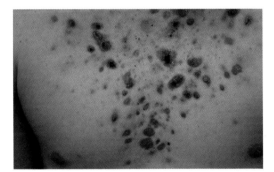

Figure 3.5. Ulceration typical of acne conglobata.

What is the treatment for acne?

MILD ACNE

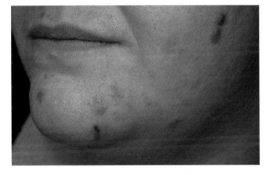

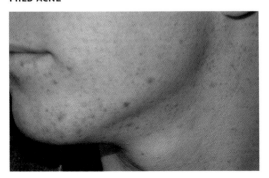

- As for mild acne plus a tetracycline, such as doxycycline 50–200 mg daily for 6 months or so.
- Erythromycin 400 mg bd or trimethoprim 300 mg daily (unapproved), if doxycycline intolerant.
- Anti-androgen therapy with long-term combination contraceptives containing

drospirenone, chlormadinone acetate, dienogest or cyproterone acetate + ethinylestradiol, other anti-androgenic oral contraceptive, and/or spironolactone may be considered in women not responding to low-dose combined oral contraceptive, particularly with polycystic ovaries.

- If trained in its use, consider isotretinoin if acne is persistent or treatment resistant.

- Start the patient on doxycycline 200 mg daily and refer to a dermatologist.
- If fever, arthralgia, bone pain, ulcerated or extensive skin lesions, arrange blood count and refer urgently.

What is the outlook for acne?

Acne tends to improve after the age of 25 years but may persist, especially in females. Treatment with isotretinoin can lead to long-term remission in many patients.

SEVERE ACNE

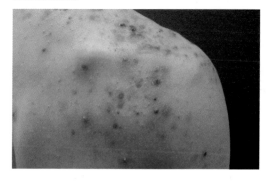

3.2 Bullous pemphigoid

What is bullous pemphigoid?

Bullous pemphigoid is an autoimmune, subepidermal blistering disease.

Who gets bullous pemphigoid?

Bullous pemphigoid often presents in people over 80 years of age, and mostly affects people over 50. It can occur in younger adults, but it is rare in infants and children.

- Bullous pemphigoid occurs equally in males and females.
- There are HLA associations indicating genetic predisposition to the disease.
- It is more prevalent in elderly patients with neurological disease, particularly stroke, dementia and Parkinson disease.
- There may be an association with internal malignancy in some patients.
- A drug, an injury, or skin infection can trigger the onset of disease.

What causes bullous pemphigoid?

Bullous pemphigoid is the result of an attack on the basement membrane of the epidermis by IgG +/– IgE immunoglobulins (antibodies) and activated T lymphocytes (white blood cells). The target is the protein BP180 (also called Type XVII collagen), or less frequently BP230 (a plakin). These proteins are within the NC16A domain of collagen XVII. They are associated with the hemidesmosomes, which are structures that ensure the epidermal keratinocyte cells stick to the dermis to make a waterproof seal.

The binding of the autoantibodies to the proteins and/or release of cytokines from the T cells leads to complement activation, recruitment of neutrophils and the release of proteolytic enzymes. These destroy the hemidesmosomes and cause the formation of subepidermal blisters.

The association of the skin disease with neurological disease is thought to relate to the presence of collagen XVII in the central nervous system and in skin hemidesmosomes.

What are the clinical features of bullous pemphigoid?

Bullous pemphigoid causes severe itch and (usually) large, tense bullae (fluid-filled blisters), which rupture forming crusted erosions (*Fig. 3.7*).

Other variable features include:
- non-specific rash for several weeks before blisters appear.
- eczematous areas (*Fig. 3.8a*).
- urticated erythematous plaques (*Fig. 3.8b*).
- annular or targetoid lesions (*Fig. 3.8c*).
- prurigo nodules.
- clear or cloudy, yellowish or blood-stained blister fluid.
- post-inflammatory pigmentation.
- milia in healed areas.

Bullous pemphigoid may be localised to one area, or widespread on the trunk and proximal limbs.
- It frequently affects the skin around skin folds.
- Blisters inside the mouth and in genital sites are uncommon.

Some patients have a diagnosis of bullous pemphigoid made despite not having any bullae (non-bullous pemphigoid). This can affect any body site.

Complications of bullous pemphigoid

Bullous pemphigoid can be a serious disease, particularly when widespread or resistant to treatment. Morbidity and mortality result from:
- bacterial skin infection and sepsis.
- complications of treatment.
- underlying and associated diseases.

How is bullous pemphigoid diagnosed?

When typical bullae are present, the diagnosis is suspected clinically. In most cases, the

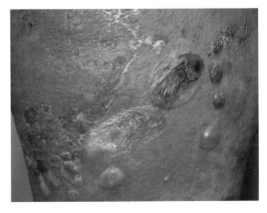

Figure 3.7. Bullous pemphigoid.

diagnosis will be confirmed by a skin biopsy of an early blister. The diagnosis can also be made from non-blistered, inflamed skin.

Pathological examination shows a split under the epidermis. A dermal neutrophilic infiltrate is usual but not always present. Eosinophils may be prominent.

Direct immunofluorescence staining of a skin biopsy, taken adjacent to a blister, highlights antibodies along the basement membrane that lies between the epidermis and dermis.

Blood tests include an indirect immunofluorescence test for circulating pemphigoid BP180 antibodies. Other tests relate to planning and monitoring treatment.

What is the treatment for bullous pemphigoid?

Bullous pemphigoid of limited extent can be treated with high-potency topical steroid, doxycycline and nicotinamide. If the pemphigoid is very widespread, hospital admission may be arranged to dress blisters and erosions.

Medical treatment involves:
- ultrapotent topical steroid to treat limited disease (e.g. clobetasol proprionate).
- moderate potency topical steroids and emollients to relieve itch and dryness.
- systemic steroids.
- steroid-sparing medications.
- antibiotics for secondary bacterial infection.
- analgesics.

Most patients with bullous pemphigoid are treated with steroid tablets, usually prednisone. The dose is adjusted until the blisters have stopped appearing, which usually takes several weeks. The dose of prednisone is then slowly reduced over many months or years. As systemic steroids have many undesirable side-effects, other medications are added to ensure the lowest possible dose (aiming for 5–10 mg prednisone daily). These other medications may include:
- tetracycline antibiotics, e.g. doxycycline.
- nicotinamide.
- dapsone.
- methotrexate.
- azathioprine.
- mycophenolate.
- intravenous immunoglobulin.
- rituximab.

Assessment and monitoring

As systemic treatment may be required for long periods, the extent and severity of the disease should be recorded carefully at baseline and at follow-up appointments. The following aspects may be considered:
- Body sites affected (skin and mucous membranes).
- Type of lesion – transient and non-transient.

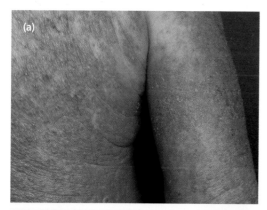

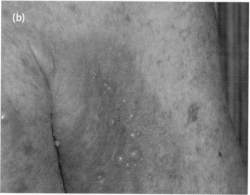

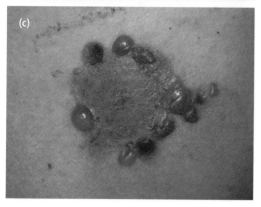

Figure 3.8. (a) Eczematous areas, (b) urticated erythematous plaques, (c) annular or targetoid lesions.

- Numbers of lesions – blisters, urticarial weals, eczematous plaques.
- Severity of itch.
- Observation point – initial phase, active treatment, reducing treatment, maintenance phase on minimal treatment, or complete remission off treatment.
- Current treatment.

The Bullous Pemphigoid Disease Area Index (BPDAI) has separate scores for skin and mucous membrane activity.

Blood pressure, body weight, DEXA bone scan, and blood tests are required to monitor therapy, because medications used for bullous pemphigoid may have serious side-effects in some patients.

How can bullous pemphigoid be prevented?

Unknown at present.

What is the outlook for bullous pemphigoid?

Treatment is usually needed for several years. In many cases, the pemphigoid eventually completely clears up and the treatment can be stopped. If it recurs, it can be restarted.

3.3 Chilblains

What are chilblains?

Chilblains are itchy and/or tender red or purple bumps that occur as a reaction to cold. Chilblains are also known as pernio or perniosis. They are a localised form of vasculitis.

Severe cold injury can also damage the small bones in the digits, leading to microgeodic disease, swelling and, sometimes, bone fracture.

Who gets chilblains?

Chilblains most often affect children and the elderly in damp, temperate climates.

- Chilblains in children may recur each winter for a few years and then clear up.
- Chilblains in elderly people have a tendency to get worse every year unless precipitating factors are avoided.

What is the cause of chilblains?

Chilblains occur several hours after exposure to the cold. Cold causes constriction of the small arteries and veins in the skin. The chilblains are sometimes aggravated by sun exposure, because rewarming results in leakage of blood into the tissues and swelling of the skin.

Chilblains are less common in countries where the cold is more extreme because the air is drier and people have specially designed living conditions and clothing.

Chilblains are more likely to develop in those with poor peripheral circulation, noted by blue-red mottled skin on the limbs (acrocyanosis).

CONTRIBUTING FACTORS

Other factors contributing to chilblains include:

- familial tendency to chilblains.
- peripheral vascular disease, due to diabetes, smoking, hyperlipidaemia.
- low body weight, or malnutrition, e.g. anorexia nervosa.
- hormonal changes – chilblains can improve during pregnancy.
- connective tissue disease, particularly lupus erythematosus (chilblain lupus, *Fig. 3.9*) or, in association with Raynaud phenomenon, systemic sclerosis.
- bone marrow disorders.

What are the clinical features of chilblains?

Each chilblain comes up over a few hours as an itchy red swelling and subsides over the next 7–14 days or longer. In severe cases, blistering, pustules, scabs and ulceration can occur. Occasionally the lesions may be ring-shaped. Chilblains may become thickened and persist for months (*Fig. 3.10*).

Common sites for chilblains are:

- backs and sides of the fingers and toes.
- heels.
- lower legs.
- thighs (*Fig. 3.11*).
- wrists of babies.
- over a fatty lump (lipoma).
- nose.
- ears.

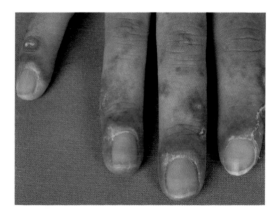

Figure 3.9. Ragged cuticles, periungual telangiectasia and chilblains associated with connective tissue disease.

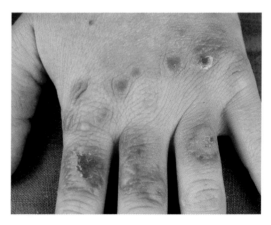

Figure 3.10. Chilblains.

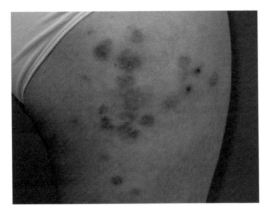

Figure 3.11. Chilblains on the thighs.

What is the treatment for chilblains?

Unfortunately, chilblains respond poorly to treatment. The following may be useful:

- topical corticosteroid cream applied accurately for a few days to relieve itch and swelling.
- antibiotic ointment or oral antibiotics for secondary infection.

Can chilblains be prevented?

People with a tendency to chilblains must keep their hands and feet warm to reduce the risk.

- Nicotine constricts the blood vessels, so smokers must stop smoking.
- Home and workplace should be well insulated without draughts, and heated in winter.
- Warm clothing should include gloves, thick woollen socks and comfortable protective footwear.
- Cotton-lined waterproof gloves are protective for wet work.
- Soaking hands in warm water for several minutes warms them for up to several hours.
- Vigorous indoor exercise keeps the body warm for a period afterwards.
- Medicines that constrict blood vessels should be minimised, including caffeine, decongestants and diet aids.
- Vasodilator medications such as nifedipine are taken throughout the winter months. Side-effects may include flushing and headache.

3.4 Cutaneous lupus erythematosus

What is lupus erythematosus?

Lupus erythematosus (LE) is an autoimmune connective tissue disorder that can affect one or several organs. Circulating autoantibodies and immune complexes are due to loss of normal immune tolerance and are pathogenic. Clinical features of LE are highly variable. LE nearly always affects the skin to some degree.

What is cutaneous lupus erythematosus?

Cutaneous LE comprises several chronic and relapsing LE-specific and LE-nonspecific inflammatory conditions. There can be some overlap.

- LE-specific cutaneous LE has been classified as acute, subacute, chronic and intermittent. Lesions may be localised or generalised. In LE-specific cutaneous LE, lesions are often induced by exposure to sunlight.
- LE-nonspecific cutaneous LE may relate to systemic LE or other autoimmune disease.

Who gets cutaneous lupus erythematosus?

Cutaneous LE most often affects young to middle-aged adult women (aged 20–50 years) but children, the elderly, and males may be affected.

Important predisposing factors for cutaneous LE include:
- female gender.
- genes: ≥25 risk loci have been identified and there are HLA associations.
- skin of colour.

What causes lupus erythematosus?

LE is classified as autoimmune, as it is associated with pathogenic antibodies directed against components of cell nuclei in various tissues. UVB irradiation causes keratinocyte necrosis, immune system activation and antibody formation.

Factors that aggravate LE include:
- sun exposure.
- cigarette smoking.
- hormones.
- viral infection.
- certain drugs.

What are the specific features of cutaneous lupus erythematosus?

There are various types of cutaneous LE. The Revised Cutaneous Lupus Erythematosus Disease Area and Severity Index (RCLASI) can be used to assess disease activity and damage.

ACUTE CUTANEOUS LUPUS ERYTHEMATOSUS

Acute cutaneous LE affects at least 50% of patients with systemic lupus erythematosus (SLE). Many are sick, young, fair-skinned females.

Specific features of acute cutaneous LE may include:
- malar eruption or 'butterfly rash' (erythema and oedema of cheeks, sparing nasolabial folds) lasting hours to days, see *Fig. 3.12*.
- erythematous papular rash on arms, sometimes forming large plaques and spreading widely, see *Fig. 3.13*.
- photosensitivity (a rash on all recently sun-exposed skin).
- cheilitis and mouth ulcers, see *Fig. 3.14*.
- blisters (bullous LE) and erosions.

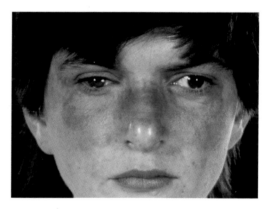

Figure 3.12. Malar eruption of systemic LE.

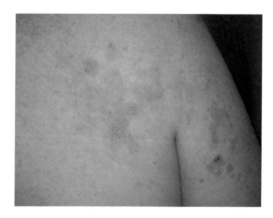

Figure 3.13. Erythematous papular rash in systemic LE.

SLE may also affect joints, kidneys, lungs, heart, liver, brain, blood vessels (vasculitis) and blood cells. It may be accompanied by antiphospholipid syndrome.

SUBACUTE CUTANEOUS LUPUS ERYTHEMATOSUS

About 15% of patients with cutaneous LE have subacute cutaneous LE. One-third of cases are due to previous drug exposure.

Features of subacute cutaneous LE include:
- precipitation or aggravation by sun exposure.
- non-itchy psoriasis-like papulosquamous rash on the upper back, chest and upper arms, see *Fig. 3.15*.
- annular or polycyclic plaques that clear centrally.
- absence of scarring on resolution.

Up to 50% of patients with subacute cutaneous LE may also have a mild form of SLE, resulting in arthralgia or arthritis and low blood counts. Severe SLE is rare in patients with subacute cutaneous LE.

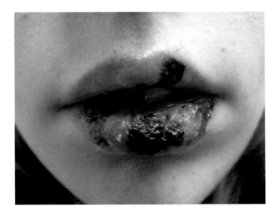

Figure 3.14. Mouth ulcers in systemic LE.

Drug-induced subacute cutaneous LE. More than 100 drugs have been associated with the onset of subacute cutaneous LE. They include:
- terbinafine.
- tumour necrosis factor alpha (TNF-α) inhibitors.
- anticonvulsants.
- proton pump inhibitors.

NEONATAL CUTANEOUS LUPUS ERYTHEMATOSUS

Neonatal cutaneous LE arises within 2 months of birth from mothers with known or subclinical subacute cutaneous LE.

Features of neonatal cutaneous LE may include:
- an annular erythematous rash, which slowly resolves over 6 months.
- rash is most often periorbital, see *Fig. 3.16*.
- photosensitivity.
- blood count abnormalities – haemolytic anaemia, leucopenia, thrombocytopenia.
- hepatobiliary disease.
- persistent congenital heart block.

A paediatrician should assess all babies born to mothers with subacute LE (or carrying the antibody for this condition) at birth. Mortality in babies with heart block is up to 20%, despite pacemaker implantation.

INTERMITTENT CUTANEOUS LUPUS ERYTHEMATOSUS

Intermittent cutaneous LE (*Fig. 3.17*), more often known as lupus tumidus, is a dermal form of lupus.

Features of lupus tumidus include:
- affects sun-exposed sites.

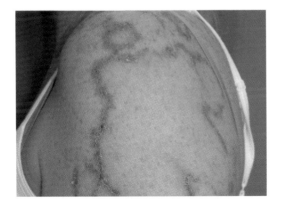

Figure 3.15. Psoriasis-like annular rash of subacute cutaneous LE.

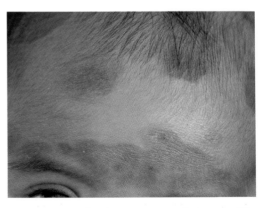

Figure 3.16. Annular plaques in neonatal cutaneous LE.

- erythematous, urticaria-like patches and plaques with a smooth surface, see *Figs 3.17* and *3.18.*
- round or annular shapes.
- clears during the winter months.
- non-scarring.

Lupus tumidus is similar to Jessner lymphocytic infiltrate, in which diagnostic criteria for lupus are absent.

CHRONIC CUTANEOUS LUPUS ERYTHEMATOSUS
Chronic cutaneous LE accounts for 80% of presentations with cutaneous LE. About 25% of patients with chronic cutaneous LE also have systemic LE.

Discoid LE is the most common form of chronic cutaneous LE. It is more prevalent in patients with skin of colour, who are at greater risk of postinflammatory hyperpigmentation and hypertrophic scarring.

- Discoid LE is confined to the skin above the neck in most patients, but can spread below the neck to affect upper back, V of neck, forearms and backs of hands.
- Scalp, ears, cheeks, nose are the most common sites, see *Fig. 3.19.*
- Most patients have photosensitivity.
- New lesions are destructive, erythematous scaly plaques with follicular prominence.
- Scalp discoid LE presents as red, scaly and bald plaques, see *Fig. 3.20.*
- Slow healing leads to postinflammatory pigmentation and white scars.
- Hair growth may partially or completely recover with treatment. Cicatricial (scarring) alopecia can be permanent.

Hypertrophic LE is a variant of discoid LE in which there are thickened and warty plaques resembling viral warts or skin cancers. It can occur on palms and/or soles (palmoplantar LE, a form of acquired keratoderma).

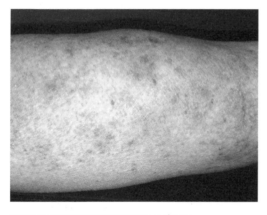

Figure 3.17. Intermittent cutaneous lupus erythematosus.

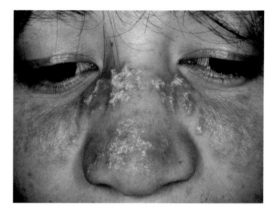

Figure 3.19. Discoid LE.

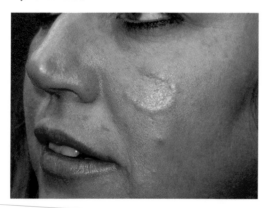

Figure 3.18. Erythematous plaques of lupus tumidus.

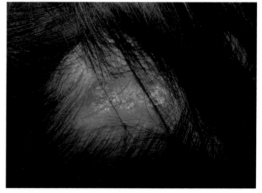

Figure 3.20. Scalp discoid LE.

Mucosal LE presents with plaques, ulcers and scaling of the lips. Mucosal lesions may predispose to squamous cell carcinoma.
- Lips and inside the mouth, see *Fig. 3.21*.
- Lower eyelid with madarosis (loss of eyelashes).
- Rarely, vulva/penis.

Lupus profundus affects subcutaneous tissue and may also be called 'lupus panniculitis'.
- Lupus profundus may develop at any age, including childhood.
- It may involve face, buttocks, limbs or anywhere.
- Firm deep and tender nodules persist for some months, see *Fig. 3.22*.
- Lesions resolve leaving dented, atrophic scars (lipoatrophy).

What are the non-specific cutaneous features of lupus erythematosus?

LE non-specific cutaneous features are most often associated with SLE. They include:
- diffuse hair thinning, see *Fig. 3.23*.
- urticaria.
- Raynaud phenomenon – abnormal blanching of fingers and toes in response to cold weather, followed by numbness and slow rewarming by the fingers which go blue then red, see *Fig. 3.24*.
- chilblains – painful erythematous nodules on fingers and toes during cooler months, see *Fig. 3.25*.
- dilated periungual capillaries, ragged cuticles and nail dystrophy, see *Fig. 3.9*.
- digital ulcers and pitting scars.
- thrombophlebitis.
- papular and nodular mucinosis on cheeks, upper chest, upper arms or back.

- vasculitis – small vessel vasculitis, urticarial vasculitis and less often, vasculitis of medium and large vessels, see *Fig. 3.26*.
- livedo reticularis and antiphospholipid syndrome, see *Fig. 3.27*.

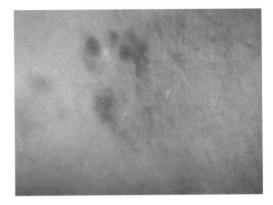

Figure 3.22. Lupus profundus.

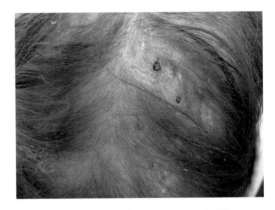

Figure 3.23. Diffuse hair thinning in systemic LE.

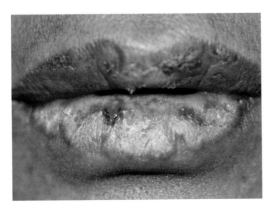

Figure 3.21. Mucosal LE.

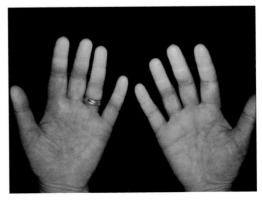

Figure 3.24. Raynaud phenomenon.

Complications of cutaneous lupus erythematosus

Chronic cutaneous LE causes facial deformity and scarring. Active and burned-out disease can lead to social isolation and depression.

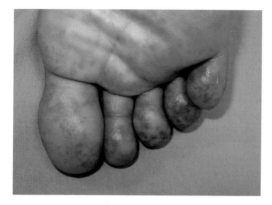

Figure 3.25. Lupus chilblains.

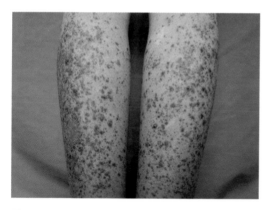

Figure 3.26. Vasculitis.

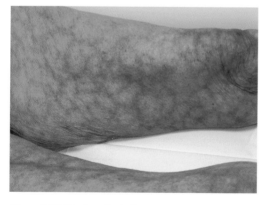

Figure 3.27. Livedo reticularis.

Systemic LE may involve heart, lung and brain with significant morbidity and mortality. Vasculitis involving internal organs can be serious.

How is cutaneous lupus erythematosus diagnosed?

Diagnostic features are more likely to be found in LE-specific than in LE-nonspecific cutaneous LE.

- SLE is associated with high titre antinuclear antibodies.
- About 70% of patients with subacute LE and intermittent cutaneous LE have antiRo/La extractable nuclear antigens (ENA).
- The severity of LE may be reflected in the titre of ANA and/or ENA.
- ANA and ENA are often negative in a patient with chronic cutaneous LE.
- Mild anaemia or leucopenia may be present in cutaneous patients who do not have SLE.

Skin biopsy may be diagnostic, showing a lichenoid tissue reaction and features specific to the kind of cutaneous LE. Direct immunofluorescence tests may show positive antibody deposition along the basement membrane (lupus band test).

How can cutaneous lupus erythematosus be prevented?

- Carefully protect all exposed skin from sun exposure with covering clothing and SPF50+ broad-spectrum sunscreens (see *www.dermnetnz.org/topics/topical-sunscreen-agents*, photosensitivity).
- Smoking cessation is essential – it is best to avoid nicotine replacement as nicotine in any form may exacerbate cutaneous LE.
- If subacute LE is drug-induced, stop the responsible medication.

What is the treatment for cutaneous lupus erythematosus?

The aim of treatment for cutaneous LE is to prevent flares, improve appearance and to prevent scarring.

Local therapy

- Potent or ultrapotent topical steroids are applied to chronic discoid LE plaques.
- Calcineurin inhibitors, pimecrolimus cream or tacrolimus ointment can be used instead of topical steroids.

- Intralesional corticosteroids can be injected into small lesions resistant to topical therapy.
- Topical retinoids, calcipotriol and imiquimod have also been reported to be helpful in a few patients.
- Cosmetic camouflage may be used to disguise unsightly plaques.

SYSTEMIC THERAPY

Treatment for cutaneous and systemic LE may include:

- antimalarials especially hydroxychloroquine.
- immune modulators such as methotrexate, mycophenolate, dapsone, ciclosporin.
- retinoids, i.e. isotretinoin, acitretin.
- systemic corticosteroids.

Severe disease may require more aggressive treatment:

- cyclophosphamide.
- thalidomide.
- photopheresis.
- intravenous immunoglobulin.
- monoclonal antibodies targeting T cells, B cells and cytokines – rituximab.

PROCEDURES

- Phototherapy using UVA1 may be used to treat skin lesions of cutaneous LE.
- Photodynamic therapy has been reported to clear chronic cutaneous LE.
- Vascular laser can reduce telangiectasia.
- Surgery may improve appearance of disfiguring scars.

What is the outlook for cutaneous lupus erythematosus?

The prognosis for cutaneous LE is variable.

- The skin involvement in SLE tends to mirror systemic involvement. SLE can have significant morbidity and mortality when affecting kidneys, heart and brain.
- Drug-induced SCLE clears within a few weeks of withdrawal of the responsible drug.
- Untreated chronic cutaneous LE tends to persist, but severity is lessened by strict sun protection and avoidance of nicotine.

3.5 Drug eruptions

3.5.1 General

What is a drug eruption?

A drug eruption is an acute or subacute adverse cutaneous reaction to a drug or medicine.

There are several different types of drug eruption, which range from a clinically mild and unnoticed rash to a severe cutaneous adverse reaction (SCAR) that may be life threatening.

The most common drug eruptions are:

- morbilliform or exanthematous drug eruption (see *Section 3.5.3*; *Fig. 3.28*).
- urticaria and/or angioedema (see *Section 3.22*; *Fig. 3.29*).

The most serious drug eruptions are rare:

- drug hypersensitivity syndrome (see *Section 3.5.2*; *Fig. 3.30*).
- Stevens–Johnson syndrome/toxic epidermal necrolysis (SJS/TEN, see *Section 3.5.4*; *Fig. 3.31*).

There are many other cutaneous adverse reactions including:

- acute generalised exanthematous pustulosis (pustular psoriasis-like), see *Fig. 3.32*.
- serum sickness (urticaria, fever, arthralgia, lymphadenopathy), see *Fig. 3.33*.
- hypersensitivity vasculitis (palpable purpura), see *Section 3.23*; *Fig. 3.34*.
- fixed drug eruption (single or multiple recurring blistered plaques), see *Fig. 3.35*.

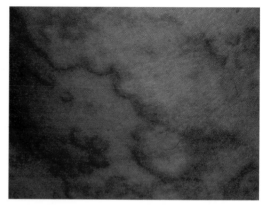

Figure 3.29. Urticaria.

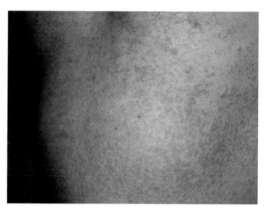

Figure 3.30. Morbilliform rash associated with drug hypersensitivity syndrome.

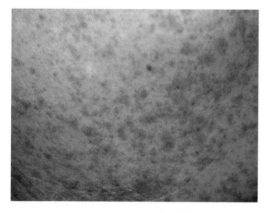

Figure 3.28. Morbilliform drug eruption.

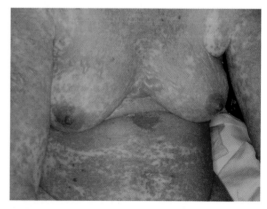

Figure 3.31. SJS/TEN.

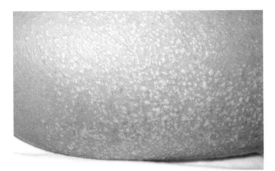

Figure 3.32. Bullous adverse reaction to amoxicillin.

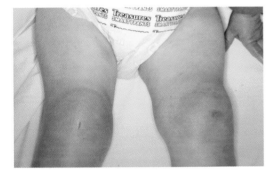

Figure 3.33. Reaction to ceflacor.

- lichenoid drug eruption (lichen planus-like reaction), see *Fig. 3.36.*
- phototoxicity (exaggerated sunburn) or photoallergy (eczema in sun-exposed sites), see *Fig. 3.37.*
- immunobullous disease (important to recognise, as drug withdrawal leads to clearance).
- drug-induced erythema multiforme, see *Fig. 3.38.*
- drug-induced lupus erythematosus, see *Fig. 3.39.*

Drugs can also cause:
- drug-induced stomatitis, see *Fig. 3.40.*
- pigmentary changes, see *Fig. 3.41.*
- precipitation of a skin problem that is ordinarily not caused by a drug (e.g. psoriasis triggered by lithium), see *Fig. 3.42.*
- hair loss (*Fig. 3.43*) or increase (*Fig. 3.44*).
- nail pigmentation or dystrophy, see *Fig. 3.45.*
- allergic contact dermatitis, see *Fig. 3.46.*
- systemic contact dermatitis, see *Fig. 3.47.*

Certain classes of drugs have their own spectra of reactions, particularly:
- hormones.
- chemotherapy agents.

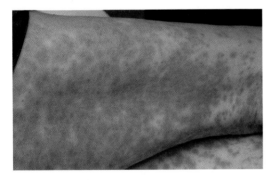

Figure 3.34. Hypersensitivity vasculitis of unknown cause.

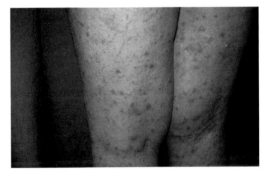

Figure 3.36. Lichenoid reaction to hydroxychloroquine.

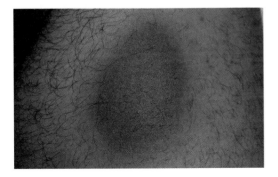

Figure 3.35. Fixed drug eruption due to paracetamol.

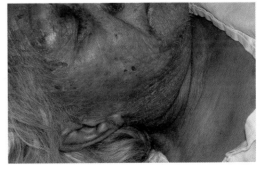

Figure 3.37. Photosensitive reaction to frusemide.

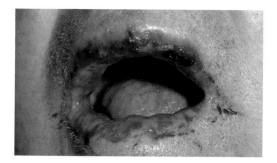

Figure 3.38. Mucositis induced by topical imiquimod applied to chest.

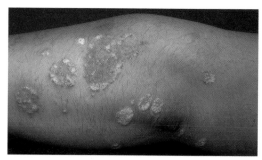

Figure 3.42. Psoriasis triggered by lithium.

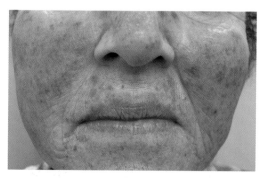

Figure 3.39. Drug-induced subacute lupus erythematosus.

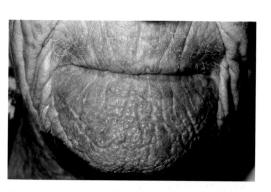

Figure 3.40. Stomatitis caused by topical prochlorperazine.

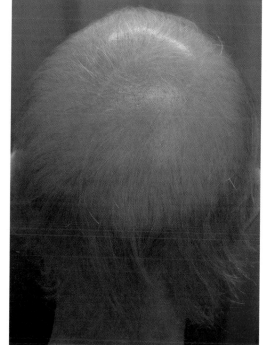

Figure 3.43. Hair loss caused by chemotherapy.

Figure 3.41. Pigmentary changes caused by minocycline.

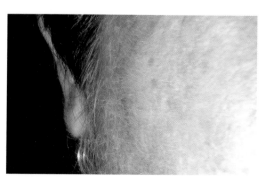

Figure 3.44. Hypertrichosis due to ciclosporin.

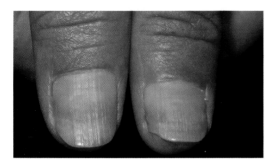

Figure 3.45. Onycholysis due to doxycycline.

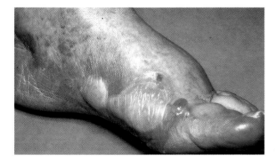

Figure 3.46. Allergic contact dermatitis due to topical neomycin.

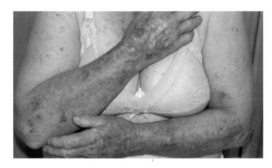

Figure 3.47. Reaction to thiomersal in vaccine.

- anticoagulants.
- biologics.
- epidermal growth factor inhibitors.

Who gets drug eruptions?

On average about 2% of prescriptions of a new medication lead to a drug eruption.
- Allergic reactions to some drugs are more common in females than in males.
- There are genetic factors that predispose people to drug eruptions. These may include differences in drug metabolism.

- Underlying viral infections and diseases can influence reactions.
- Previous allergic drug reaction or drug intolerance increases the risk of reaction to another drug. The more drugs prescribed, the more likelihood of allergy.
- Cross-reactions can occur relating to previous sensitivity to different medications, sunscreens, cosmetics, foods or insect bites.

It should be noted that some symptoms are falsely attributed to a medication when due to another cause.

What causes drug eruptions?

There are several causes of drug eruptions.
- True allergy: this is due to an immunological mechanism.
  - Immediate reactions occur within an hour of exposure to the drug and are mediated by IgE antibodies (urticaria, anaphylaxis).
  - Delayed reactions occur between 6 hours and several weeks of first exposure to the drug. They may be mediated by IgG antibody, immune complex or cytotoxic T cells.
- Predictable reactions explicable by pharmacology.
- Drug intolerance, i.e. dose-related reactions.
- Pseudoallergy, i.e. an urticarial reaction assumed to be allergy but actually due to direct release of mast cell mediators by the drug (opioids, NSAIDs).

What are the clinical features of drug eruptions?

Each drug eruption has its own characteristics (see detailed topic pages).

Additional systemic symptoms accompanying drug eruption may include:
- fever.
- malaise.
- other organ involvement (in SCAR).

Complications of drug eruptions

Incorrect attribution of drug eruption can deprive the patient of a useful medication, or lead to recurrence when the drug is taken at a later date.

Patients with SCAR may die from it.

SJS/TEN can cause permanent scarring leading to blindness and deformity.

How are drug eruptions diagnosed?

A careful history, skin and general physical examination are necessary to diagnose a drug eruption and to assess its severity.

- Determine any previous exposure to the medication(s) under suspicion.
- Review the medical record to determine the relationship between onset of symptoms and commencing medication(s).
- Some medications (such as antibiotics and antiepileptic drugs) are more likely than others (such as cardiac medications) to cause drug eruptions.
- Medications may need to be stopped and later reintroduced to see whether symptoms recur. This is not safe if the patient had SJS/TEN or anaphylaxis.

Blood tests generally include blood count, liver function and kidney function. Eosinophilia may or may not be present, and is non-specific unless of recent onset.

It is sometimes difficult to determine which drug is responsible for a rash, if any.

- Skin prick/intradermal tests can be undertaken by allergy specialist/immunologist to check for immediate reactions to penicillin and a few other drugs. However, tests are not available to confirm most drug reactions.
- Patch tests are sometimes performed using drugs thought to have caused exanthems, but can be difficult to interpret.

What is the treatment for drug eruptions?

The main thing is to identify and stop the responsible drug as soon as possible.

The use of systemic glucocorticoids for drug eruptions such as prednisone is controversial. They are unnecessary if the rash is mild. Get advice from a specialist immunologist or dermatologist if the rash is severe.

- Topical corticosteroids, e.g. betamethasone cream, are safe short-term, and may reduce symptoms.
- Emollients can be applied liberally and frequently.
- Urticaria often responds to antihistamines, but they are rarely useful for other eruptions.

Educate the patient to avoid re-exposure to the responsible medication and known drugs with which it cross-reacts.

How can drug eruptions be prevented?

As most serious drug eruptions are due to antibiotics, their use should be limited and underlying conditions should be treated in other ways whenever possible.

Patients should always be asked about previous drug allergies when prescribing a new medicine.

What is the outlook for patients with drug eruptions?

Some patients can tolerate re-exposure to a medication later on. Reasons for this may include:

- the drug was not responsible for the original symptoms.
- drug sensitivity has been lost over time.
- the underlying illness may have settled.

For those with confirmed drug allergy, an unrelated medication should be prescribed if needed and where possible. Often these are more expensive, may be less effective, and might also have side effects and risks. Cross-reactions can occur to similar medicines because of a similar chemical structure or a drug class effect.

Graduated challenges and desensitisation are sometimes carried out in specialist clinics.

Patients who have had severe adverse drug reactions should carry a wallet card and/or register with a drug allergy service, such as MedicAlert.

3.5.2 Drug hypersensitivity syndrome

What is drug hypersensitivity syndrome?

Drug hypersensitivity syndrome is a severe, unexpected reaction to a medicine, which affects several organ systems at the same time. It most commonly causes the combination of:

- high fever.
- morbilliform eruption.
- haematological abnormalities.
- lymphadenopathy.
- inflammation of one or more internal organs.

Drug hypersensitivity syndrome is sometimes also called drug reaction with eosinophilia and systemic symptoms (DRESS) and drug-induced hypersensitivity syndrome (DIHS).

The syndrome is classified as a severe cutaneous adverse reaction (SCAR). It may have overlapping features with Stevens–Johnson syndrome/toxic epidermal necrolysis and acute generalised exanthematous pustulosis (AGEP).

Who gets drug hypersensitivity syndrome?

Drug hypersensitivity syndrome is relatively rare. It mainly affects adults and is equal in incidence in males and females. Genetic susceptibility and HLA associations have been found for several causative drugs.

The most common drugs to cause this reaction are the anti-gout drug, allopurinol, a number of anti-epilepsy drugs (particularly carbamazepine, phenobarbital and phenytoin) and the sulphonamide group of antibiotics. It has been estimated that 1 in every 10 000 patients treated with an anticonvulsant will develop drug hypersensitivity syndrome.

The risk of drug hypersensitivity syndrome in patients on allopurinol depends on the dose of allopurinol. It is greater if the patient has kidney disease and if they are also taking thiazide diuretics.

It has also, rarely, been reported to be due to other medicines. It can be very difficult to determine the exact cause of drug hypersensitivity syndrome if several medicines have been commenced in preceding weeks. In about 10% of cases, the causative drug is never identified.

What causes drug hypersensitivity syndrome?

Drug hypersensitivity syndrome is a delayed T cell-mediated reaction. Tissue damage is due to cytotoxic T cells and cytokine release.

- There is a genetic predisposition to drug hypersensitivity syndrome.
- A defect in the way the liver metabolizes drugs may be responsible.
- Reactivation of human herpes virus 6 (HHV6) or Epstein–Barr virus (EBV) may also be important.

What are the clinical features of drug hypersensitivity syndrome?

Drug hypersensitivity syndrome usually develops over several days, with onset between 2 and 8 weeks after starting the responsible medicine.

A high fever of 38–40°C is usually noticed first. This is quickly followed by a widespread skin rash. Characteristics of the rash are diverse.

- Morbilliform eruption affects 80% of cases (see *Figs 3.30* and *3.50*), with varying morphology including targetoid lesions, blisters and pustules, see *Fig. 3.48*.
- Erythroderma or exfoliative dermatitis (involving >90% body surface area) may follow in about 10%.

- Facial swelling affects 30%, see *Fig. 3.49*.
- Mucosal involvement affects 25% (lips, mouth, throat, genitals).

The rash can last many weeks.

SYSTEMIC INVOLVEMENT

Symptoms may worsen after stopping the drug, and may continue for weeks or even months despite drug withdrawal. The severity of the rash does not necessarily correlate with the extent of internal organ involvement. Later symptoms depend on the internal organs affected. They may include:

- enlarged lymph nodes in several sites (75%).
- haematological disorders – raised white count (or less often, reduced white count), eosinophilia (in 30% this is >2.0×10^9/L),

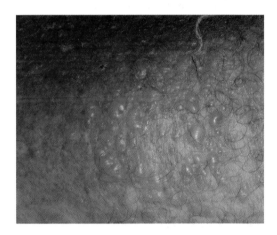

Figure 3.48. Bullous eruption.

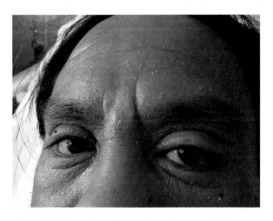

Figure 3.49. Facial swelling in drug hypersensitivity syndrome.

atypical lymphocytes, thrombocytopenia, anaemia, haemophagocytic syndrome.
- liver enlargement, hepatitis and, rarely, hepatic necrosis with liver failure; abnormal liver function tests are found in 70–90%.
- kidney disease – this affects about 10% and is usually mild (interstitial nephritis); renal failure is rare.
- inflammation of the heart (myocarditis) or heart sac (pericarditis), causing chest pain, breathlessness and lowered blood pressure.
- lung disease, causing shortness of breath and cough (interstitial pneumonitis, pleuritis, pneumonia and acute respiratory distress syndrome).
- neurological involvement, which may lead to meningitis and encephalitis, polyneuritis, causing headache, seizures, coma and palsies.
- gastrointestinal symptoms – gastroenteritis, pancreatitis, bleeding and dehydration; in severe cases, acute colitis and pancreatitis can occur, and chronic enteropathy may ensue.
- endocrine abnormalities – thyroiditis and diabetes.
- muscle disease (myositis).
- eye disease (uveitis).

Complications of drug hypersensitivity syndrome

The mortality from drug hypersensitivity syndrome is estimated at around 8%. Causes of death include:
- acute liver failure causing coagulation problems, jaundice and impaired consciousness.
- multiorgan failure.
- fulminant myocarditis.
- haemophagocytosis.

How is drug hypersensitivity syndrome diagnosed?

The diagnosis of drug hypersensitivity syndrome is based on the clinical presentation of the triad of:
- high fever.
- extensive skin rash.
- organ involvement.

It is supported by eosinophilia and abnormal liver function tests.

As drug hypersensitivity syndrome can occur up to eight weeks after first exposure to the responsible drug, a great degree of care is required when determining the responsible medicine. A temporal association between medicine use and the start of the syndrome is the strongest evidence.

The European Registry of Severe Cutaneous Adverse Reactions to Drugs and Collection of Biological Samples (RegiSCAR) has produced diagnostic criteria to assist in the diagnosis of drug hypersensitivity syndrome. RegiSCAR inclusion criteria for potential cases require at least three of the following:
- hospitalisation.
- reaction suspected to be drug related.
- acute skin rash.
- fever above 38°C.
- enlarged lymph nodes at two sites.
- involvement of at least one internal organ.
- blood count abnormalities such as low platelets, raised eosinophils or abnormal lymphocyte count.

Attempts to confirm which drug has caused drug hypersensitivity syndrome may include patch tests. Patch testing has been reported to be most successful for antiepileptic drugs, with 50% positive reactions. It is not useful for allopurinol, with 0% positive reactions. Lymphocyte transformation testing is available in some centres, where specialist interpretation may reveal the causative drug in the majority of cases.

INVESTIGATIONS

After taking a careful history and performing skin and general examination, the following tests may be requested.

Skin biopsy usually shows dense infiltration of inflammatory cells, including lymphocytes and eosinophils, extravasated erythrocytes and oedema.

Blood tests may include:
- blood count and coagulation studies.
- biochemical tests – at least liver function, renal function, muscle enzymes.
- viral serology – hepatitis B, C, EBV, CMV, HHV-6.
- endocrine function – thyroid, glucose levels.

Urinalysis is undertaken to assess renal damage.

Cardiac and pulmonary evaluation may include electrocardiograph (ECG), echocardiogram and chest X-ray. Scans may be performed to evaluate liver, kidney and brain depending on symptoms and the results of initial tests.

What is the treatment for drug hypersensitivity syndrome?

Treatment consists of immediate withdrawal of all suspect medicines, followed by careful monitoring and supportive care. It is very important for patients presenting with a high fever and a rash, where a diagnosis of drug hypersensitivity syndrome is considered, to have blood tests as soon as possible.

Systemic steroids (e.g. prednisone) are generally used in the more severe cases of drug hypersensitivity syndrome involving significant exfoliative dermatitis, pneumonitis and/or hepatitis. However, the benefits of corticosteroids are unknown as controlled clinical trials are lacking. Once effective, they should be withdrawn very slowly as the syndrome can recur as the dose reduces.

Additional treatment may include intravenous immunoglobulins, plasmapheresis, and immunomodulatory drugs such as cyclophosphamide, ciclosporin, mycophenolate and rituximab.

Supportive treatment for the skin rash may include:
- dressings.
- topical corticosteroids.
- emollients.
- oral antihistamines.

Fluid, electrolytes and calorie intake may need attention. A warm environment and expert nursing care are required. Secondary infections may require antibiotics.

How can drug hypersensitivity syndrome be prevented?

Patients who develop drug hypersensitivity syndrome must avoid taking the causative medicine(s) again.

Cross-reactions are common between the three main aromatic anticonvulsant drugs (phenytoin, carbamazepine and phenobarbitone), and patients who have experienced drug hypersensitivity syndrome with any one of these medicines must avoid all three.

Because genetic factors are suspected in drug hypersensitivity syndrome, first-degree relatives should be alerted to their elevated risk of developing hypersensitivity reactions to the same medicine(s).

What is the outlook for drug hypersensitivity syndrome?

Most patients fully recover from drug hypersensitivity within weeks to months. Relapse after initial improvement is common.

Patients recovering from drug hypersensitivity syndrome are thought to be at risk of developing autoimmune diseases.

3.5.3 Morbilliform drug eruption

What is morbilliform drug eruption?

Morbilliform drug eruption is the most common form of drug eruption (*Fig. 3.50*). Many drugs can trigger this allergic reaction, but antibiotics are the most common group. The eruption may resemble exanthems (*Section 2.3.3*) caused by viral and bacterial infections.
- A morbilliform skin rash in an adult is usually due to a drug.
- In a child, it is more likely to be viral in origin.

Morbilliform drug eruption is also called maculopapular drug eruption, exanthematous drug eruption and maculopapular exanthem.

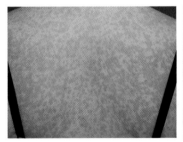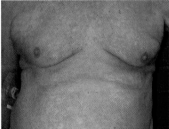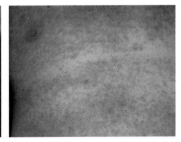

Figure 3.50. Morbilliform drug eruptions.

Who gets morbilliform drug eruption?

About 2% of prescriptions of new drugs cause a drug eruption. About 95% of these are morbilliform drug eruptions.

They mainly affect people prescribed beta-lactam antibiotics (penicillins, cephalosporins), sulphonamides, allopurinol, antiepileptic drugs and non-steroidal anti-inflammatory drugs (NSAIDs). Numerous other drugs have been reported to cause morbilliform drug eruptions, including herbal and natural therapies.

Predisposing factors include:
- previous drug eruption or strong family history of drug eruptions.
- underlying viral infection, particularly acute Epstein–Barr virus (EBV, infectious mononucleosis) and human herpes virus 6 and 7.
- immunodeficiency including human immunodeficiency virus (HIV), cystic fibrosis, autoimmune disorders.
- multiple medications.

What causes morbilliform drug eruption?

Morbilliform drug eruption is a form of allergic reaction. It is mediated by cytotoxic T cells and classified as a Type IV immune reaction. The target of attack may be a drug, a metabolite of the drug, or a protein bonded to the drug. Inflammation follows the release of cytokines and other effector immune cells.

What are the clinical features of morbilliform drug eruption?

On the first occasion, the skin rash usually appears 1–2 weeks after starting the drug, but it may occur up to 1 week after stopping it. On re-exposure to the causative (or related) drug, skin lesions appear within 1–3 days. It is very rare for a drug that has been taken for months or years to cause a morbilliform drug eruption.

Morbilliform drug eruption usually first appears on the trunk and then spreads to the limbs and neck. The distribution is bilateral and symmetrical.
- The primary lesion is a pink–red flat macule or papule.
- Annular, targetoid, urticarial or polymorphous morphology may occur.
- Lesions mostly blanch with pressure but may be non-blanchable (purpuric), especially on the lower legs.
- Discrete lesions may merge together to form large erythematous patches or plaques.

- Axilla, groin, hands and feet are usually spared.
- Paradoxical prominent rash in axillae and groins may be due to symmetrical drug-related intertriginous and flexural exanthema (SDRIFE).
- Mucous membranes, hair and nails are not affected in uncomplicated drug eruptions.

The rash may be associated with a mild fever and itch. As it improves, the redness dies away and the surface skin peels off.

What are the complications of morbilliform drug eruption?

In the early phase, it may not be possible to clinically distinguish an uncomplicated morbilliform eruption from other more serious forms of drug reaction, for example:
- drug hypersensitivity syndrome, also called drug reaction with eosinophilia and systemic symptoms (DRESS).
- Stevens–Johnson syndrome/toxic epidermal necrolysis (SJS/TEN).
- acute generalised exanthematous pustulosis (AGEP).

Patients with the following symptoms/signs should be hospitalised for specialist assessment and supportive care:
- erythroderma (whole-body involvement).
- high fever or significant malaise.
- any mucosal involvement.
- skin tenderness.
- blistering.
- pustules.
- palpable purpura.
- evidence of other organ involvement (e.g. liver, kidneys, lungs, blood).

How is morbilliform drug eruption diagnosed?

A strong clinical suspicion of morbilliform drug eruption depends on:
- typical exanthematous rash.
- recently introduced medication.

To identify the possible causative drug, a drug calendar, including all prescribed and over-the-counter products, may be helpful. The starting date of each new drug is documented together with the onset of the rash. The calendar must extend back at least 2 weeks and up to one month. Drugs can then be classified as unlikely or likely causes based on:

- time relative to onset of the rash.
- the specific drug; some drugs can be excluded as rarely causing allergy.
- patient's past experience with other drugs in the same class.

There are no routine tests to make the diagnosis or to identify the culprit drug. Differential diagnosis includes measles, rubella, scarlet fever, non-specific toxic erythema associated with infection, Kawasaki disease, connective tissue disease and acute graft-versus-host disease.

Tests are not usually necessary if the cause has been identified and stopped, the rash is mild and the patient is well. They may include:
- routine blood count, liver and kidney function tests, C-reactive protein.
- serology for infections that can cause similar rashes.
- possible skin biopsy, which shows interface dermatitis, mixed perivascular infiltration and other histopathological features.

Eosinophilia is supportive but not diagnostic. Further investigations will depend on clinical features, progress of the patient, and the results of the initial tests.

What is the treatment for morbilliform drug eruption?

The most important thing is to identify the causative drug and if possible, stop it. If the reaction is mild, and the drug is essential and not replaceable, obtain a specialist opinion whether it is safe to continue the drug before doing so.
- Monitor the patient carefully in case of complications.
- Apply emollients and potent topical steroid creams.
- Consider wet wraps for very red, inflamed skin.
- Antihistamines are often prescribed, but in general they are not very helpful.

How can morbilliform drug eruption be prevented?

It is not possible to completely prevent morbilliform eruptions. Prescribers must be vigilant. Their incidence may be reduced by:
- minimising prescriptions for antibiotics.
- educating the patient about the cause of their rash and the danger of re-exposure to the same medication.
- adding the reaction to the medical record alerts.

What is the outlook for morbilliform drug eruption?

If the causative drug is ceased, the rash begins to improve within 48 hours and clears within 1–2 weeks.

If the drug is continued, the rash may:
- resolve despite continued exposure to the drug.
- persist without change.
- progress to erythroderma.

3.5.4 Stevens–Johnson syndrome/ toxic epidermal necrolysis

What is SJS/TEN?

Stevens–Johnson syndrome (SJS) and toxic epidermal necrolysis (TEN) are now believed to be variants of the same condition, distinct from erythema multiforme. SJS/TEN is a very rare, acute, serious and potentially fatal skin reaction in which there is sheet-like skin and mucosal loss. Using current definitions, this SCAR is nearly always caused by medications.

Who gets SJS/TEN?

SJS/TEN is a very rare complication of medication use (estimated at 1–2/million each year for SJS, and 0.4–1.2/million each year for TEN).
- Anyone on medication can develop SJS/TEN unpredictably.
- It can affect all age groups and all races.
- It is slightly more common in females than in males.
- It is 100 times more common in association with human immunodeficiency virus infection (HIV) especially if AIDS is present.

Genetic factors are important:
- HLA associations in some races to anticonvulsants and allopurinol.
- polymorphisms to specific genes, e.g. *CYP2C* coding for cytochrome P450 in patients reacting to anticonvulsants.

More than 200 medications have been reported in association with SJS/TEN.
- It is more often seen with drugs with long half-lives compared to even a chemically similar related drug with a short half-life. A half-life of a medication is the time that half of the delivered dose remains circulating in the body.

- The medications are usually systemic (taken by mouth or injection) but TEN has been reported after topical use.
- No drug is implicated in about 20% of cases.
- SJS/TEN has rarely been associated with vaccination and infections such as mycoplasma and cytomegalovirus. Infections are generally associated with mucosal involvement and less severe cutaneous disease than when drugs are the cause.

The drugs that most commonly cause SJS/TEN are:

- sulphonamides – cotrimoxizole.
- beta-lactam – penicillins, cephalosporins.
- anticonvulsants – lamotrigine, carbamazepine, phenytoin, phenobarbitone.
- allopurinol.
- paracetamol (acetaminophen).
- nevirapine (non-nucleoside reverse-transcriptase inhibitor).
- non-steroidal anti-inflammatory drugs (NSAIDs) (oxicam type mainly).

What causes SJS/TEN?

SJS/TEN is a rare and unpredictable reaction to medication. The mechanism has still not been understood and is complex.

Drug-specific CD8+ cytotoxic lymphocytes can be detected in the early blister fluid. They have some natural killer cell activity and can probably kill keratinocytes by direct contact. Cytokines implicated include perforin/granzyme, Fas-L and tumour necrosis factor (TNF) alpha.

There are probably two major pathways involved:

- Fas-Fas ligand pathway of apoptosis has been considered a pivotal step in the pathogenesis of TEN. The Fas ligand (FasL), a form of tumour necrosis factor, is secreted by blood lymphocytes and can bind to the Fas 'death' receptor expressed by keratinocytes.
- Granule-mediated exocytosis via perforin and granzyme B, resulting in cytotoxicity (cell death). Perforin and granzyme B can be detected in early blister fluid and it has been suggested that levels may be associated with disease severity.

What are the clinical features of SJS/TEN?

The adverse drug reaction SJS/TEN usually develops within the first week of antibiotic therapy but up to 2 months after starting an anticonvulsant. For most drugs the onset is within a few days up to 1 month.

Before the rash appears, there is usually a prodromal illness of several days' duration resembling an upper respiratory tract infection or 'flu-like illness. Symptoms may include:

- fever >39°C.
- sore throat, difficulty swallowing.
- runny nose and cough.
- sore red eyes, conjunctivitis.
- general aches and pains.

There is then an abrupt onset of a tender/painful red skin rash, starting on the trunk and extending rapidly over hours to days onto the face and limbs (but rarely affecting scalp, palms or soles). The maximum extent is usually reached by 4 days.

The skin lesions may be:

- macules – flat, red and diffuse (measles-like spots) or purple (purpuric) spots.
- diffuse erythema.
- targetoid – as in erythema multiforme, see *Fig. 3.51*.
- blisters – flaccid (i.e. not tense).

The blisters then merge to form sheets of skin detachment, exposing red, oozing dermis (see *Fig. 3.31*). The Nikolsky sign is positive in areas of skin redness. This means that blisters and erosions appear when the skin is rubbed gently.

Mucosal involvement is prominent and severe, although not forming actual blisters. At least two mucosal surfaces are affected, including:

- eyes (conjunctivitis, less often corneal ulceration, anterior uveitis,

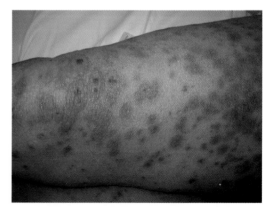

Figure 3.51. Targetoid skin lesions.

panophthalmitis) – red, sore, sticky, photosensitive eyes, see *Fig. 3.52*.
- lips/mouth (cheilitis, stomatitis) – red crusted lips, painful mouth ulcers, see *Fig. 3.53*.
- pharynx, oesophagus – causing difficulty eating.
- genital area and urinary tract – erosions, ulcers, urinary retention, see *Fig. 3.54*.
- upper respiratory tract (trachea and bronchi) – causing cough and respiratory distress.
- gastrointestinal tract – causing diarrhoea.

The patient is very ill, extremely anxious and in considerable pain. In addition to skin/mucosal involvement, other organs may be affected, including liver, kidneys, lungs, bone marrow and joints. There can be overlap with DIHS and AGEP.

Complications of SJS/TEN

SJS/TEN can be fatal due to complications in the acute phase. The mortality rate is up to 10% for SJS and at least 30% for TEN.

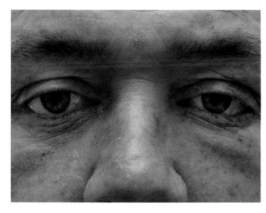

Figure 3.52. Photosensitive eyes.

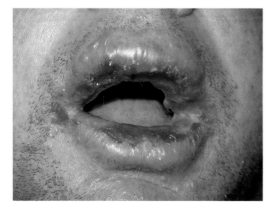

Figure 3.53. Mouth ulcers.

During the acute phase, potentially fatal complications include:
- dehydration and acute malnutrition.
- infection of skin, mucous membranes, lungs (pneumonia), septicaemia (blood poisoning).
- acute respiratory distress syndrome.
- gastrointestinal ulceration, perforation and intussusception.
- shock and multiple organ failure including kidney failure.
- thromboembolism and disseminated intravascular coagulopathy.

How is SJS/TEN diagnosed?

SJS/TEN is suspected clinically and classified based on the skin surface area detached at maximum extent.

CLASSIFICATION OF TEN – SJS
- Skin detachment <10% of body surface area (BSA).
- Widespread erythematous or purpuric macules or flat atypical targets.

CLASSIFICATION OF TEN – OVERLAP SJS/TEN
- Detachment between 10% and 30% of BSA.
- Widespread purpuric macules or flat atypical targets.

CLASSIFICATION OF TEN – TEN WITH SPOTS
- Detachment >30% of BSA.
- Widespread purpuric macules or flat atypical targets.

CLASSIFICATION OF TEN – TEN WITHOUT SPOTS
- Detachment of >10% of BSA.

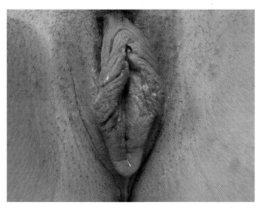

Figure 3.54. Genital ulcers.

- Large epidermal sheets and no purpuric macules.

The category cannot always be defined with certainty on initial presentation. The diagnosis may therefore change during the first few days in hospital.

INVESTIGATIONS

If the test is available, elevated levels of serum granulysin taken in the first few days of a drug eruption may be predictive of SJS/TEN.

Skin biopsy is usually required to confirm the clinical diagnosis and to exclude staphylococcal scalded skin syndrome (SSSS) and other generalised rashes with blisters. The histopathology shows keratinocyte necrosis, full thickness epidermal/epithelial necrosis, and minimal lymphocytic inflammation. The direct immunofluorescence test on the skin biopsy is negative, indicating the disease is not due to deposition of antibodies in the skin.

Blood tests do not help to make the diagnosis but are essential to make sure fluid and vital nutrients have been replaced, to identify complications and to assess prognostic factors (see *below*). Abnormalities may include the following:

- Anaemia occurs in virtually all cases.
- Leucopenia especially lymphopenia is very common (90%).
- Neutropenia if present, is a bad prognostic sign.
- Eosinophilia and atypical lymphocytosis do not occur (unlike drug hypersensitivity syndrome).
- Raised liver enzymes in 50%; approximately 10% develop overt hepatitis with hypoalbuminaemia, raised glucose.
- Mild proteinuria occurs in about 50%. Some changes in kidney function occur in the majority.

Patch testing rarely identifies the culprit in SJS/TEN following recovery, and is not recommended.

SCORTEN

SCORTEN is an illness severity score that has been developed to predict mortality in SJS and TEN cases. One point is scored for each of seven criteria present at the time of admission. The SCORTEN criteria are:

- age >40 years.
- presence of a malignancy (cancer).
- heart rate >120.
- initial percentage of epidermal detachment >10%.
- serum urea level >10 mmol/L.
- serum glucose level >14 mmol/L.
- serum bicarbonate level <20 mmol/L.

The risk of dying from SJS/TEN depends on the score.

SCORTEN predicted mortality rates
SCORTEN 0–1:   >3.2%
SCORTEN 2:   >12.1%
SCORTEN 3:   >35.3%
SCORTEN 4:   >58.3%
SCORTEN ≥5:   >90%

What is the treatment for SJS/TEN?

Care of a patient with SJS/TEN requires:

- cessation of suspected causative drug(s) – the patient is less likely to die and complications are less if the culprit drug is stopped on or before the day that blisters/erosions appear.
- hospital admission – preferably immediately to an intensive care and/or burns unit with specialist nursing care, as this improves survival, reduces infection and shortens hospital stay.
- consider fluidised air bed.
- nutritional and fluid replacement (crystalloid) by intravenous and nasogastric routes – reviewed and adjusted daily.
- temperature maintenance – as body temperature regulation is impaired, patient should be in a warm room (30–32°C).
- pain relief – as pain can be extreme.
- sterile handling and reverse isolation procedures.

Skin care:

- examine daily for extent of detachment and for infection (take swabs for bacterial culture).
- topical antiseptics e.g. silver nitrate, chlorhexidine (but not silver sulphadiazine as it is a sulpha drug).
- dressings such as gauze with petrolatum, non-adherent nanocrystalline-containing silver gauze or biosynthetic skin substitutes can reduce pain.

- avoid using adhesive tapes and unnecessary removal of dead skin; leave the blister roof as a 'biological dressing'.

Eye care:
- daily assessment by ophthalmologist.
- frequent eye drops/ointments (antiseptic, antibiotic, cortisone).

Mouth care:
- mouthwashes.
- topical oral anaesthetic.

Genital care:
- if ulcerated, prevent vaginal adhesions using intravaginal steroid ointment, soft vaginal dilators.

Lung care:
- consider aerosols, bronchial aspiration, physiotherapy.
- may require intubation and mechanical ventilation if trachea and bronchi are involved.

Urinary care:
- catheter because of genital involvement and immobility.
- culture urine for bacterial infection.

General:
- psychiatric support for extreme anxiety and emotional lability.
- physiotherapy to maintain joint movement and reduce risk of pneumonia.
- regular assessment for staphylococcal or Gram-negative infection.
- appropriate antibiotic should be given if infection develops; prophylactic antibiotics are not recommended and may even increase the risk of sepsis.
- consider heparin to prevent thromboembolism (blood clots).

The role of systemic corticosteroids remains controversial. Some clinicians prescribe high doses of corticosteroids for a short time at the start of the reaction, e.g. prednisone 1–2 mg/kg/day for 3–5 days. However, concerns have been raised that they may increase the risk of infection, impair wound healing and other complications, and they have not been proven to have any benefit. They are not effective later in the course of the illness.

Case reports and small patient series have reported benefit from active adjuvant treatments delivered during the first 24–48 hours of illness.

As SJS/TEN is fortunately a rare condition, controlled trials of therapies in large numbers of patients are difficult.
- Ciclosporin 3–5 mg/kg/day.
- Anti-TNF-α monoclonal antibodies, e.g. infliximab, etanercept.
- Cyclophosphamide.
- Intravenous immunoglobulin (IVIG) 2–3 g/kg given over 2–3 days.
- Plasmapheresis.

Thalidomide, trialled because of its anti-TNF-α effect, increased mortality, and should not be used.

How can SJS/TEN be prevented?

People who have survived SJS/TEN must be educated to avoid taking the causative drug or structurally related medicines as SJS/TEN may recur. Cross-reactions can occur between:
- anticonvulsants: carbamazepine, phenytoin, lamotrigine and phenobarbital.
- beta-lactam antibiotics: penicillin, cephalosporin and carbapenem.
- NSAIDs.
- sulphonamides: sulphamethoxazole, sulphadiazine, sulphapyridine.

In the future, we may be able to predict who is at risk of SJS/TEN using genetic screening.

Allopurinol should be prescribed for good indications (e.g. gout with hyperuricaemia) and commenced at low dose (100 mg/day), as SJS/TEN is more likely at doses >200 mg/day.

What is the outlook for SJS/TEN?

The acute phase of SJS/TEN lasts 8–12 days.

Re-epithelialisation of denuded areas takes several weeks, and is accompanied by peeling of the less severely affected skin. Survivors of the acute phase have increased ongoing mortality, especially if aged or sick.

Long-term sequelae include:
- pigment change – patchwork of increased and decreased pigmentation.
- skin scarring, especially at sites of pressure or infection.
- loss of nails with permanent scarring (pterygium) and failure to regrow.
- scarred genitalia – phimosis (constricted foreskin which cannot retract) and vaginal adhesions (occluded vagina).
- joint contractures.
- lung disease – bronchiolitis, bronchiectasis, obstructive disorders.

Eye problems can lead to blindness:
- dry and/or watery eyes, which may burn and sting when exposed to light.
- conjunctivitis – red, crusted, or ulcerated conjunctiva.
- corneal ulcers, opacities and scarring.
- symblepharon – adhesion of conjunctiva of eyelid to eyeball.
- ectropion or entropion – turned-out or turned-in eyelid.
- trichiasis – inverted eyelashes.
- synechiae – iris sticks to cornea.

It may take weeks to months for symptoms and signs to settle.

3.6 Eczema/dermatitis

3.6.1 General

Dermatitis/eczema can be defined by its histological characteristics: spongiosis and variable epidermal acanthosis with a superficial perivascular lympho-histiocytic infiltrate.

Clinical features depend on the acuity of the eruption, which is nearly always itchy.

- Acute eczema – erythematous papules and plaques, oedema, vesicles and bullae, see *Fig. 3.55*.
- Subacute eczema – erythematous plaques, dryness, see *Fig. 3.56*.
- Chronic eczema – dryness, skin thickening, hyperpigmentation (in darker skin types), see *Fig. 3.57*.
- Secondary findings – excoriations, lichenification (thickened skin, increased skin markings), bacterial (*Fig. 3.58*) or viral infection (*Fig. 3.59*).

Common types of dermatitis/eczema include:
- atopic eczema, see *Fig. 3.60*.
- seborrhoeic eczema, see *Fig. 3.61*.
- discoid eczema, see *Fig. 3.62*.
- asteatotic eczema, see *Fig. 3.63*.
- otitis externa, see *Fig. 3.64*.
- venous eczema, see *Fig. 3.65*.
- contact eczema, see *Fig. 3.66*.
- pompholyx, see *Fig. 3.67*.
- lichen simplex, see *Fig. 3.68*.
- disseminated secondary eczema, see *Fig. 3.69*.

How is eczema/dermatitis diagnosed?

Different forms of eczema/dermatitis are distinguished by age of onset, affected body

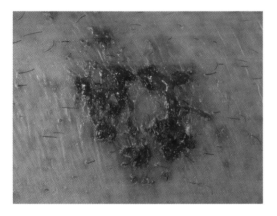

Figure 3.55. Acute eczema.

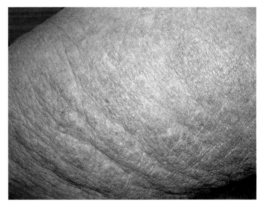

Figure 3.57. Chronic eczema.

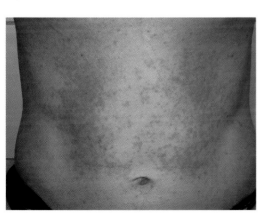

Figure 3.56. Subacute eczema.

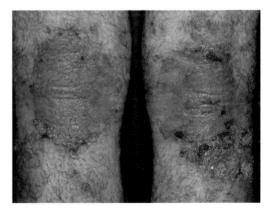

Figure 3.58. Staphylococcus aureus infection in eczema.

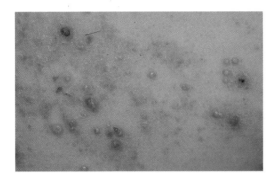

Figure 3.59. Eczema associated with molluscum contagiosum.

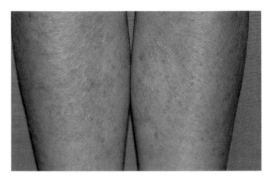

Figure 3.63. Asteatotic eczema.

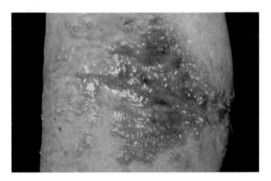

Figure 3.60. Acute atopic eczema.

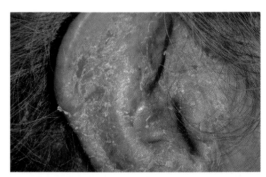

Figure 3.64. Otitis externa.

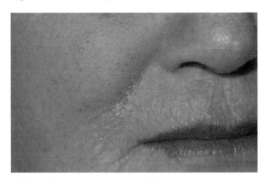

Figure 3.61. Seborrhoeic eczema.

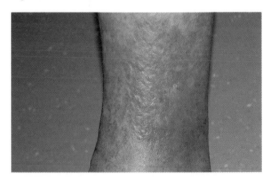

Figure 3.65. Venous eczema.

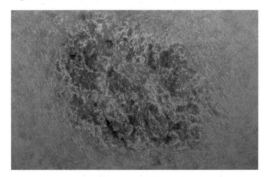

Figure 3.62. Discoid eczema.

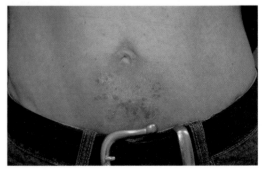

Figure 3.66. Contact eczema.

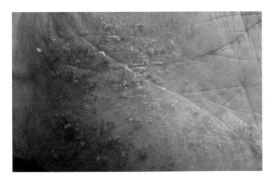

Figure 3.67. Pompholyx.

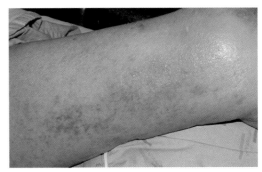

Figure 3.69. Disseminated secondary eczema.

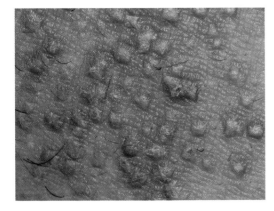

Figure 3.68. Lichen simplex.

sites, known causes and other clinical features; see *Table 3.1*. Biopsy is not helpful. Combinations can occur, especially in patients with atopy.

What tests should be done?

In most cases, dermatitis is diagnosed clinically. Tests may include:
- swabs for bacteria and herpes viruses.
- patch tests to identify contact allergen.
- scrapings to exclude fungal infection.
- skin biopsy to confirm presence of dermatitis.

How is eczema/dermatitis treated?
- Known causes should be addressed, where possible (see *individual topic pages*).
- Minimise contact with irritants: friction, soap, detergents, solvents, acids, alkalis.
- Apply bland emollients and skin protectants (barrier cream, gloves – changed frequently).
- Short courses of topical steroids (2–4 weeks): potency depends on site and severity; vehicle depends on site and acuity.

- Topical calcineurin inhibitors may be used where or when topical corticosteroids are contraindicated (e.g. eyelids).
- Oral antibiotics for secondary infection.
- Oral steroids (prednisone or prednisolone) for severe acute eczema/dermatitis.
- Specialists may treat intractable eczema/dermatitis with phototherapy, methotrexate, azathioprine, ciclosporin and other second-line agents.

3.6.2 Asteatotic eczema

What is asteatotic eczema?

Asteatosis means lack of fat; asteatotic eczema refers to a type of eczema/dermatitis related to very dry skin (xerosis). It is also known as eczema craquelé because of its cracked appearance (*Fig. 3.70*). The lower leg is the most common site for asteatotic eczema, but it can arise on any body site.

What causes asteatotic eczema?

Asteatotic eczema is mainly due to water loss from the stratum corneum. This occurs because of a breakdown of the skin barrier due to genetic predisposition and injury by environmental factors such as low humidity, excessive bathing, soaps and detergents.

Who gets asteatotic eczema?

Asteatotic eczema can occur in anyone with very dry skin.
- It most often affects older people.
- It is also a complication of inherited and acquired forms of ichthyosis.
- Systemic causes include hypothyroidism (myxoedema), malnutrition (zinc, fatty acids), cachexia and lymphoma.

Table 3.1. Diagnosis of eczema/dermatitis.

Type of eczema	Age of onset	Body site	Known causes	Other features
Atopic (see *Section 3.6.3*)	Before 5 years in 90%	Depends on age: *Infants*: cheeks, extensor limbs *Childhood*: flexures *Adult*: face, hands	Genetic Barrier function defects *Staphylococcus aureus*	Associated with asthma, hay fever, food allergy
Seborrhoeic (see *Section 3.6.12*)	First year of life or post-adolescence	Scalp Skin folds of face, ears Sometimes other flexures	Immunological reaction to *Malassezia*	Thin, ill-defined, salmon-pink plaques with yellowish scale
Discoid (see *Section 3.6.5*)	Any age	Lower limbs Upper limbs Trunk	Skin injury *Staphylococcus aureus*	Round or oval plaques
Asteatotic (see *Section 3.6.2*)	Most often observed in elderly	Lower legs	Xerosis (dry skin) Thyroid deficiency	Dry or crusted plaques with swelling
Otitis externa	Any age	Ear	Infection Trauma Contact factors Psoriasis	
Venous (see *Section 3.6.13*)	Middle-aged to elderly	Lower legs	Venous insufficiency	Signs include leg oedema or lipodermatosclerosis and haemosiderin deposition
Contact (see *Section 3.6.4*)	Any age	Any Hand dermatitis	Irritant (friction, soap, detergent, solvent, acid, alkali) and/or allergen (metal, fragrance, adhesive, preservative or other)	Worst affected areas in direct contact with causative agent Often unilateral, or if bilateral, asymmetrical, with sharp borders. Patch testing used to detect or confirm allergy
Pompholyx (see *Section 3.6.11*)	Young adults	Palms and soles	Sweating due to hot environment or stressful event	Crops of intensely itchy vesicles
Lichen simplex (see *Section 3.6.8*)	Mainly adults	Genitals Nape of neck Forearms Lower legs	Chronic itch, from pre-existing skin disease or neuropathy	Often solitary plaque but may be bilateral or widespread
Disseminated secondary eczema (see *Section 3.6.6*)	Any	Distal limbs Trunk	Localised inflammatory reaction, e.g. tinea infection, venous	Non-specific generalised symmetrical papulovesicular eruption

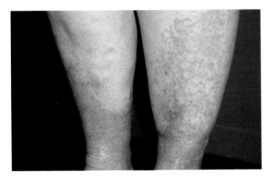 

Figure 3.70. Asteatotic eczema.

- Drugs can cause asteatotic eczema, particularly retinoids (acitretin, isotretinoin), diuretics and protein kinase inhibitors.

What are the clinical features of asteatotic eczema?

- Asteatotic eczema is characterised by diamond-shaped plates of skin, which are separated by red bands, forming a reticular pattern resembling crazy paving.
- One or both shins are most often affected.
- It may rarely spread to other sites.

How is asteatotic eczema diagnosed?

Asteatotic eczema is diagnosed by its typical clinical appearance in association with dry skin. In unusual or severe cases, perform a careful history and examination and arrange screening investigations including thyroid function and blood count.

What is the treatment for asteatotic eczema?

In most cases, asteatotic eczema rapidly improves with the following treatments:
- Reduction in bathing, avoidance of soaps and detergents.
- Liberal applications of emollients.
- Short course of mild topical corticosteroid cream or ointment.

3.6.3 Atopic eczema

What is atopic eczema?

Atopic eczema is a chronic relapsing form of eczema/dermatitis. It is characterised by pruritus, scratching, and acute, subacute and chronic eczematous lesions (see *Figs 3.71–3.76*). It may have a severe impact on quality of life due to disrupted sleep, poor performance at school or work, and unsightliness.

Affected individuals often have a personal or family history of asthma, hay fever and/or type 1 food allergy (anaphylactoid reactions). Ophthalmic associations include keratoconus, keratoconjunctivitis, and anterior cataracts.

What causes atopic eczema?

Eczema is not completely understood. Genetic and environmental factors impacting on epidermal barrier function and adaptive immune function are involved.

Genetic mutations of various proteins are under investigation. Filaggrin mutations are found in 50%, accounting for a defective skin barrier and increased transepidermal water loss – dry skin. Deficiencies in ceramides and antimicrobial peptides are documented. Eczema involves a type 2 cytokine inflammatory response, with activation of interleukin (IL)-4 and IL-13.

The rising incidence of atopic eczema in industrialised countries during the 20th century is unexplained.

Who gets atopic eczema?

The lifetime prevalence of atopic eczema is 20%. It affects males and females equally. Atopic eczema begins in 90% between 3 months and 5 years of age. It persists into adult life in at least one quarter of cases.

What are the clinical features of atopic eczema?

There are age-specific patterns of affected body sites.
- Facial, neck, and extensor involvement in infants and children, see *Fig. 3.77*.
- Flexural and nipple lesions in any age group (current or previous), see *Fig. 3.78*.
- Groin and axillary regions are generally spared.

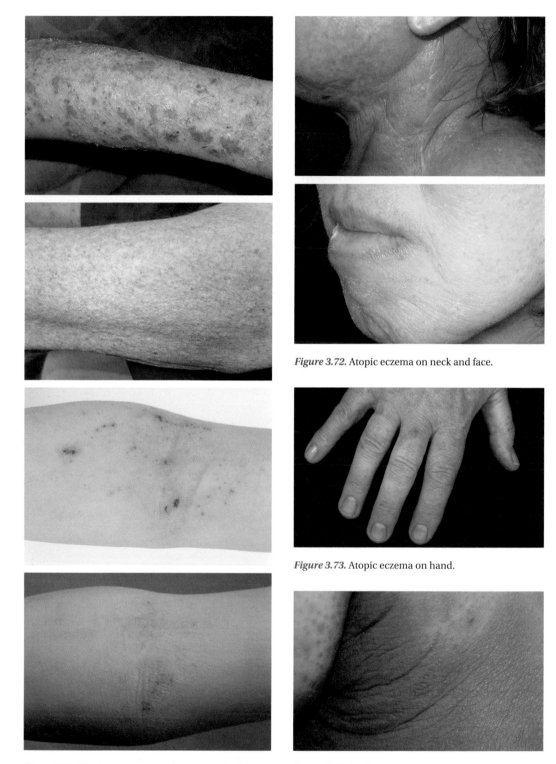

Figure 3.72. Atopic eczema on neck and face.

Figure 3.73. Atopic eczema on hand.

Figure 3.71. Atopic eczema on arms.

Figure 3.74. Atopic eczema.

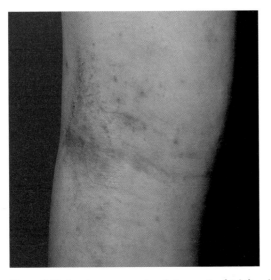
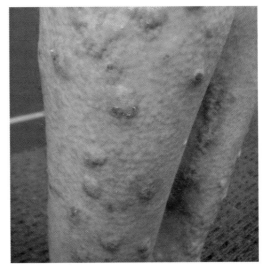

Figure 3.75. Atopic eczema and nodular prurigo (right) on legs.

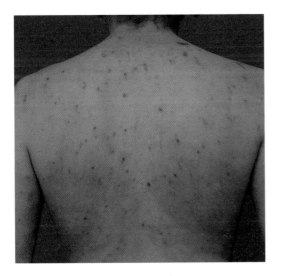

Figure 3.76. Atopic eczema on trunk.

- Pityriasis alba (hypopigmented patches) affects face and upper arms of children and adolescents, see *Fig. 3.79*.
- Eczematous cheilitis is common in children and adults.
- Hand dermatitis and face/neck dermatitis are the common patterns in adults, see *Fig. 3.80*.

Other features may include:
- dry skin (xerosis or ichthyosis vulgaris).
- increased skin markings on palms and soles, see *Fig. 3.81*.

- double skinfold under lower eyelid (Dennie–Morgan fold), and eyelids may be darkened, see *Fig. 3.82*.
- white dermographism (white marks or weals at sites of scratching), see *Fig. 3.83*.
- lifelong sensitive skin.

Flares of acute eczema are localised or widespread. They are characterised by erythematous papules and vesicles, ill-defined or circumscribed plaques, excoriations, oozing and crust formation (*Fig. 3.84*).

Subacute eczema is erythematous (*Fig. 3.85*).

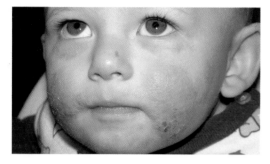

Figure 3.77. Facial involvement in a child.

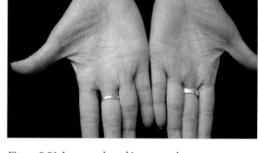

Figure 3.81. Increased markings on palms.

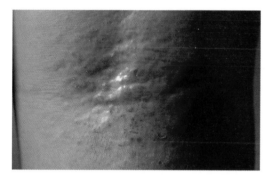

Figure 3.78. Flexural eczema.

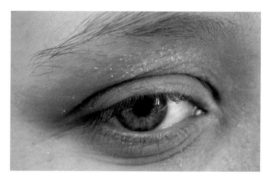

Figure 3.82. Darkened, flaky and lichenified eyelids.

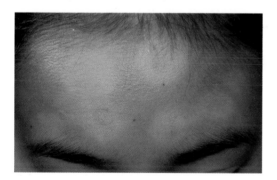

Figure 3.79. Pityriasis alba.

Figure 3.83. White dermographism.

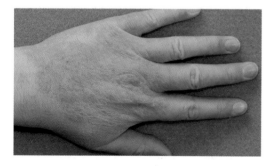

Figure 3.80. Hand dermatitis.

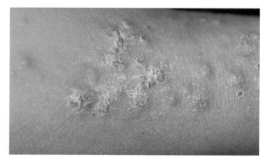

Figure 3.84. Pustules and crusted papules in acute infected eczema.

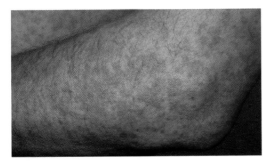

Figure 3.85. Subacute eczema.

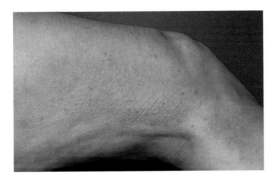

Figure 3.86. Plaques.

Acute eczematous flares may resolve or become chronic eczema. This can be localised or widespread, with itchy, scratched or rubbed, thickened or lichenified, dry or scaly, plaques (*Fig. 3.86*).

Flares may be provoked by any of the following factors:

- bacterial infection – *Staphylococcus aureus*.
- contact with irritants – hot water, soaps, toiletries, detergents and wool.
- contact urticaria due to type 1 allergens – dust, pet hair, certain foods (citrus fruit, tomatoes).
- humid/hot temperatures, or excessive air conditioning.
- psychosocial stressors.
- uncommonly, certain foods to which the individual is allergic.

Severe eczema is characterised by widespread involvement, repeated infection, and persistence of symptoms despite treatment. Severity can be graded according to several scoring systems such as SCORAD and EASI; online or smartphone apps make the calculations easier.

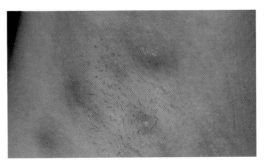

Figure 3.87. Furunculosis in a patient with atopic dermatitis.

What are the complications of atopic eczema?

Complications can include:

- erythroderma – whole-body eczema resulting in fluid loss, unstable thermoregulation and cardiac decompensation.
- bacterial infection – impetiginisation, cellulitis, folliculitis and furunculosis (see *Fig. 3.87*).
- viral infection – herpes simplex (eczema herpeticum, *Fig. 3.88*), widespread molluscum contagiosum or viral warts.
- nodular prurigo – intensely itchy, treatment-resistant nodules (*Fig. 3.89*).

How is atopic eczema diagnosed?

Diagnosis of atopic eczema depends on consistent clinical features (itch, body sites affected, eczematous morphology, chronic or relapsing course).

Atopy implies elevated IgE levels, but these are not always present. Testing is not advocated, as it does not alter management.

Skin swabs for bacterial and viral culture may be warranted if first-line treatment is not effective.

The prevalence of contact allergy in atopics is similar to non-atopics. Patch tests should be performed if there is suspicion of contact allergy.

What is the treatment for atopic eczema?

Treatment depends on the phase of the eczema. Patient and caregiver education is an important part of management.

AT ALL TIMES

- Minimise known exacerbating factors: consider environmental temperature, clothing.
- Hydrate in warm bath with soap-alternative, followed by emollient.
- Apply bland emollient whenever itchy or skin is dry.

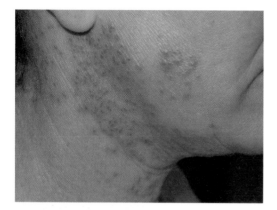

Figure 3.88. Eczema herpeticum.

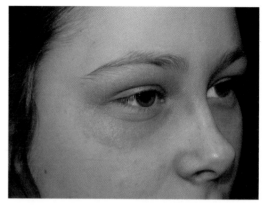

Figure 3.90. Irritant reaction to chlorinated water under swimming goggles.

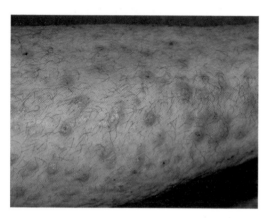

Figure 3.89. Nodular prurigo.

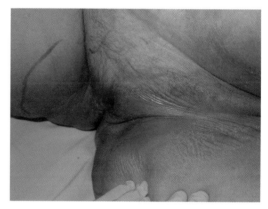

Figure 3.91. Irritant reaction to incontinence of urine.

Mild eczema

- Intermittent low-potency topical corticosteroid creams (acute or subacute eczema) or ointments (chronic eczema, dry skin).
- Topical calcineurin inhibitors can be used on face, eyelids and skin folds.

Moderate flares

- Intermediate and high-potency topical corticosteroid creams for 1–3 weeks.
- Treat skin infection with anti-staphylococcal antibiotic, e.g. flucloxacillin.
- Bleach baths may reduce incidence and severity of bacterial infections.
- Oral antifungal agents to reduce *Malassezia* can be tried, if head and neck dermatitis with exaggerated flaking is prominent.

Severe eczema

- Hot, red, weeping skin may be treated using wet dressings or bandages over corticosteroid creams.

- Short courses of oral prednisone are indicated for very widespread acute eczema but repeated use should be avoided.
- Sedating antihistamines at bedtime may improve sleep.
- Refer for phototherapy or systemic immunomodulatory agents such as methotrexate, ciclosporin or azathioprine.
- Biologic agents are being developed for atopic dermatitis. The first monoclonal antibody approved by the FDA for atopic dermatitis was dupilumab, a monoclonal antibody that targets interleukin (IL)-4 and IL-13.

3.6.4 Contact eczema

What is contact eczema?

Contact eczema is classified as:
- irritant contact eczema (*Figs 3.90* and *3.91*).
- allergic contact eczema (*Figs 3.92* and *3.93*).

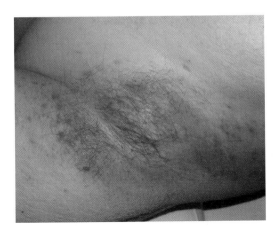

Figure 3.92. Contact allergy to blue fabric dye.

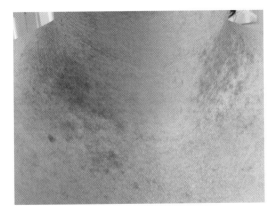

Figure 3.93. Contact allergy to nickel in jewelery.

Irritant and allergic contact eczema can co-exist. There are acute and chronic forms of contact eczema. It can affect any site of the body, but is particularly prevalent on the hands, where it is usually of mixed aetiology. Mucosal surfaces can have similar reactions: contact stomatitis and contact cheilitis.

What causes contact eczema?

Endogenous predisposition relates to malfunction of epidermal proteins such as filaggrin, ceramides, claudins, antimicrobial factors and proteases.

Irritant contact dermatitis is due to direct injury to the skin by an irritant – any agent that is capable of producing cell damage if applied for sufficient time and in sufficient concentration. Irritants damage the barrier function of the skin by denaturing keratin and lipids and by increasing transepidermal

water loss. Cumulative irritants include friction, trauma, wet-work, sweat, soaps, detergents, rubber gloves, vegetables, garden plants and many other materials.

Allergic contact dermatitis affects previously sensitised individuals and is immunological in origin. There are numerous potential contact allergens; they are small molecules. The most common allergens are nickel, fragrances, rubber accelerants, preservatives, adhesives and various foods and plants.

Who gets contact eczema?

Contact eczema is common in children and adults of all ages. Predisposing factors include:
- past or current atopic eczema.
- occupational exposure to irritants.

What are the clinical features of contact eczema?

Contact dermatitis affects the areas in direct contact with an irritant or allergen; it is not always possible to determine the cause or causes from the clinical features or distribution, which may be unilateral or bilateral and tends to be asymmetrical. Bizarre patterns may occur. The distribution, configuration and morphology depend on the agent responsible.
- Acute eczema: localised circumscribed erythematous papules, vesicles and plaques, see *Fig. 3.94*.
- Chronic eczema: localised or widespread itchy, scratched or rubbed, thickened or lichenified, dry or scaly, fissured and poorly circumscribed plaques, see *Fig. 3.95*.

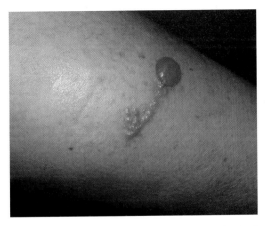

Figure 3.94. Acute eczema; linear pattern is suggestive of plant origin.

Hand eczema

Hand eczema is usually related to occupational or routine household activities. It affects about 10% of the population at one time or other, and is more common in females. Hand eczema is particularly prevalent in hairdressers, cleaners, caregivers, nurses and food handlers. It is often multifactorial. Clinical examples include:

- ring eczema – possible irritant dermatitis from soap and water or allergic dermatitis due to contact with nickel-containing jewellery.
- housewives' dermatitis – dry dorsum of hands and inflamed webspaces, see *Fig. 3.96.*
- fissured thumb and forefinger – due to degreasing agents + trauma, or garlic/onions.

How is contact eczema diagnosed?

The diagnosis and cause of contact eczema are not always obvious. If the reaction is persistent or recurrent, investigations should include referral to a dermatologist for patch testing, see *Fig. 3.97.*

Patch testing elicits evidence of contact allergy to tested potential allergens. Interpretation of the results requires training and experience. At least three visits to the clinic are necessary over 5 days or so: to apply test patches, to remove them, and to interpret the results see *Fig. 3.98.*

What is the treatment for contact eczema?

- Education of the patient is paramount.
- Avoid contact with known irritants and allergens when possible (this is not always practicable).
- Protect vulnerable skin using barrier creams and gloves (these are sometimes contraindicated).

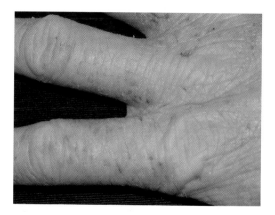

Figure 3.95. Chronic eczema.

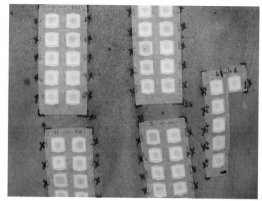

Figure 3.97. Patch testing.

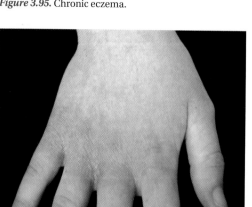

Figure 3.96. Housewives' dermatitis.

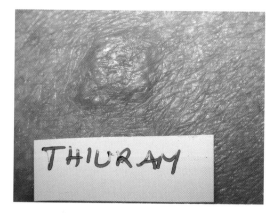

Figure 3.98. Positive patch to thiuram, a rubber accelerant.

- Apply emollients frequently where possible, especially overnight.
- Treat active eczema with topical steroid. Ultrapotent corticosteroid creams are necessary for palmar dermatitis.
- Short courses of systemic corticosteroids (prednisone or prednisolone) are appropriate for severe flares.
- Refer patients with persistent contact dermatitis to a specialist for phototherapy or immunomodulatory treatment.

3.6.5 Discoid eczema

What is discoid eczema?

Discoid eczema is a common type of eczema/dermatitis, in which there are scattered, roundish patches of eczema. They can be intensely itchy. The rash is also called nummular dermatitis.

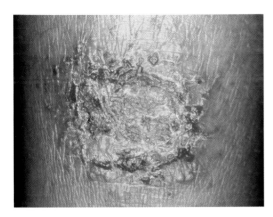

Figure 3.99. Discoid eczema.

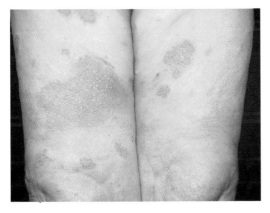

Figure 3.100. Discoid pattern of secondary eczematisation in patient with venous disease.

What causes discoid eczema?

The cause of discoid eczema is unknown. Some cases are associated with *Staphylococcus aureus* infection, see *Fig. 3.99*.

The eruption can be precipitated by:
- localised injury, such as scratch, insect bite or thermal burn.
- localised skin infection, such as impetigo or wound infection.
- contact dermatitis.
- dry skin.
- varicose veins (varicose eczema).
- another skin problem.

Who gets discoid eczema?

Discoid eczema can affect children and adults. It is slightly more prevalent in adult males than females. In males over the age of 50 years, there is an association with chronic alcoholism.

Discoid eczema can occur in atopic eczema, asteatotic eczema and secondary eczematisation; see *Fig. 3.100*.

What are the clinical features of discoid eczema?

There are two forms of discoid eczema:
- exudative acute discoid eczema – oozy papules, vesicles and plaques, see *Fig. 3.101*.

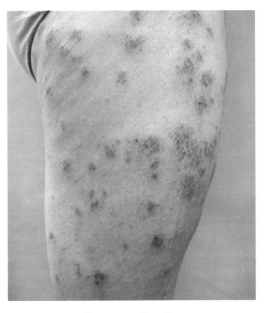

Figure 3.101. Exudative acute discoid eczema.

- dry discoid eczema – subacute or chronic erythematous, dry plaques, see *Fig. 3.102*.

Both forms of discoid eczema are usually more prevalent on the limbs than the trunk, but the rash may be widespread. Although often bilateral, the distribution is often asymmetrical, see *Fig. 3.103*.

Individual plaques are well circumscribed, mostly 1–3 cm in diameter and inflamed. They are mostly round or oval in shape. The skin between the patches is usually normal, but may be dry and irritable. Post-inflammatory pigmentation is common in darker skin types.

How is discoid eczema diagnosed?

In most cases, the appearance of discoid eczema is quite characteristic.
- Bacterial swabs may reveal *Staphylococcus aureus* colonisation or infection.
- Scrapings are commonly taken for mycology, as discoid eczema can look very similar to tinea corporis.
- Patch testing is generally negative.

What is the treatment for discoid eczema?

Treatments may include:
- medium- to high-potency topical corticosteroid ointments for 2–4 weeks.
- tar preparations and topical calcineurin inhibitors.
- emollients – essential in dry skin; they can also be used to soothe itchy skin and reduce dependence on topical steroids.
- oral anti-staphylococcal antibiotics for secondary infection; long-term antibiotics are sometimes required.

- short-term systemic corticosteroids, e.g. prednisone or prednisolone, for severe or extensive flare-up.

Refer patients with persistent or severe discoid eczema for phototherapy or immunomodulatory treatment.

3.6.6 Disseminated secondary eczema

What is disseminated secondary eczema?

Disseminated secondary eczema is an acute, generalised eczema/dermatitis that arises in response to a prior localised inflammatory skin disease.

It is also called an id reaction, autosensitisation dermatitis and autoeczematisation.

What causes disseminated secondary eczema?

The cause of disseminated secondary eczema is unknown. Theories have suggested it is an immune response to autologous skin antigens and/or to circulating infectious antigens or cytokines.

Who gets disseminated secondary eczema?

Disseminated secondary eczema can occur in children and adults, but is more often diagnosed in the elderly with a neglected primary rash on the lower leg.

The most common types of eczema/dermatitis that precede disseminated secondary eczema – an eczematid – are:

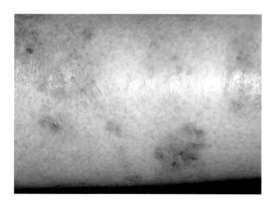

Figure 3.102. Dry discoid eczema.

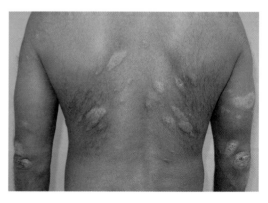

Figure 3.103. Bilateral but asymmetrical distribution in discoid eczema.

- chronic venous eczema, see *Fig. 3.104*.
- acute contact eczema, see *Fig. 3.105*.
- acute or chronic discoid eczema, see *Fig. 3.106*.

Infections preceding disseminated secondary eczema include:
- inflammatory dermatophyte infection, e.g. tinea pedis (*Fig. 3.107*), flaring because of occlusive footwear, or kerion due to zoophilic infection – a dermatophytid.
- bacterial infection, e.g. impetiginised wound or thermal burn – a bacterid.
- viral infection, e.g. molluscum contagiosum.
- arthropod infestation, e.g. scabies or pediculosis – a pediculid.

What are the clinical features of disseminated secondary eczema?

Disseminated secondary eczema presents as an acute, symmetrical, generalised acute eczema. It tends to be extremely itchy, disturbing sleep.

- Hands, forearms, lower legs, thighs and trunk are commonly affected, see *Fig. 3.108*.
- Morphology varies and includes papulovesicles, crusted plaques (discoid eczema), follicular papules, morbilliform eruption, targetoid lesions and pompholyx, see *Fig. 3.109*.
- Occasionally, the patient may feel unwell with fever and anorexia.

Non-eczematous id reactions include erythema nodosum, Sweet syndrome, guttate psoriasis and immunobullous disease.

How is disseminated secondary eczema diagnosed?

The clinical features of disseminated secondary eczema are characteristic. Finding the cause depends on taking a careful history of the initial site of a skin problem. This is sometimes difficult to obtain, because the patient may not

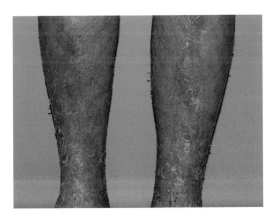

Figure 3.104. Venous eczema.

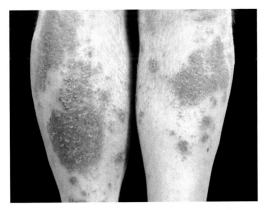

Figure 3.106. Discoid eczema.

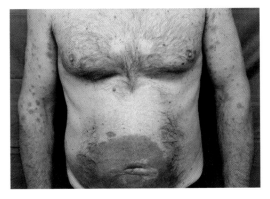

Figure 3.105. Disseminated eczema following dermatitis at site of umbilical hernia repair.

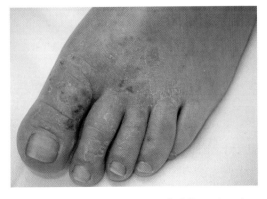

Figure 3.107. Tinea pedis that provoked disseminated secondary eczema.

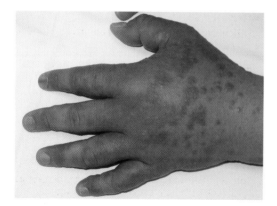

Figure 3.108. Disseminated secondary eczema.

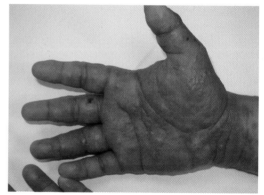

Figure 3.109. Pompholyx.

associate a chronic minor rash with their current widespread and symptomatic eruption.

Additional investigations to be considered include:

- dermatoscopy of hair shafts for nits and of burrows for scabies mites.
- swabs of crusted areas or pustules for bacteriology.
- scrapings of scaly annular or hairless plaques for mycology.
- skin biopsy of primary lesion and/or secondary rash (histology is spongiotic dermatitis).
- blood count in an unwell patient.
- referral for patch tests, if there is suspicion of contact allergy.

Patch testing should not be undertaken during the acute phase of disseminated secondary eczema, but may be planned in several months when it has settled.

What is the treatment for disseminated secondary eczema?

The primary rash needs to be treated vigorously. This may require systemic therapy, e.g. antibiotics for bacterid or oral antifungal for confirmed dermatophytid.

The secondary eczema is often extensive and highly symptomatic. Treatment may entail:

- referral for specialist assessment and treatment, including admission to hospital.
- wet dressings or bandaging for exudative eczematous plaques.
- potassium permanganate 1:10 000 soaks for localised oozing, infected areas.
- potent topical corticosteroid creams for 1–3 weeks.

- systemic corticosteroids, e.g. prednisone or prednisolone for several weeks.
- oral sedating antihistamines at night.

3.6.7 Hand dermatitis

What is hand dermatitis?

Hand dermatitis is a common group of acute and chronic eczematous disorders that affect the dorsal and palmar aspects of the hand.

Hand dermatitis is also known as hand eczema.

Who gets hand dermatitis?

Hand dermatitis is common (especially in young adult females) and accounts for 20–35% of all dermatitis. It may occur at any age, including during childhood. It is particularly prevalent in people with a history of atopic eczema.

Hand dermatitis is particularly common in industries involving cleaning, catering, metalwork, hairdressing, healthcare, painting and mechanical work. This is mainly due to the contact with irritants, but specific contact allergies can contribute.

What causes hand dermatitis?

Hand dermatitis often results from a combination of causes, including:

- genetic and unknown factors (constitutional hand dermatitis).
- injury (contact irritant dermatitis).
- immune reactions (contact allergic dermatitis).

Hand dermatitis is frequently caused or aggravated by work, when it is known as occupational dermatitis.

Irritants include water, detergents, solvents, acids, alkalis, cold, heat and friction. These damage the outer stratum corneum, removing lipids and disturbing the skin's barrier function. Water loss and inflammation lead to further impairment of barrier function.

Contact allergy is a delayed hypersensitivity reaction with elicitation and memory phases involving T lymphocytes and release of cytokines.

What are the clinical features of hand dermatitis?

Hand dermatitis may affect the backs of the hands, the palms or both. It can be very itchy, often burns, and is sometimes painful. It has acute, relapsing and chronic phases.

Acute hand dermatitis presents with:
- red macules, papules and plaques, see *Fig. 3.110*.

- swelling.
- blistering and weeping, see *Fig. 3.111*.
- fissuring, see *Fig. 3.112*.

Features of chronic hand dermatitis include:
- dryness and scale, see *Fig. 3.113*.
- lichenification, see *Fig. 3.114*.

There are various causes and clinical presentations of hand dermatitis.

ATOPIC HAND DERMATITIS
Atopic hand dermatitis depends on constitutional weakness of the skin barrier function and is triggered by contact with irritants. It may affect one or both dorsal hands and palms. It may manifest as a discoid pattern of eczema. Patients may also have eczema in other sites including feet, hands, flexures.

NUMMULAR DERMATITIS
Nummular dermatitis or discoid eczema tends to affect the dorsal surfaces of the hands and fingers as circumscribed plaques; see *Fig. 3.115*. Other sites of the body may or may not be affected.

VESICULAR HAND DERMATITIS
Vesicular hand dermatitis is also known as pompholyx, cheiropompholyx and dyshidrotic eczema. Intensely itchy crops of skin-coloured blisters arise on the palms and the sides of the hands and fingers. Similar symptoms often affect the feet. It is likely this form of dermatitis is triggered by emotional factors via sweating.

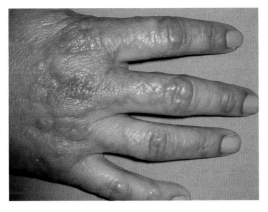

Figure 3.110. Red plaques of acute hand dermatitis.

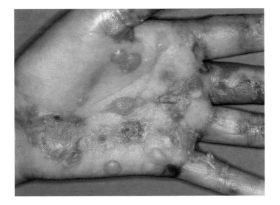

Figure 3.111. Blistering in acute hand dermatitis.

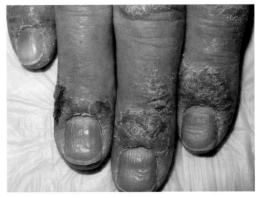

Figure 3.112. Fissuring, crusting and nail dystrophy in vesicular hand dermatitis.

CHRONIC RELAPSING VESICULOSQUAMOUS DERMATITIS

Chronic relapsing vesiculosquamous dermatitis is a common pattern of palmar and finger dermatitis, in which episodes of acute vesicular dermatitis are followed by chronic scaling and fissuring.

HYPERKERATOTIC HAND DERMATITIS

Hyperkeratotic hand dermatitis is a chronic, dry, non-inflammatory palmar dermatitis. It can appear similar to palmar psoriasis, but is less red and less well circumscribed; see *Fig. 3.116*.

FINGERTIP DERMATITIS

Fingertip dermatitis can be isolated to one or several fingers.

IRRITANT CONTACT DERMATITIS

The hands are the most common site for irritant contact dermatitis, and it is often due to wet work and repeated exposure to low-grade irritants. The finger-webs are the first place to be affected, but inflammation can extend to fingers, the backs of the hands and the wrists. Irritant contact dermatitis often spares the palms.

- Acute irritant dermatitis is due to injury by potent irritants such as acids and alkalis, often in an occupational setting.
- Repeated exposure to low-grade irritants such as water, soaps, and detergents leads to chronic cumulative irritant dermatitis.

ALLERGIC CONTACT DERMATITIS

Allergic contact dermatitis may be difficult to distinguish from constitutional forms of hand dermatitis and irritant contact dermatitis. There are about 30 common allergens and innumerable uncommon or rare ones. Common allergens include nickel, fragrances, rubber accelerators (in gloves) and

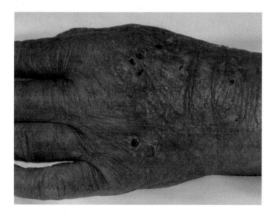

Figure 3.113. Dryness and scale in chronic hand dermatitis.

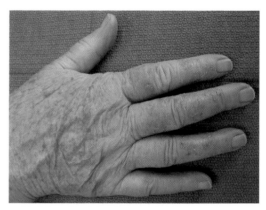

Figure 3.115. Nummular dermatitis.

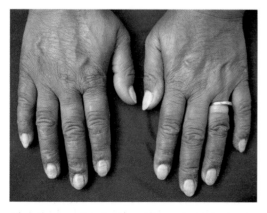

Figure 3.114. Lichenification in chronic hand dermatitis.

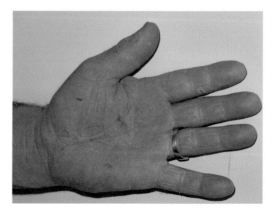

Figure 3.116. Hyperkeratotic hand dermatitis.

p-phenylenediamine (permanent hair dye). Clues to contact allergy depend on the allergen, but may include:
- periodic flare-ups associated with certain tasks or places hours to days earlier.
- irregular, asymmetrical distribution of rash.
- sharp border to the rash, e.g. at wrist corresponding with cuff of rubber glove.

Complications of hand dermatitis
- Bacterial infection can result in pustules, crusting and pain.
- Dermatitis at the ends of the fingers may result in nail dystrophy, see *Fig. 3.117*.
- Dermatitis can spread to affect other sites, particularly the forearms and feet.

How is hand dermatitis diagnosed?
Hand dermatitis is usually straightforward to diagnose and classify by history and examination, considering:
- acute, relapsing or chronic course.
- past history of skin disease.
- dermatitis on other sites.

Various scoring systems have been proposed to assess severity of hand dermatitis. The simplest 3-item system is used for non-vesicular forms of hand dermatitis, assessing erythema, scale and induration.
Differential diagnosis includes:
- contact urticaria, e.g. to latex gloves (immediate redness, itching and swelling that resolves within an hour).
- protein contact dermatitis, most often affecting caterers (combination of urticaria and dermatitis induced by reactions to meat and some vegetables, particularly potatoes).
- psoriasis (symmetrical, well circumscribed, red, scaly plaques).
- tinea (unilateral or asymmetrical, peripheral scale, slowly expanding edge).

Patients with chronic hand dermatitis may have patch tests to detect contact allergens (*Section 6.1*).

What is the treatment for hand dermatitis?
Patients with all forms of hand dermatitis should be most particular to:
- minimise contact with irritants – even water.
- when washing hands, use non-soap cleanser, rinse carefully, and ensure hands are completely dry afterwards.
- completely avoid touching allergens that have been identified by patch testing.
- wear task-appropriate protective gloves.
- apply thick emollients before work/school and reapply after washing or when the skin dries out (this may be 10–20 times in a day).

Vinyl gloves are less likely than rubber gloves to cause allergic reactions.
- They must be scrupulously clean and should have no holes.
- They should not be worn for long periods.
- Sweating under the gloves aggravates dermatitis.
- Lined gloves or inner cotton gloves improve comfort.

Topical steroids reduce inflammation.
- Use a potent topical steroid on dermatitis on the backs of the hands and an ultrapotent topical steroid on palms.
- Cream formulation is usually best for vesicular hand dermatitis, and ointment for chronic dermatitis.
- They should be applied to areas of active dermatitis once or twice daily for several weeks, then discontinued or frequency/potency reduced.
- Short-term occlusion increases potency and is warranted if standard applications have not been effective.

Secondary infection may require oral antibiotic, usually flucloxacillin.
Severe acute flares of hand dermatitis are treated with prednisone for 2–4 weeks. Chronic

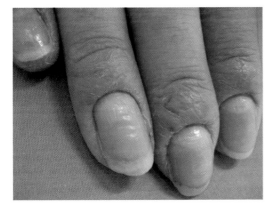

Figure 3.117. Nail dystrophy and paronychia associated with hand dermatitis.

intractable hand dermatitis may be treated with second-line agents such as azathioprine, methotrexate, ciclosporin, alitretinoin or phototherapy.

How can hand dermatitis be prevented?

Contact irritant hand dermatitis can be prevented by careful protective measures and active treatment. It is very important that people with atopic dermatitis (eczema) are made aware of the risk of hand dermatitis, particularly when considering what occupation to pursue.

What is the outlook for hand dermatitis?

With careful management, hand dermatitis usually recovers completely. A few days off work may be helpful. When occupational dermatitis is severe, it may not be possible to work for weeks or months. Occasionally a change of occupation is necessary.

3.6.8 Lichen simplex

What is lichen simplex?

Lichen simplex is a localised area of chronic, lichenified eczema. There may be a single or multiple plaques. It is also called neurodermatitis.

Who gets lichen simplex?

Lichen simplex occurs in adult males and females. It is unusual in children.

It is more common in people with anxiety and/or obsessive compulsive disorder.

What causes lichen simplex?

Although the mechanism is not understood, lichen simplex follows repetitive scratching and rubbing, which arises because of chronic localised itch. The primary itch can be due to:

- atopic eczema.
- contact eczema.
- venous eczema.
- psoriasis.
- lichen planus.
- dermatophyte infection.
- insect bite.
- neuropathy (radiculopathy).

Pruritus due to radiculopathy appears to be due to hyperexcitable sensory afferent nerve fibres following nerve injury.

What are the clinical features of lichen simplex?

A solitary plaque of lichen simplex is circumscribed, somewhat linear or oval in shape, and markedly thickened. It is intensely pruritic. Other features may include:

- exaggerated skin markings.
- dry or scaly surface.
- leathery induration.
- broken-off hairs.
- hyperpigmentation.
- excoriations.

Lichen simplex is often solitary and unilateral, usually affecting the patient's dominant side. Multiple plaques can also arise, with bilateral and symmetrical or asymmetrical distribution. The location of lichen simplex is not random, as some body sites are particularly commonly affected.

- Occipital and nuchal areas.
- Perineum and scrotum in men (see *Fig. 3.118*); labia majora in women (see *Fig. 3.119*).
- Wrists and extensor surfaces of the forearms.
- Anterior or medial lower legs, see *Fig. 3.120*.

How is lichen simplex diagnosed?

Clinical appearance is generally typical. At times, it may be helpful to do some investigations.

- Skin scrapings for possible dermatophyte infection.
- Skin biopsy (acanthosis, mild chronic inflammatory infiltration, nerve hypertrophy and sometimes, features of underlying dermatosis).

In the absence of a primary dermatosis or infection, consider neuropathy. Does the patient have a history of spinal injury, disease or symptoms? In severe cases, the following tests may be performed but they have a low diagnostic yield.

- Spinal imaging: X-ray, CT scan, MRI scan.
- Electrophysiological nerve conduction studies.

What is the treatment for lichen simplex?

The patient requires an explanation that their itchy patch of skin is, at least in part, due to scratching and rubbing and that treatment will address the symptoms and any underlying cause.

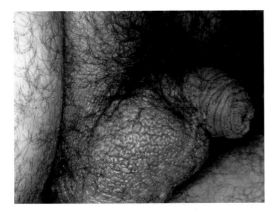

Figure 3.118. Lichen simplex on the scrotum.

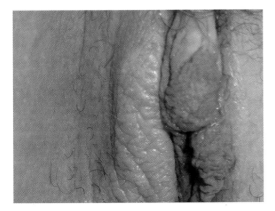

Figure 3.119. Lichen simplex affecting labia majora.

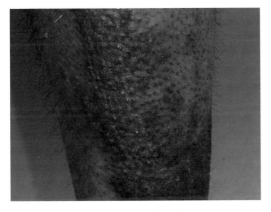

Figure 3.120. Lichen simplex on lower leg.

Symptomatic treatment may include:
- potent topical steroids until the plaque is resolved (4–6 weeks).
- occlusion for a few hours after application may enhance efficacy.

- reduce potency or frequency of topical steroids once lichenification resolved.
- intralesional corticosteroid injections into thickened plaque every 4–6 weeks.
- moisturisers to relieve dryness and reduce desire to scratch.
- cooling creams containing menthol.
- sedating antihistamine or tricyclic at night.

The primary condition needs treating, e.g.:
- antifungal agents for dermatophyte infection.
- phototherapy and immunomodulatory medications for inflammatory dermatoses.
- tricyclic antidepressants (amitriptyline, nortriptyline, doxepin) or antiepileptic medications (valproate, lamotrigine, gabapentin) for radiculopathy.

3.6.9 Nappy rash

What is nappy rash?

Nappy rash affects the skin under a nappy or diaper. It is also called napkin or diaper dermatitis. It affects the groin, perineum, genital and/or perianal areas in male and female babies.

Who gets nappy rash?

Nappy rash most often affects babies aged 3 to 15 months of age, especially those wearing traditional cloth nappies (50%). It is much less prevalent in babies wearing modern breathable and multilayered disposable nappies.

Nappy rash also affects older children and adults who are incontinent.

What causes nappy rash?

Nappy rash follows damage to the normal skin barrier and is primarily a form of irritant contact dermatitis.
- Urine and occlusion leads to overhydration and skin maceration.
- Faecal bile salts and enzymes break down stratum corneum lipids and proteins.
- A mixture of urine and faeces creates ammonium hydroxide, raising pH.
- The wet skin is colonised by microorganisms, particularly candida.
- Mechanical friction from limb movement may increase discomfort.

Differential diagnosis of nappy rashes includes:
- *Candida albicans* infection.
- impetigo.

- infantile seborrhoeic dermatitis.
- atopic dermatitis.
- psoriasis.
- miliaria.
- rare disorders.

Nappy rash is not due to:
- allergy to the nappies.
- toxins in the nappies.
- washing powders.
- dermatophyte fungal infections (tinea).

What are the clinical features of nappy rash?

One or more forms of nappy rash may be present.
- Irritant napkin dermatitis: well-demarcated variable erythema, oedema, dryness and scaling. Affected skin is in contact with the wet nappy and tends to spare the skin folds; see *Fig. 3.121*.

- Chafing: erythema and erosions where the nappy rubs, usually on waistband or thighs.
- *Candida albicans*: erythematous papules and plaques with small satellite spots or superficial pustules, see *Fig. 3.122*.
- Impetigo (*Staphylococcus aureus* and/or *Streptococcus pyogenes*): irregular blisters and pustules.
- Infantile seborrhoeic dermatitis: cradle cap and bilateral salmon pink patches, often desquamating, in skin folds; see *Fig. 3.123*.
- Atopic dermatitis: bilateral scratched, dry plaques anywhere, but uncommon in nappy area; family history common.
- Psoriasis: persistent, well-circumscribed, symmetrical, shiny, red, scaly or macerated plaques; other sites may be involved; family history common.
- Secondary spread or autoeczematisation: rash in distal sites associated with severe nappy rash.

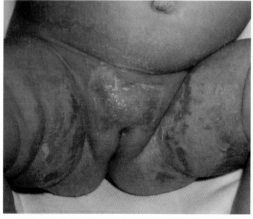

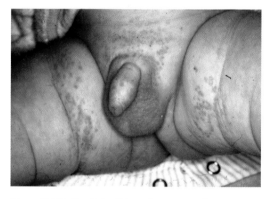

Figure 3.122. Candida albicans in nappy rash.

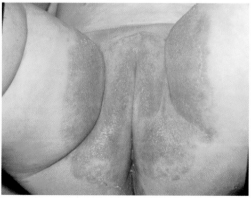

Figure 3.121. Nappy rash.

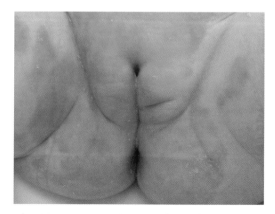

Figure 3.123. Infantile seborrhoeic dermatitis in nappy rash.

What tests should be done?

In most cases no tests are necessary. Skin swabs may be useful to confirm yeast or bacterial infection.

What is the treatment for nappy rash?

GENERAL MEASURES

Explain how and why nappy rash arises. Emphasise the need to keep baby dry and use barrier protection. Explain that nappy rash is much less common with disposable nappies compared to cloth varieties.

Disposable nappies:
- are available in different shapes and sizes depending on age and gender.
- keep the skin dry and clean.
- maintain optimal skin pH.
- should be changed when wet or soiled.
- contain cellulose pulp and superabsorbent polymers.
- may include petrolatum-based moisturising lotion to support skin barrier.
- have fasteners, backsheets and stretch which reduce leakage.
- are non-toxic and biologically inert.
- do not contain allergens such as natural rubber latex or disperse dyes.
- lead to less household exposure to faecal matter.

If using cloth nappies, suggest nappy liners to keep the skin dry and avoid plastic pants.

At nappy changes:
- gently clean the baby's skin with water and a soft cloth.
- wet wipes are convenient but expensive and can lead to contact allergy to preservatives used to stop them going mouldy.
- aqueous cream or other non-soap cleanser can be used if necessary.
- pat dry gently and allow to air dry.
- apply protective ointment containing petrolatum and/or zinc oxide.

Other suggestions:
- give evening fluids early to reduce wetting at night.
- minimise acidic foods such as orange juice or stewed rhubarb.

PRESCRIPTION TREATMENTS
- Hydrocortisone cream applied once or twice daily to inflamed areas for 1–2 weeks.
- Topical antifungal cream twice daily to affected areas, if suspicious of *Candida albicans* infection.

3.6.10 Pityriasis alba

What is pityriasis alba?

Pityriasis alba is a low-grade type of eczema/dermatitis that primarily affects children.

The name refers to its appearance: *pityriasis* refers to its characteristic fine scale, and *alba* to its pale colour (hypopigmentation).

Who gets pityriasis alba?

Pityriasis alba is common worldwide with a prevalence in children of around 5%.
- It mainly affects children and adolescents aged 3 to 16 years, but may also arise in older and younger people.
- It affects boys and girls equally.
- It is more prominent, and may also be more prevalent, in dark skin compared to white skin.

What causes pityriasis alba?

The cause of pityriasis alba is unknown.
- It often coexists with dry skin and atopic dermatitis.
- It often presents following sun exposure, perhaps because tanning of surrounding skin makes affected areas more prominent.

Researchers have not reached any conclusions about the relationship of pityriasis alba to the following:
- ultraviolet radiation.
- excessive or inadequate bathing.
- low levels of serum copper.
- possibly, malassezia yeasts (which produce a metabolite, pityriacitrin, that inhibits tyrosinase).

What are the clinical features of pityriasis alba?

Classic pityriasis alba usually presents with 1–20 patches or thin plaques.
- Most lesions occur on the face, especially on cheeks and chin (*Fig. 3.124*).
- They may also arise on neck, shoulders and upper arm and are uncommon on other sites of the body (*Fig. 3.125*).
- Size varies from 0.5 to 5 cm in diameter.
- They are round, oval or irregular in shape.
- Pityriasis alba may have well-demarcated or poorly defined edges.

- Itch is minimal or absent.
- Hypopigmentation is more noticeable in summer, especially in dark-skinned children.
- Dryness and scaling is more noticeable in winter, when environmental humidity tends to be lower.

Typically, each area of pityriasis alba goes through several stages:

1. Slightly scaly pink plaque with just palpable papular surface.
2. Hypopigmented plaque with fine surface scale.
3. Then post-inflammatory hypopigmented macule without scale.
4. Resolution.

Complications of pityriasis alba

None are known.

How is pityriasis alba diagnosed?

Pityriasis alba can be confused with several other disorders that cause hypopigmentation (see *Section 4.8*).

To exclude these, investigations may include:
- Wood lamp examination – hypopigmentation does not enhance, and there is no fluorescence in pityriasis alba.
- scrapings for mycology – microscopy and fungal culture are negative in pityriasis alba.
- skin biopsy is rarely required, but may reveal mildly spongiotic dermatitis and reduction in melanin.

What is the treatment for pityriasis alba?

No treatment is necessary for asymptomatic pityriasis alba.
- A moisturising cream may improve the dry appearance.
- Hydrocortisone cream may reduce redness and itch.
- Pimecrolimus cream and tacrolimus ointment may be as effective as hydrocortisone and have been reported to speed recovery of skin colour.

How can pityriasis alba be prevented?

The development or prominence of pityriasis alba can be reduced by avoiding exposure to sunlight.

What is the outlook for pityriasis alba?

Pityriasis clears up after a few months, or in some cases persists for up to two or three years. The colour gradually returns completely to normal.

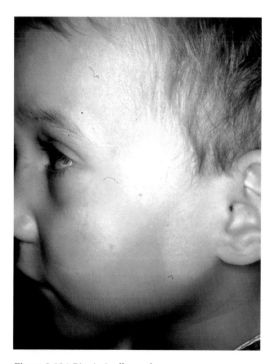

Figure 3.124. Pityriasis alba on face.

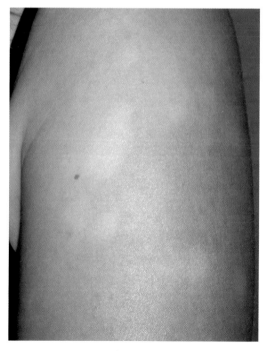

Figure 3.125. Pityriasis alba on upper arm.

3.6.11 Pompholyx

What is pompholyx?

Pompholyx is a form of hand/foot eczema characterised by vesicles or bullae (blisters). It is a form of vesicular dermatitis of hands and feet, also called vesicular endogenous eczema, and may be the same condition as dyshidrotic eczema. It is sometimes subclassified as cheiropompholyx (hands) and pedopompholyx (feet).

Who gets pompholyx?

Pompholyx most often affects young adults.
- It is more common in females than males.
- Many of them report palmoplantar hyperhidrosis.
- There is a personal or family history of atopic eczema in 50%.

What causes pompholyx?

Pompholyx is multifactorial. In many cases it appears to be related to sweating, as flares often occur during hot weather, humid conditions, or following emotional upset. Other contributing factors include:
- genetics.
- contact with irritants such as water, detergents, solvents and friction.
- association with contact allergy to nickel and other allergens.
- inflammatory dermatophyte infections (when it is known as a dermatophytid).
- adverse reaction to drugs, most often immunoglobulin therapy.

What are the clinical features of pompholyx?

Pompholyx presents as recurrent crops of deep-seated vesicles and bullae on the palms and soles (*Fig. 3.126*). They cause intense itch and/or a burning sensation. The blisters peel off and the skin then appears erythematous, dry and fissured.

When involving the distal finger adjacent or proximal to the nail fold, it can result in paronychia and nail dystrophy with irregular pitting and ridges.

What are the complications of pompholyx?

Secondary bacterial infection with *Staphylococcus aureus* and/or *Streptococcus pyogenes* is common in pompholyx, and results in pain, swelling and pustules on the hands and feet.

How is pompholyx diagnosed?

The clinical presentation is typical.
- Check carefully for dermatophyte infection (e.g. unilateral athlete's foot); if suspicious, take scrapings for mycology.
- Patch testing is indicated in chronic or atypical cases.
- Skin biopsy is rarely necessary. It shows spongiotic eczema.

What is the treatment for pompholyx?

Pompholyx is challenging to treat. Topical therapy is relatively ineffective because of the thick horny layer of skin of palms and soles.

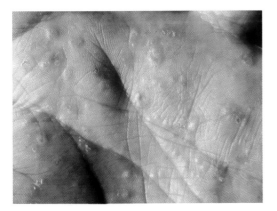
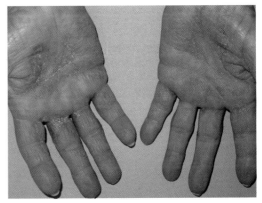

Figure 3.126. Pompholyx on hands.

GENERAL MEASURES

- Wet dressings to dry up blisters, using dilute potassium permanganate, aluminium acetate or acetic acid.
- Cold packs.
- Soothing emollient lotions and creams.
- Potent antiperspirants applied to palms and soles at night.
- Well-fitting footwear, with two pairs of socks to absorb sweat and reduce friction.

PRESCRIPTION MEDICINES

- Ultrapotent topical corticosteroid creams to new blisters under occlusion.
- Short courses of systemic corticosteroids, e.g. prednisone or prednisolone, for flare-ups.
- Oral antistaphylococcal antibiotics for secondary infection.
- Topical and oral antifungal agents for confirmed dermatophyte infection.
- In patients with hyperhidrosis, a trial of probanthine or oxybutynin is worth trying.
- In severe cases, immune modulating medicines are indicated. These include methotrexate, mycophenolate mofetil, azathioprine and ciclosporin.
- Where available, alitretinoin is used for resistant chronic disease.

OTHER OPTIONS

- Superficial radiotherapy.
- Botulinum toxin injections.
- Phototherapy and photochemotherapy.

What is the outlook for pompholyx?

Pompholyx generally gradually subsides and resolves spontaneously. It may recur, and in some patients is recalcitrant.

3.6.12 Seborrhoeic eczema

What is seborrhoeic eczema?

Seborrhoeic eczema is a common chronic or relapsing form of eczema/dermatitis that mainly affects the scalp and face. There are infantile and adult forms of seborrhoeic eczema. It is sometimes associated with psoriasis (sebopsoriasis).

What causes seborrhoeic eczema?

The cause of seborrhoeic eczema is not completely understood. It is associated with proliferation of various species of the skin commensal *Malassezia* in its yeast form. Its metabolites cause an eczematous inflammatory reaction. Differences in skin barrier function may account for individual presentations.

Who gets seborrhoeic eczema?

Infantile seborrhoeic eczema affects babies under the age of 3 months and usually resolves by one year of age.

Adult seborrhoeic eczema tends to begin in late adolescence. Prevalence is greatest in young adults and in the elderly. It is more common in males than in females.

The following factors are sometimes associated with severe adult seborrhoeic eczema:

- oily skin.
- familial tendency to seborrhoeic eczema or a family history of psoriasis.
- immunosuppression: organ transplant recipient, human immunodeficiency virus (HIV) infection and others.
- neurological and psychiatric diseases – Parkinson disease, tardive dyskinesia and depression.

What are the clinical features of seborrhoeic eczema?

INFANTILE SEBORRHOEIC ECZEMA

Infantile seborrhoeic eczema causes cradle cap (diffuse greasy scaling), see *Fig. 3.127*. The rash may spread to affect axillary and inguinal skin folds (a form of nappy rash) and sometimes generalises, see *Fig. 3.128*.

- There are salmon-pink patches that may flake or peel.

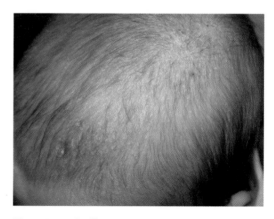

Figure 3.127. Cradle cap.

- It is not especially itchy, so the baby often appears undisturbed by the rash, even when generalised.

ADULT SEBORRHOEIC ECZEMA

Seborrhoeic eczema affects the scalp (*Fig. 3.129*), face (nasolabial folds, behind ears, within eyebrows; *Fig. 3.130*) and upper trunk.

Typical features include:
- winter flares, improving in summer following sun exposure.
- minimal pruritus (usually, but severe pruritus occasionally occurs).
- combination oily and dry mid-facial skin.
- pityriasis capitis (dandruff) with ill-defined localised scaly patches or diffuse scale throughout the scalp.
- blepharitis: scaly, red eyelid margins.
- salmon-pink, thin, scaly and ill-defined plaques in skin folds, symmetrically distributed on face.

- petaloid or annular flaky patches on anterior chest (*Fig. 3.131*) and on hairline (see *Fig. 3.132*).
- rash in axillae (*Fig. 3.133*), submammary sites, inguinal folds and genital creases (*Fig. 3.134*).
- superficial folliculitis on cheeks and upper trunk.

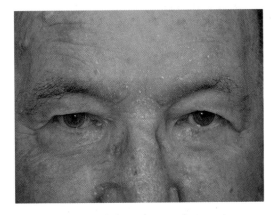

Figure 3.130. Seborrhoeic eczema on face.

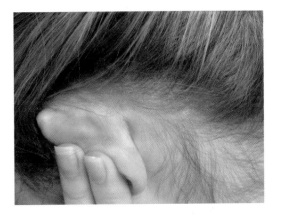

Figure 3.128. Generalised infantile seborrhoeic eczema.

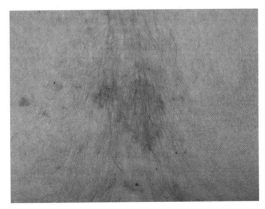

Figure 3.131. Seborrhoeic eczema on anterior chest.

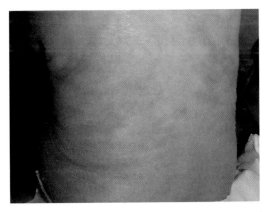

Figure 3.129. Seborrhoeic eczema on scalp.

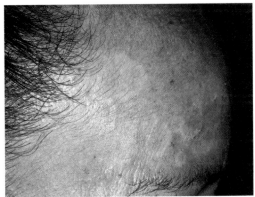

Figure 3.132. Annular flaky patches on hairline.

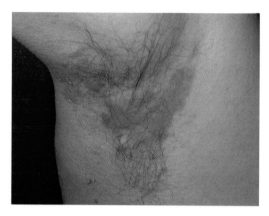

Figure 3.133. Rash in axilla.

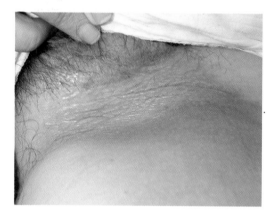

Figure 3.134. Rash in genital creases.

Extensive seborrhoeic eczema affecting scalp, neck and trunk is sometimes called pityriasiform seborrhoeide.

How is seborrhoeic eczema diagnosed?

Seborrhoeic eczema is diagnosed by its clinical appearance and behaviour. As *Malassezia* is a commensal, its presence on microscopy of skin scrapings is not diagnostic. Skin biopsy may be helpful but is rarely indicated.

What is the treatment for seborrhoeic eczema?

Treatment of seborrhoeic eczema often involves several of the following options:
- Keratolytics can be used to remove scale when necessary, e.g. salicylic acid, lactic acid, urea, propylene glycol.
- Topical antifungal agents are applied to reduce *Malassezia* e.g. ketoconazole or ciclopirox shampoo and/or cream. Note, some strains of

Malassezia are resistant to azole antifungals. Try zinc pyrithione or selenium sulphide.
- Topical corticosteroids are prescribed for 1–3 weeks to reduce the inflammation of an acute flare.
- Topical calcineurin inhibitors (pimecrolimus cream, tacrolimus ointment) are indicated if topical corticosteroids are often needed, as they have fewer adverse effects on facial skin.

In resistant cases, oral itraconazole and/or doxycycline may be useful.

3.6.13 Venous eczema

What is venous eczema?

Venous eczema is a common form of eczema/dermatitis that affects one or both lower legs in association with venous insufficiency. It is also called gravitational or stasis dermatitis.

Who gets venous eczema?

Venous eczema is most often seen in middle-aged and elderly patients – it is reported to affect 20% of those over 70 years. It is associated with:
- history of deep venous thrombosis in affected limb.
- history of cellulitis in affected limb.
- chronic oedema of lower leg.
- varicose veins.
- venous ulceration.

What causes venous eczema?

Venous eczema appears to be due to fluid collecting in the tissues and activation of the innate immune response.

What are the clinical features of venous eczema?

Venous eczema can form discrete plaques or become confluent and circumferential. Features include:
- itchy red, blistered and crusted plaques; or dry, fissured and scaly plaques on one or both lower legs, see *Fig. 3.135*.
- orange–brown macular pigmentation due to haemosiderin deposition, see *Fig. 3.136*.
- atrophie blanche (white irregular scars surrounded by enlarged capillaries), see *Fig. 3.137*.
- "champagne bottle" shape of lower leg (distal narrowing) and induration (lipodermatosclerosis), see *Fig. 3.138*.

Complications can include:

- secondary eczema spread to other parts of the body, see *Fig. 3.139*.
- contact irritant or allergic dermatitis to topical dressings and medicaments, see *Fig. 3.140*.
- secondary infection with *Staphylococcus aureus* (impetiginisation, see *Fig. 3.141*) or *Streptococcus pyogenes* (cellulitis).
- ulceration triggered by minor injury, leg swelling or infection, see *Fig. 3.142*.

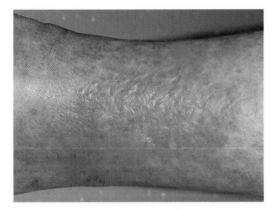

Figure 3.135. Dry plaques of venous eczema.

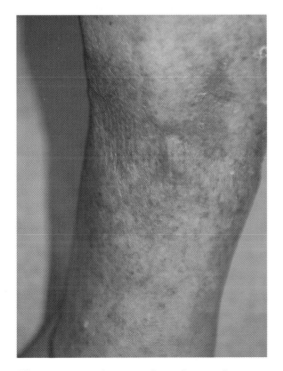

Figure 3.136. Macular orange–brown haemosiderin pigmentation.

How is venous eczema diagnosed?

Diagnosis of venous eczema is clinical.

Patch tests may be undertaken if there is suspicion of contact allergy.

What is the treatment for venous eczema?

Regular exercise, elevation of lower legs, and compression therapy to reduce swelling and improve venous return are essential. Protect affected skin from injury.

The eczema is treated with:

- wet dressings for acute exudative eczema.
- emollients for dry skin.
- antibiotics for secondary infection.
- daily potent topical steroids during acute phase followed by less potent or less frequent applications during maintenance phase.

Refer to a vascular surgeon for assessment of underlying venous insufficiency. Treatment may

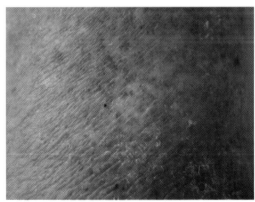

Figure 3.137. Atrophie blanche.

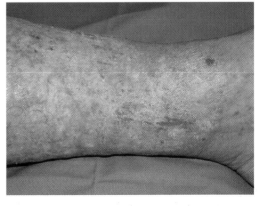

Figure 3.138. Lipodermatosclerosis and venous eczema.

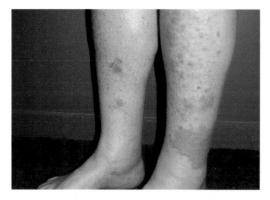

Figure 3.139. Secondary eczema that began on the ankles.

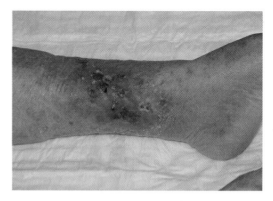

Figure 3.141. Impetiginisation of venous eczema.

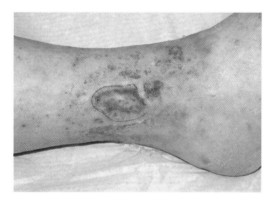

Figure 3.140. Reaction to dressings around venous ulcer.

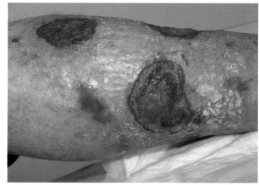

Figure 3.142. Venous ulceration, lipodermatosclerosis and eczema.

include surgery, endovenous laser ablation or sclerotherapy of ectatic veins.

How can venous eczema be prevented?

Venous eczema cannot be completely prevented but the number and severity of flare-ups can be reduced by the following measures.
- Avoid prolonged standing or sitting with legs down.
- Wear compression socks or stockings.
- Avoid and treat leg swelling.
- Apply emollients frequently and regularly to dry skin.
- Avoid soap; use water alone or non-soap cleansers when bathing.

What is the outlook for venous eczema?

Venous eczema tends to be a recurring or chronic lifelong disorder. Treat recurrence promptly with topical steroids.

3.7 Erythema multiforme

What is erythema multiforme?

Erythema multiforme is a hypersensitivity reaction usually triggered by infections, most commonly herpes simplex virus (HSV). It presents with a skin eruption characterised by a typical target lesion. There may be mucous membrane involvement. It is acute and self-limiting, usually resolving without complications.

Erythema multiforme is divided into major and minor forms and is distinct from Stevens–Johnson syndrome (SJS)/toxic epidermal necrolysis (TEN).

Who gets erythema multiforme?

Erythema multiforme most commonly affects young adults (20–40 years of age); however, all age groups can be affected. There is a male predominance but no racial bias.

There is a genetic tendency to erythema multiforme. Certain tissue types are more often found in people with herpes-associated erythema multiforme (HLA-DQw3) and recurrent erythema multiforme (HLA-B15, -B35, -A33, -DR53, -DQB1*0301).

What triggers erythema multiforme?

INFECTIONS

Infections are probably associated with at least 90% of cases of erythema multiforme.

The single most common trigger for developing erythema multiforme is herpes simplex virus (HSV) infection, usually herpes labialis (cold sore on the lip; see *Fig. 3.143*) and less often genital herpes. HSV type 1 is more commonly associated than type 2. The herpes infection usually precedes the skin eruption by 3–14 days.

Mycoplasma pneumonia (a lung infection caused by the bacteria *Mycoplasma pneumoniae*) is the next most common trigger.

Many different virus infections have been reported to trigger erythema multiforme including:

- parapoxvirus (orf and milkers' nodules).
- herpes varicella-zoster (chickenpox, shingles).
- adenovirus.
- hepatitis viruses.
- human immunodeficiency virus (HIV).
- cytomegalovirus.
- viral vaccines.

Dermatophyte fungal infections (tinea) have also been reported in association with erythema multiforme.

DRUGS   *PAN BS*

Medications are probably an uncommon cause (<10%) of erythema multiforme. If this diagnosis is being seriously considered then alternative drug eruptions should be excluded (see *Section 3.5*).

Many drugs have been reported to trigger erythema multiforme, including barbiturates, non-steroidal anti-inflammatory drugs, penicillins, sulphonamides, phenothiazines and anticonvulsants.

Clinical features of erythema multiforme

GENERAL SYMPTOMS

There are usually no prodromal symptoms in erythema multiforme minor. However, erythema multiforme major may be preceded by mild symptoms such as fever or chills, weakness or painful joints.

SKIN LESIONS

Typically in erythema multiforme, few to hundreds of skin lesions erupt within a

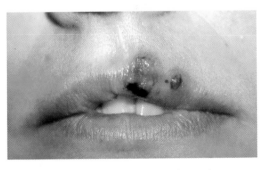

Figure 3.143. Herpes labialis, a trigger for erythema multiforme.

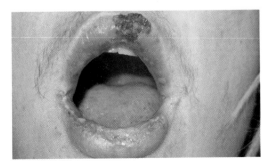

Figure 3.144. Mucosal lesions in erythema multiforme.

24-hour period. The lesions are first seen on the backs of hands (see *Fig. 3.145*) and/or tops of feet, and then spread along the limbs towards the trunk. The upper limbs (see *Fig. 3.147*) are more commonly affected than the lower; palms and soles may be involved (*Fig. 3.146*). The face, neck and trunk are common sites. Skin lesions are often grouped on elbows and knees. There may be an associated mild itch or burning sensation.

The initial lesions are sharply demarcated, round, red/pink macules, which become papules and gradually enlarge to form plaques up to several centimetres in diameter. The centre of the papule/plaque darkens in colour and develops epidermal changes such as blistering or crusting. Lesions usually evolve over 72 hours.

The typical target lesion (also called iris lesion) of erythema multiforme has a sharp margin, regular round shape and three concentric colour zones.
- The centre is dusky or dark red with a blister or crust.
- The next ring is a paler pink and is raised due to oedema (fluid swelling).
- The outermost ring is bright red.
- Atypical target lesions show just two zones and/or an indistinct border.

The eruption is polymorphous (many forms), hence the 'multiforme' in the name. Lesions may be at various stages of development with both typical and atypical targets present at the same time. A full skin examination may be required to find typical targets, as these may be few in number.

Lesions show the Köbner (isomorphic) phenomenon, meaning they can develop at sites of preceding (but not concurrent or subsequent) skin trauma.

There is no associated swelling of face, hands or feet, despite these being common sites of rash distribution. However the lips are often swollen, especially in erythema multiforme major.

MUCOUS MEMBRANE INVOLVEMENT

Mucosal lesions, if present, typically develop a few days after the skin rash begins.

In erythema multiforme minor, mucous membrane involvement is absent or mild. Mucosal changes, if present, consist initially of redness of the lips and inside cheek. Sometimes blisters develop and quickly break to form erosions and ulcers.

In erythema multiforme major, one or more mucous membranes are typically affected, most often the oral mucosa:
- most commonly lips, inside the cheeks, tongue.
- less commonly floor of the mouth, palate, gums.

Other mucosal sites affected may include:
- eye.
- anus and genitals.
- trachea/bronchi.
- gastrointestinal tract.

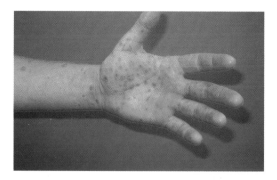

Figure 3.146. Erythema multiforme lesions on palm of hand.

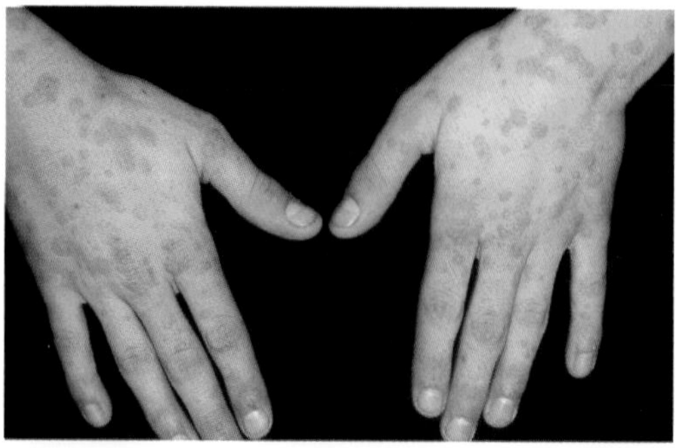

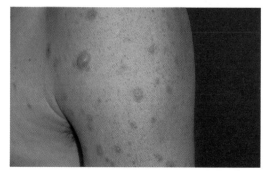

Figure 3.147. Skin lesions in erythema multiforme on arm.

Figure 3.145. Erythema multiforme lesions on back of hands.

Mucosal lesions consist of swelling and redness with blister formation. The blisters break quickly to leave large, shallow, irregular shaped, painful ulcers that are covered by a whitish pseudomembrane. Typically the lips are swollen with haemorrhagic crusts, see *Fig. 3.144*. The patient may have difficulty speaking or swallowing due to pain.

With mycoplasma pneumonia, the mucous membranes may be the only affected sites (mucositis). This can be severe and require hospitalisation due to difficulty in eating and drinking. Whether this is a limited form of erythema multiforme has not been determined.

RECURRENT ERYTHEMA MULTIFORME
Erythema multiforme can be recurrent, with multiple episodes per year for many years. This is believed to be nearly always due to HSV-1 infection.

How is the diagnosis of erythema multiforme made?

Erythema multiforme is a clinical diagnosis, although skin biopsy may be required to exclude other conditions. The histology of erythema multiforme is characteristic but not diagnostic. It varies with the age of the lesion, its appearance, and which part is biopsied.

Other tests may be done looking for infections commonly seen in association with erythema multiforme, such as mycoplasma.

Treatment of erythema multiforme

For the majority of cases, no treatment is required, as the rash settles by itself over several weeks without complications.

Treatment directed to any possible cause may be required such as oral aciclovir (not topical) for HSV or antibiotics (e.g. erythromycin) for mycoplasma. If a drug cause is suspected then the possible offending drug should be ceased.

Supportive/symptomatic treatment may be necessary:
- Itch – oral antihistamines and/or topical corticosteroids may help.
- Oral pain – mouthwashes containing local anaesthetic and antiseptic reduce pain and secondary infection.

- Eye involvement should be assessed and treated by an ophthalmologist.
- Erythema multiforme major may require hospital admission for supportive care, particularly if severe oral involvement restricts drinking.

The role of oral corticosteroids remains controversial, as no controlled studies have shown any benefit. However, for severe disease 0.5–1 mg/kg/day prednis(ol)one is often used early in the disease process.

Recurrent erythema multiforme is usually treated initially with continuous oral aciclovir for 6 months at a dose of 10 mg/kg/day in divided doses (e.g. 400 mg twice daily), even if HSV has not been an obvious trigger for the patient's erythema multiforme. This has been shown to be effective in placebo-controlled double blind studies. However, erythema multiforme may recur when the aciclovir is stopped. Other antiviral drugs such as valciclovir (500–1000 mg/day) and famciclovir (250 mg twice daily) should be tried if aciclovir has not helped; check for availability of these drugs as they are not used in all countries.

Other treatments (used continuously) that have been reported to help suppress recurrent erythema multiforme include:
- dapsone 100–150 mg/day.
- antimalarial drugs, e.g. hydroxychloroquine.
- azathioprine 100–150 mg/day.
- others – thalidomide, ciclosporin, mycophenolate mofetil, photochemotherapy (PUVA).

What is the outlook for erythema multiforme?

Erythema multiforme minor usually resolves spontaneously without scarring over 2 to 3 weeks. Erythema multiforme major can take up to 6 weeks to resolve. Erythema multiforme does not progress to SJS/TEN.

There may be residual mottled skin discoloration. Significant eye involvement in erythema multiforme major may result in serious eye problems, including blindness, as may occur with SJS/TEN.

3.8 Erythroderma

What is erythroderma?

Erythroderma is the term used to describe intense and usually widespread reddening of the skin due to inflammatory skin disease. It often precedes or is associated with exfoliation (skin peeling off in scales or layers), when it may also be known as exfoliative dermatitis (ED). Idiopathic erythroderma is sometimes called the "red man syndrome".

Who gets erythroderma and what is the cause?

Erythroderma is rare. It can arise at any age and in people of all races. It is about three times more common in males than in females. Most have a pre-existing skin disease or a systemic condition known to be associated with erythroderma. About 30% of cases of erythroderma are idiopathic.

Erythrodermic atopic dermatitis most often affects children and young adults, but other forms of erythroderma are more common in middle-aged and elderly people.

The most common skin conditions to cause erythroderma are:

- drug eruption – with numerous diverse drugs implicated (see *Fig. 3.148*). See *Section 3.5*.

- dermatitis, especially atopic dermatitis (see *Fig. 3.149*).
- psoriasis, especially after withdrawal of systemic steroids or other treatment (see *Fig. 3.150*).
- pityriasis rubra pilaris (see *Fig. 3.151*).

Other skin diseases that less frequently cause erythroderma include:

- other forms of dermatitis – contact dermatitis (allergic or irritant), stasis dermatitis and, in babies, seborrhoeic dermatitis or

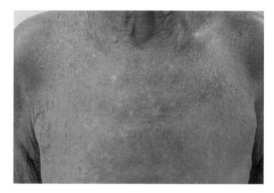

Figure 3.149. Erythroderma caused by atopic dermatitis.

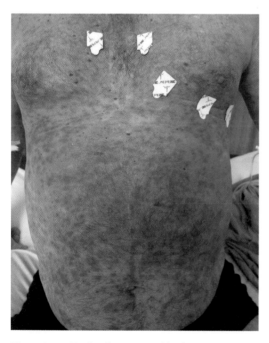

Figure 3.148. Erythroderma caused by drug eruption.

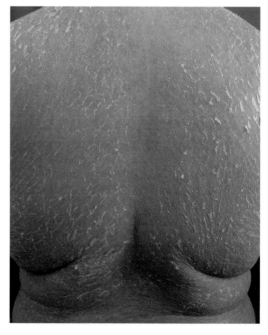

Figure 3.150. Erythroderma caused by psoriasis.

staphylococcal scalded skin syndrome (see *Fig. 3.152*).

- blistering diseases – pemphigus and bullous pemphigoid (see *Fig. 3.153*).
- Sézary syndrome (the erythrodermic form of cutaneous T-cell lymphoma; see *Fig. 3.154*).
- several very rare congenital ichthyotic conditions (epidermolytic ichthyosis; see *Fig. 3.155*).

Erythroderma may be a symptom or sign of a systemic disease. These may include:

- haematological malignancies, e.g. lymphoma, leukaemia.
- internal malignancies, e.g. carcinoma of rectum, lung, Fallopian tubes, colon.
- graft-versus-host disease.
- human immunodeficiency virus (HIV) infection.

It is not known why some skin diseases in some people progress to erythroderma. The pathogenesis is complicated, involving keratinocytes and lymphocytes, and their interaction with adhesion molecules and cytokines. The result is a dramatic increase in turnover of epidermal cells.

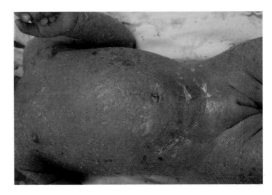

Figure 3.152. Staphylococcal scalded skin syndrome.

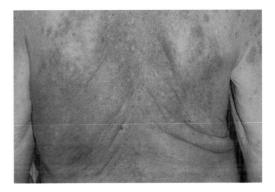

Figure 3.153. Bullous pemphigoid, which progressed to erythroderma.

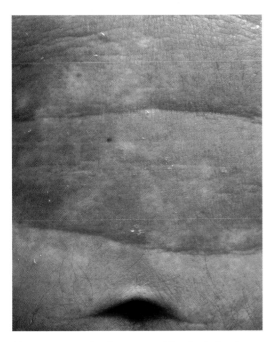

Figure 3.151. Erythroderma caused by pityriasis rubra pilaris.

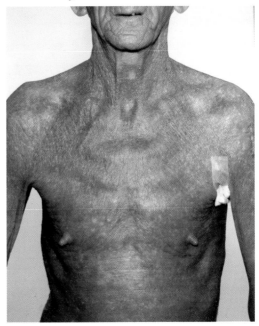

Figure 3.154. Sézary syndrome.

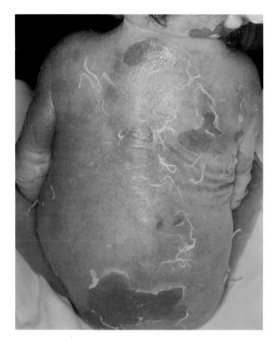

Figure 3.155. Epidermolytic ichthyosis.

What are the clinical features of erythroderma?

Erythroderma is often preceded by morbilliform drug eruption, dermatitis, or plaque psoriasis. Generalised erythema can develop quite rapidly in acute erythroderma, or more gradually over weeks to months in chronic erythroderma.

SIGNS AND SYMPTOMS OF ERYTHRODERMA

Generalised erythema and oedema affects 90% or more of the skin surface.

- The skin feels warm to the touch.
- Itch is usually troublesome, and is sometimes intolerable. Rubbing and scratching leads to lichenification.
- Eyelid swelling may result in ectropion (*Fig. 3.156*).
- Scaling begins 2–6 days after the onset of erythema, as fine flakes or large sheets.
- Thick scaling may develop on scalp with varying degrees of hair loss including complete baldness.
- Palms and soles may develop yellowish, diffuse keratoderma (*Fig. 3.157*).
- Nails become dull, ridged, and thickened or develop onycholysis and may shed (onychomadesis).
- Lymph nodes become swollen (generalised dermatopathic lymphadenopathy).

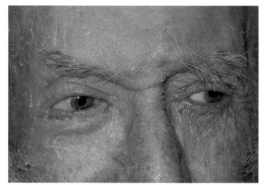

Figure 3.156. Ectropion in erythroderma.

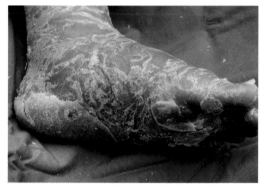

Figure 3.157. Keratoderma.

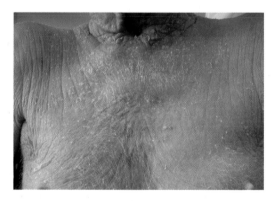

Figure 3.158. Serous ooze (atopic dermatitis).

Clues may be present as to the underlying cause.

- Serous ooze, resulting in clothes and dressings sticking to the skin and an unpleasant smell, is characteristic of atopic erythroderma (see *Fig. 3.158*).
- Persistence of circumscribed scaly plaques in certain sites such as elbows and knees suggests psoriasis.

- Islands of sparing, follicular prominence, orange hue to keratoderma are typical of pityriasis rubra pilaris (see *Fig. 3.159*).
- Subungual hyperkeratosis, crusting on palms and soles, and burrows are indicative of crusted scabies (see *Fig. 3.160*).
- Sparing of abdominal creases (deckchair sign) is typical of papuloerythroderma of Ofuji.

Systemic symptoms may be due to the erythroderma or to its cause.
- Lymphadenopathy, hepatosplenomegaly, abnormal liver dysfunction and fever may suggest a drug hypersensitivity syndrome or malignancy.
- Leg oedema may be due to inflamed skin, high output cardiac failure and/or hypoalbuminaemia.

Complications of erythroderma

Erythroderma often results in acute and chronic local and systemic complications. The patient is unwell with fever, temperature dysregulation and losing a great deal of fluid by transpiration through the skin.
- Heat loss leads to hypothermia.
- Fluid loss leads to electrolyte abnormalities and dehydration.
- Red skin leads to high-output heart failure.
- Secondary skin infection may occur (impetigo, cellulitis).
- General unwellness can lead to pneumonia.
- Hypoalbuminaemia from protein loss and increased metabolic rate causes oedema.
- Long-standing erythroderma may result in pigmentary changes (brown and/or white skin patches).

How is erythroderma diagnosed?

Erythroderma is readily diagnosed when erythema affects >90% of the body. The underlying cause is generally determined by a careful history. Further investigations may be unhelpful or may reflect the cause or the result of the erythroderma.
- Blood count may show anaemia, white cell count abnormalities, and eosinophilia. Marked eosinophilia should raise suspicions for lymphoma.
- >20% circulating Sézary cells suggests Sézary syndrome.
- C-reactive protein may or may not be elevated.

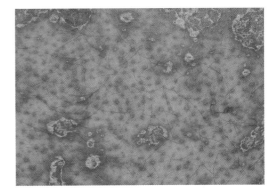

Figure 3.159. Pityriasis rubra pilaris.

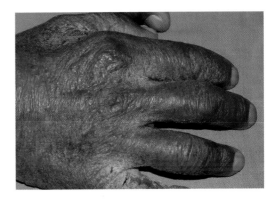

Figure 3.160. Crusted scabies.

- Proteins may reveal hypoalbuminaemia and abnormal liver function.
- Polyclonal gamma globulins are common, and raised immunoglobulin E (IgE) is typical of idiopathic erythroderma.

Skin biopsies from several sites may be taken if the cause is unknown. They tend to show non-specific inflammation on histopathology. Diagnostic features may be present, however.

Direct immunofluorescence is of benefit if an autoimmune blistering disease or connective tissue disease is considered.

What is the treatment for erythroderma?

Erythroderma is potentially serious, even life-threatening, and most patients require hospitalisation for monitoring and to restore fluid and electrolyte balance, circulatory status and body temperature.

The following general measures apply:
- discontinue all unnecessary medications.
- monitor fluid balance and body temperature.

- maintain skin moisture with wet wraps, other types of wet dressings, emollients and mild topical steroids.
- antibiotics are prescribed only for bacterial infection.
- antihistamines may reduce severe itch and can provide some sedation.
- specific treatment for identified underlying skin disease should be started, e.g. topical and systemic steroids for atopic dermatitis; acitretin or methotrexate for psoriasis.

How can erythroderma be prevented?

In most cases, erythroderma cannot be prevented.

- People with known drug allergy should be made aware that they should avoid the drug forever, and if their reaction was severe, wear a drug alert bracelet. All medical records should be updated if there is an adverse reaction to a medication, and referred to whenever starting a new drug.

- Patients with severe skin diseases should be informed if they are at risk of decompensating. They should be educated about the risks of discontinuing their medication.

What is the outlook for erythroderma?

Prognosis of erythroderma depends on the underlying disease process. If the cause can be removed or corrected, prognosis is generally good.

If erythroderma is the result of a generalised spread of a primary skin disorder such as psoriasis or dermatitis, it usually clears with appropriate treatment of the skin disease but may recur at any time.

The course of idiopathic erythroderma is unpredictable. It may persist for a long time with periods of acute exacerbation.

3.9 Granuloma annulare

What is granuloma annulare?

Granuloma annulare (GA) is a common skin condition in which there are smooth discoloured plaques. They are usually thickened and annular in configuration. Granuloma annulare is more correctly known as necrobiotic papulosis. There are several clinical patterns.

Who gets granuloma annulare?

Granuloma annulare affects the skin of children, teenagers or young adults (or older adults, less commonly).

What is the cause of granuloma annulare?

Granuloma annulare is a delayed hypersensitivity reaction to some component of the dermis. Inflammation is mediated by tumour necrosis factor alpha (TNF-α). The reason that this occurs is unknown.

Localised granuloma annulare is sometimes associated with autoimmune thyroiditis but it does not clear up with thyroid replacement. Extensive granuloma annulare is sometimes associated with diabetes mellitus, hyperlipidaemia, and, rarely, with lymphoma, HIV infection and solid tumours.

What are the clinical features of granuloma annulare?

Granuloma annulare can occur on any site of the body and is occasionally quite widespread. It only affects the skin and is considered harmless. Granuloma annulare may cause no symptoms, but affected areas are often tender when knocked. The plaques tend to slowly change shape, size and position.

LOCALISED GRANULOMA ANNULARE

The localised form is the most common type of granuloma annulare in children. One or more skin-coloured bumps occur in rings in the skin over joints, particularly the knuckles. The centre of each ring is often a little depressed. Localised granuloma annulare usually affects the fingers or the backs of both hands, but is also common on top of the foot or ankle, and over one or both elbows (*Fig. 3.161*).

GENERALISED GRANULOMA ANNULARE

Generalised granuloma annulare usually presents in adults, as widespread skin-coloured, pinkish or slightly mauve-coloured patches. The disseminated type is composed of small papules, usually arranged symmetrically in rings 10 cm or more in diameter. They are often found around the skin folds of the trunk (armpits, groin, see *Fig. 3.162*).

DEEP OR SUBCUTANEOUS GRANULOMA ANNULARE

Subcutaneous granuloma annulare most often occurs in children and presents as rubbery lumps. They appear on scalp margins, fingertips and shins. Subcutaneous granuloma annulare is also called pseudo-rheumatoid nodules because the subcutaneous lesions look rather like rheumatoid nodules. However, they arise in people who do not suffer from rheumatoid arthritis.

PERFORATING GRANULOMA ANNULARE

Perforating granuloma annulare describes plaques in which damaged collagen is eliminated

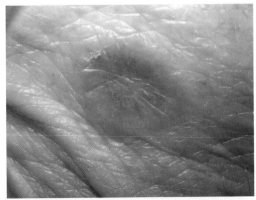

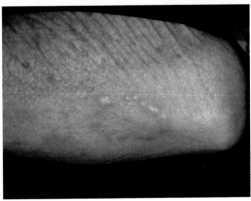

Figure 3.161. Localised granuloma annulare on back of hand and on elbow.

through the epidermis (*Fig. 3.163*). Perforating granuloma annulare is usually localised to the hands but plaques may occasionally arise on any body site, especially within scars. Dermoscopy helps to confirm the presence of perforations in small papules arising within otherwise typical

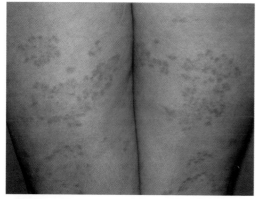

Figure 3.162. Generalised granuloma annulare.

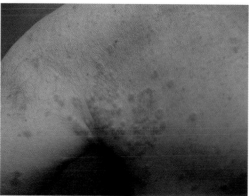

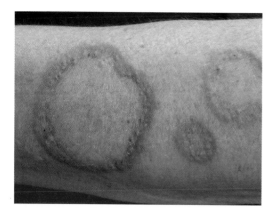

Figure 3.163. Perforating granuloma annulare.

plaques of granuloma annulare. Perforating lesions are frequently itchy or tender.

ATYPICAL GRANULOMA ANNULARE

Atypical granuloma annulare describes:
- granuloma annulare in unusual sites, such as face, palms and ears.
- granuloma annulare with photosensitive distribution.
- unusually severe or symptomatic granuloma annulare.

INTERSTITIAL GRANULOMATOUS DERMATITIS

Interstitial granulomatous dermatitis is a pathological finding noted in some patients with extensive granuloma annulare or other disorders with similar clinical presentation.

How is granuloma annulare diagnosed?

Most often granuloma annulare is recognised clinically because of its characteristic appearance. Sometimes, however, the diagnosis is not obvious, and other conditions may be considered. Skin biopsy usually shows necrobiotic degeneration of dermal collagen surrounded by an inflammatory reaction. It is not a true granuloma.

What treatment is available for granuloma annulare?

In most cases of granuloma annulare, no treatment is required because the patches disappear by themselves in a few months, leaving no trace. However, sometimes they persist for years. Treatment is not always successful.

LOCAL THERAPY

Options to consider include:
- topical corticosteroid ointment under occlusion.
- intralesional steroid injections.
- destruction by cryotherapy or laser ablation.
- imiquimod cream.
- topical calcineurin inhibitors (tacrolimus and pimecrolimus).

SYSTEMIC THERAPY

Systemic therapy may be considered in widespread granuloma annulare. The following treatments have been reported to help at least some cases of disseminated granuloma annulare.

None of these can be relied upon to clear it, and there are some potential adverse effects.

- Systemic steroids.
- Isotretinoin.
- Methotrexate.
- Potassium iodide.
- Dapsone.
- Hydroxychloroquine.
- Pentoxifylline.
- Allopurinol.
- Antibiotics.
- Photochemotherapy (PUVA).
- UVA1 phototherapy.
- Photodynamic therapy.
- Ciclosporin.
- TNF-α inhibitors (infliximab, adalimumab).

What is the outlook for granuloma annulare?

Localised granuloma annulare tends to clear up within a few months or years, although it may recur. Generalised and atypical variants are more persistent, sometimes lasting decades.

3.10 Hidradenitis suppurativa

What is hidradenitis suppurativa?

Hidradenitis suppurativa is an inflammatory skin disease that affects apocrine gland-bearing skin in the axillae, in the groin, and under the breasts. It is characterised by recurrent boil-like nodules and abscesses that culminate in pus-like discharge, difficult-to-heal open wounds and scarring.

The term "hidradenitis" implies that it starts as an inflammatory disorder of sweat glands, which is now known to be incorrect. Hidradenitis suppurativa is also known as "acne inversa".

Who gets hidradenitis suppurativa?

Hidradenitis often starts at puberty, and is most active between the ages of 20 and 40 years. It is three times more common in females than in males. Risk factors include:

- other family members with hidradenitis suppurativa.
- obesity and insulin resistance.
- cigarette smoking.
- follicular occlusion disorders – acne conglobata, dissecting cellulitis, pilonidal sinus.
- inflammatory bowel disease (Crohn disease).
- rare autoinflammatory syndromes associated with abnormalities of *PSTPIP1* gene.*

*PAPA syndrome (pyogenic arthritis, pyoderma gangrenosum and acne), PASH syndrome (pyoderma gangrenosum, acne, suppurative hidradenitis) and PAPASH syndrome (pyogenic arthritis, pyoderma gangrenosum, acne, suppurative hidradenitis).

What causes hidradenitis suppurativa?

Hidradenitis suppurativa is an autoinflammatory disorder. Although the exact cause is not yet understood, contributing factors include:

- friction from clothing and body folds.
- aberrant immune response to commensal bacteria.
- follicular occlusion.
- release of pro-inflammatory cytokines.
- inflammation causing rupture of the follicular wall and destroying apocrine glands and ducts.
- secondary bacterial infection.

What are the clinical features of hidradenitis suppurativa?

Hidradenitis can affect a single or multiple areas in the armpits, neck, submammary area, and inner thighs. Anogenital involvement most commonly affects the groin, mons pubis, vulva (in females), sides of the scrotum (in males), perineum, buttocks and perianal folds.

Signs include:

- open and closed comedones (*Fig. 3.164*).
- painful firm papules and larger nodules, often in the form of perpendicular pleats (see *Fig. 3.165*).
- pustules, fluctuant pseudocysts and abscesses (see *Fig. 3.166*).
- pyogenic granulomas (*Fig. 3.167*).
- draining sinuses linking inflammatory lesions.
- hypertrophic and atrophic scars (see *Fig. 3.168*).

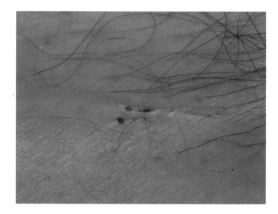

Figure 3.164. Comedones in groin.

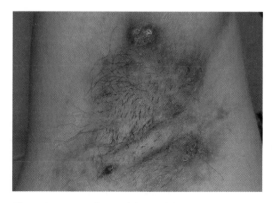

Figure 3.165. Papules, nodules and draining sinuses in axilla.

Many patients with hidradenitis suppurativa also suffer from other skin disorders, including acne, hirsutism and psoriasis.

The severity and extent of hidradenitis suppurativa is recorded at assessment and when determining the impact of a treatment. The Hurley staging system describes three distinct clinical stages:

1. Solitary or multiple, isolated abscess formation without scarring or sinus tracts.
2. Recurrent abscesses, single or multiple widely separated lesions, with sinus tract formation.
3. Diffuse or broad involvement, with multiple interconnected sinus tracts and abscesses.

Severe hidradenitis (Hurley Stage 3) has been associated with:
- male gender.
- axillary and perianal involvement.
- obesity.
- smoking.
- longer disease duration.

What is the treatment for hidradenitis suppurativa?

GENERAL MEASURES
- Weight loss; follow low-glycaemic, low-dairy diet.
- Smoking cessation: this can lead to improvement within a few months.
- Loose-fitting clothing.
- Daily antiperspirants.
- If prone to secondary infection, wash with antiseptics or take bleach baths.
- Apply hydrogen peroxide solution or medical grade honey to reduce malodour.
- Apply simple dressings to draining sinuses.
- Analgesics, such as paracetamol (acetaminophen), for pain control.

MEDICAL MANAGEMENT
Medical management of hidradenitis suppurativa is difficult. Treatment is required long term. Effective options are listed below.

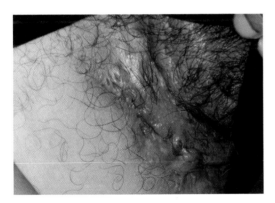

Figure 3.166. Abscess, nodules, scarring and pyogenic granuloma.

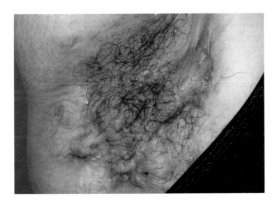

Figure 3.167. Nodules, pyogenic granulomas and scarring.

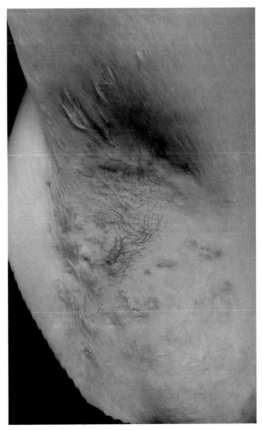

Figure 3.168. Atrophic scars.

MEDICAL MANAGEMENT – ANTIBIOTICS

- Topical clindamycin, with benzoyl peroxide to reduce bacterial resistance.
- Short course of oral antibiotics for acute staphylococcal abscesses, e.g. flucloxacillin.
- Prolonged courses (minimum 3 months) of tetracycline, metronidazole, cotrimoxazole, fluoroquinolones or dapsone for their anti-inflammatory action.
- 6–12 week courses of the combination of clindamycin (or doxycycline) and rifampicin for severe disease.

MEDICAL MANAGEMENT – ANTIANDROGENS

- Long-term oral contraceptive pill in females; antiandrogenic progesterones drospirenone or cyproterone acetate may be more effective than standard combined pills. These are more suitable than progesterone-only pills or devices.
- Response takes 6 months or longer.
- Spironolactone and finasteride have been reported to help some patients.

MEDICAL MANAGEMENT – IMMUNOMODULATORY TREATMENTS FOR SEVERE DISEASE

- Intralesional corticosteroids into nodules.
- Systemic corticosteroids short-term for flares.

- Methotrexate, ciclosporin, and azathioprine.
- TNF-α inhibitors adalimumab and infliximab, used in higher dose than required for psoriasis, are the most successful treatments to date.

MEDICAL MANAGEMENT – OTHER TREATMENTS

- Metformin in patients with insulin resistance.
- Acitretin (unsuitable for females of childbearing potential).
- Colchicine.

SURGICAL MANAGEMENT

- Incision and drainage of acute abscesses.
- Curettage and deroofing of nodules, abscesses and sinuses.
- Laser ablation of nodules, abscesses and sinuses.
- Wide local excision of persistent nodules.
- Radical excisional surgery of entire affected area.
- Laser hair removal.

3.11 Lichen planus

What is lichen planus?

Lichen planus is a chronic inflammatory skin condition affecting skin and/or mucosal surfaces. There are several clinical types of lichen planus that share similar features on histopathology:

- cutaneous lichen planus.
- mucosal lichen planus.
- lichen planopilaris.
- lichen planus of the nails.
- lichen planus pigmentosus.
- lichenoid drug eruption.

Who gets lichen planus?

Lichen planus affects about one in 100 people worldwide, mostly affecting adults over the age of 40 years. About half those affected have oral lichen planus, which is more common in women than in men. About 10% have lichen planus of the nails.

What causes lichen planus?

Lichen planus is likely a T cell-mediated autoimmune disease, in which inflammatory cells attack an unknown protein within skin and mucosal keratinocytes.

Contributing factors to lichen planus may include:

- genetic predisposition.
- physical and emotional stress.
- injury to the skin; lichen planus often appears where the skin has been scratched – isomorphic response.
- localised skin disease such as herpes zoster – isotopic response.
- systemic viral infection, such as hepatitis C (which might modify self-antigens on the surface of basal keratinocytes).
- contact factors, such as metal fillings in oral lichen planus (rare).
- drugs; gold, quinine, quinidine and others can cause a lichenoid rash.

A lichenoid inflammation is also notable in graft-versus-host disease, a complication of bone marrow transplant.

What are the clinical features of lichen planus?

Lichen planus may cause a small number or many lesions on the skin and/or mucosal surfaces.

CUTANEOUS LICHEN PLANUS

The usual presentation of the disease is classical lichen planus (see *Fig. 3.169*). Symptoms can range from none (uncommon) to intense itch.

- Papules and polygonal plaques are shiny, flat-topped and firm on palpation.
- The plaques are crossed by fine white lines called Wickham striae.
- Hypertrophic lichen planus can be scaly.
- Bullous lichen planus is rare.
- Size ranges from pinpoint to larger than a centimetre.
- Distribution may be scattered, clustered, linear or annular.
- Location can be anywhere, but most often front of the wrists, lower back, and ankles.
- Colour depends on the patient's skin type. New papules and plaques often have a purple or violet hue, except on palms and soles where they are yellowish brown.
- Plaques resolve after some months to leave greyish brown post-inflammatory macules that can take a year or longer to fade.

ORAL LICHEN PLANUS

The mouth is often the only affected area. Lichen planus often involves the inside of the cheeks and the sides of the tongue, but the gums and lips may also be involved (*Fig. 3.170*). The most common patterns are:

- painless white streaks in a lacy or fern-like pattern.
- painful and persistent erosions and ulcers (erosive lichen planus).
- diffuse redness and peeling of the gums (desquamative gingivitis).
- localised inflammation of the gums adjacent to amalgam fillings.

VULVAL LICHEN PLANUS

Lichen planus may affect labia majora, labia minora and vaginal introitus (*Fig. 3.171*). Presentation includes:

- painless white streaks in a lacy or fern-like pattern.
- painful and persistent erosions and ulcers (erosive lichen planus).
- scarring resulting in adhesions, resorption of labia minora and introital stenosis.
- painful desquamative vaginitis, preventing intercourse, and causing a mucky discharge; the eroded vagina may bleed easily on contact.

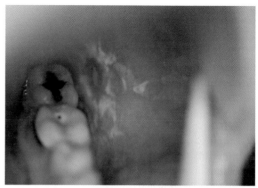

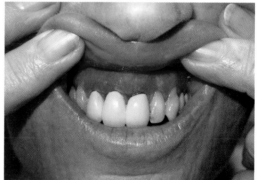

Figure 3.170. Oral lichen planus at back of tongue and on gums.

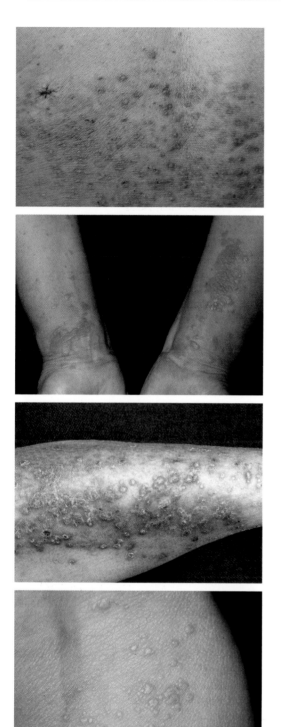

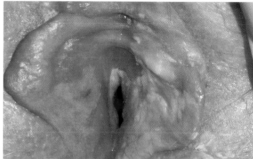

Figure 3.171. Vulval lichen planus.

PENILE LICHEN PLANUS

Penile lichen planus usually presents with classical papules in a ring around the glans (Fig. 3.172). White streaks and erosive lichen planus may occur but are less common.

OTHER MUCOSAL SITES

Erosive lichen planus uncommonly affects the lacrimal glands, eyelids, external ear canal, oesophagus, larynx, bladder and anus.

Figure 3.169. Cutaneous lichen planus.

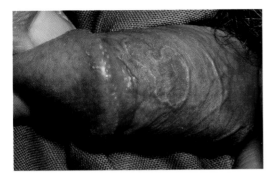

Figure 3.172. Penile lichen planus.

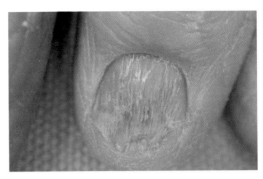

Figure 3.174. Nail lichen planus.

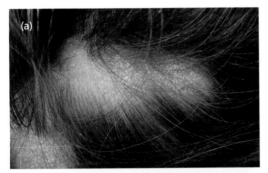

(a)

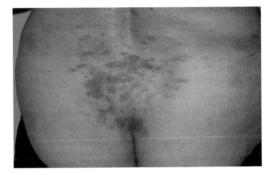

Figure 3.175. Lichen planus pigmentosus.

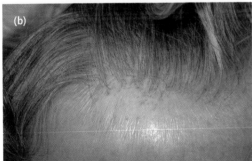

(b)

Lichen planopilaris

Lichen planopilaris presents as tiny red spiny follicular papules on the scalp or, less often, elsewhere on the body. Rarely, blistering occurs in the lesions. Destruction of the hair follicles leads to permanently bald patches characterised by sparse "lonely hairs" (see *Fig. 3.173(a)*).

- Frontal fibrosing alopecia is a form of lichen planopilaris that affects the anterior scalp, forehead (*Fig. 3.173(b)*) and eyebrows.
- Pseudopelade (*Fig. 3.173(c)*) is probably a variant of lichen planus without inflammation or scaling. Bald areas of scarring slowly appear, described as "footprints in the snow".

Nail lichen planus

Lichen planus affects one or more nails, sometimes without involving the skin surface. It is called twenty-nail dystrophy if all nails are abnormal and nowhere else is affected. Lichen planus thins the nail plate, which may become grooved and ridged (*Fig. 3.174*). The nail may darken, thicken or lift off the nail bed (onycholysis). Sometimes the cuticle is destroyed

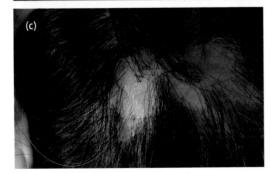

(c)

Figure 3.173. Lichen planopilaris. (a) Typical bald patch with "lonely hairs"; (b) frontal fibrosing alopecia; (c) pseudopelade.

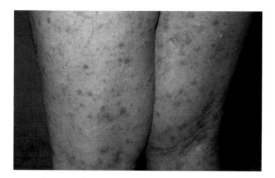

Figure 3.176. Lichenoid drug eruption to nivolumab.

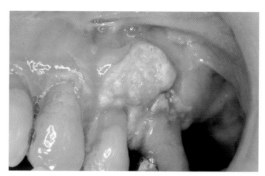

Figure 3.177. Squamous cell carcinoma of the mouth.

and forms a scar (pterygium). The nails may shed or stop growing altogether, and they may, rarely, completely disappear (anonychia).

LICHEN PLANUS PIGMENTOSUS

Lichen planus pigmentosus describes ill-defined oval, greyish brown marks on the face and neck or trunk and limbs without an inflammatory phase (*Fig. 3.175*). It can be provoked by sun exposure but can also arise in sun-protected sites such as the armpits. It has diffuse, reticulate and diffuse patterns. Lichen planus pigmentosus is similar to erythema dyschromicum perstans and may be the same disease.

Lichen planus pigmentosus may rarely affect the lips, resulting in a patchy dark pigmentation on upper and lower lips.

LICHENOID DRUG ERUPTION

Lichenoid drug eruption refers to a lichen planus-like rash caused by medications. Asymptomatic or itchy; pink, brown or purple; flat, slightly scaly patches most often arise on the trunk. The oral mucosa (oral lichenoid reaction) and other sites are also sometimes affected. Many drugs can rarely cause lichenoid eruptions. The most common are:

- gold.
- hydroxychloroquine.
- captopril.
- immunotherapy, such as PD1 checkpoint inhibitors pembrolizumab and nivolumab (see *Fig. 3.176*).
- quinine and thiazide diuretics cause photosensitive lichenoid drug eruption.

Lichenoid drug eruptions clear up slowly when the responsible medication is withdrawn.

Complications of lichen planus

Rarely, longstanding erosive lichen planus can result in squamous cell carcinoma of the mouth (see *Fig. 3.177*), vulva or penis. This should be suspected if there is an enlarging nodule or an ulcer with thickened edges. Cancer is more common in smokers, those with a past history of cancer in mucosal sites, and in those who carry oncogenic human papillomavirus.

Cancer from other forms of lichen planus is rare.

How is lichen planus diagnosed?

In most cases, lichen planus is diagnosed by observing its clinical features. A biopsy is often recommended to confirm or make the diagnosis and to look for cancer. The histopathological signs are of a "lichenoid tissue reaction" affecting the epidermis.

Typical features include:

- irregularly thickened epidermis.
- degenerative skin cells.
- liquefaction degeneration of the basal layer of the epidermis.
- band of inflammatory cells just beneath the epidermis.
- melanin (pigment) beneath the epidermis.

Direct staining by immunofluorescent techniques may reveal deposits of immunoglobulins at the base of the epidermis.

Patch testing may be recommended for patients with oral lichen planus affecting the gums, to assess for contact allergy to mercury.

What is the treatment for lichen planus?

Treatment is not always necessary. Local treatments for symptomatic cutaneous or mucosal disease are:

- potent topical corticosteroids.
- topical calcineurin inhibitors.

- topical retinoids.
- intralesional corticosteroid injections.

Systemic treatment for widespread or severe local disease often includes a 1–3 month course of oral prednisone, while commencing another agent from the following list:

- acitretin.
- hydroxychloroquine.
- methotrexate.
- azathioprine.
- mycophenolate mofetil.
- phototherapy.

In some cases of oral lichen planus affecting the gums, contact allergy to mercury in amalgam fillings on nearby teeth can be confirmed by patch testing. In these patients the lichen planus may resolve on replacing the fillings with composite material. If the lichen planus is not due to mercury allergy, removing amalgam fillings is very unlikely to result in cure.

Anecdotal success is reported from oral antibiotics and oral antifungal agents. Lichen planopilaris is reported to improve with pioglitazone.

What is the outlook for lichen planus?

Cutaneous lichen planus tends to clear within a couple of years in most people, but mucosal lichen planus is more likely to persist for a decade or longer. Spontaneous recovery is unpredictable, and lichen planus may recur at a later date.

3.12 Lichen sclerosus

What is lichen sclerosus?

Lichen sclerosus is a common chronic skin disorder that most often affects genital and perianal areas.

Older names for lichen sclerosus (LS) include lichen sclerosus et atrophicus, kraurosis vulvae (in women) and balanitis xerotica obliterans (in males).

Who gets lichen sclerosus?

Lichen sclerosus can start at any age, although it is most often diagnosed in women over 50. Pre-pubertal children can also be affected.

- Lichen sclerosus is 10 times more common in women than in men.
- 15% of patients know of a family member with lichen sclerosus.
- It may follow or co-exist with another skin condition, most often lichen simplex, psoriasis, erosive lichen planus, vitiligo or morphoea.
- People with lichen sclerosus often have a personal or family history of other autoimmune conditions such as thyroid disease (about 20% of patients), pernicious anaemia, or alopecia areata.

What causes lichen sclerosus?

The cause of lichen sclerosus is not fully understood, and may include genetic, hormonal, irritant and infectious components.

Lichen sclerosus is classified as an autoimmune disease. Autoimmune diseases are associated with antibodies to a specific protein.

- Extracellular matrix protein-1 (ECM-1) antibodies have been detected in 60–80% of women with vulval lichen sclerosus.
- Antibodies to other unknown proteins may account for other cases, explaining differing presentations of lichen sclerosus and response to treatment.

Male genital lichen sclerosus is rare in men circumcised in infancy. It has been suggested that it may be caused by chronic, intermittent damage by urine occluded under the foreskin.

What are the clinical features of lichen sclerosus?

Lichen sclerosus presents as white crinkled or thickened patches of skin that have a tendency to scar (*Fig. 3.178*). Peripheral erythema is sometimes present.

VULVAL LICHEN SCLEROSUS

Lichen sclerosus primarily involves the non-hair bearing, inner areas of the vulva (*Fig. 3.179*).

- It can be localised to one small area or extensively involve the perineum, labia minora (inner lips) and clitoral hood.
- It can spread onto the surrounding skin of the labia majora and inguinal fold and, in 50% of women, to anal and perianal skin.
- Lichen sclerosus never involves vaginal mucosa.

Lichen sclerosus can be extremely itchy and/or sore.

- Sometimes bruises, blood blisters and ulcers appear after scratching, or from minimal friction (e.g. tight clothing, sitting down; see *Fig. 3.180*).
- Urine can sting and irritate.

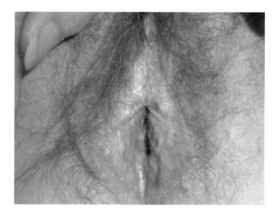

Figure 3.178. Lichen sclerosus.

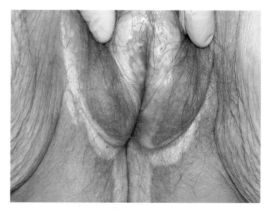

Figure 3.179. Vulval lichen sclerosus.

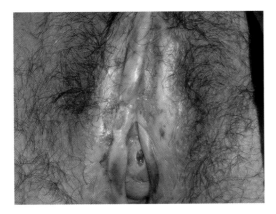

Figure 3.180. Ulcers in lichen sclerosus.

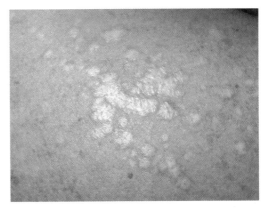

Figure 3.182. Extragenital lichen sclerosus.

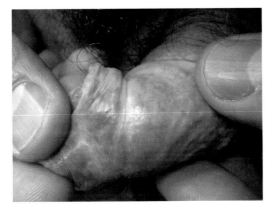

Figure 3.181. Penile lichen sclerosus.

- Sexual intercourse can be very uncomfortable and may result in painful fissuring of the posterior fourchette at the entrance to the vagina.
- It may cause discomfort or bleeding when passing bowel motions, and aggravate any tendency to constipation, particularly in children.

Lichen sclerosus causes adhesions and scarring.
- The clitoris may be buried (phimosis).
- The labia minora resorb/shrink.
- The entrance to the vagina tightens (introital stenosis).

PENILE LICHEN SCLEROSUS
In men, lichen sclerosus usually affects the tip of the penis (glans), which becomes white, firm and scarred (*Fig. 3.181*).
- The urethra may narrow (meatal stenosis), resulting in a thin or crooked urinary stream.

- The foreskin may become difficult to retract (phimosis).
- Sexual function may be affected, because of painful erections or embarrassment.

EXTRAGENITAL LICHEN SCLEROSUS
Extragenital lichen sclerosus refers to lichen sclerosus at other sites (*Fig. 3.182*).
- Extragenital lichen sclerosus affects 10% of women with vulval disease.
- Only 6% of men and women with extragenital lichen sclerosus do not have genital lichen sclerosus at the time of diagnosis.

One or more white dry plaques may be found on the inner thigh, buttocks, lower back, abdomen, under the breasts, neck, shoulders and armpits.
- Lichen sclerosus resembles cigarette paper, as the skin is dry, wrinkled and thin (atrophic).
- Hair follicles may appear prominent, containing dry plugs of keratin.
- Bruises, blisters and ulcers may appear without noticeable trauma.

Extragenital lichen sclerosus is generally not itchy or sore.

What are the complications of lichen sclerosus?

Lichen sclerosus of anogenital sites is associated with an increased risk of vulval, penile or anal cancer (squamous cell carcinoma, SCC).
- Cancer is estimated to affect up to 5% of patients with vulval lichen sclerosus.
- Cancer is more likely if the inflammatory disease is uncontrolled.

- Invasive SCC presents as an enlarging lump, or a sore that fails to heal.
- High-grade squamous intraepithelial lesions (SIL) associated with lichen sclerosus may be HPV-associated (usual type), or differentiated.

Extragenital lichen sclerosus does not appear to predispose to cancer.

How is lichen sclerosus diagnosed?

An experienced clinician can often diagnose lichen sclerosus by its appearance. Skin biopsy is frequently recommended.

- Biopsy may confirm the suspected diagnosis of lichen sclerosus.
- Another skin condition may be diagnosed or coexist with lichen sclerosus.
- A focal area may undergo biopsy to assess for cancer or SIL.

Biopsy may also be recommended at follow-up, to evaluate areas of concern or to explain poor response to treatment.

What is the treatment for lichen sclerosus?

Patients with lichen sclerosus are best to consult a doctor with a special interest in the condition for accurate diagnosis and treatment recommendations.

They are advised to become familiar with the location and appearance of their lichen sclerosus.

- Women may use a mirror when applying topical therapy.
- Photographs may help in monitoring activity and treatment.

GENERAL MEASURES FOR GENITAL LICHEN SCLEROSUS

- Wash gently once or twice daily.
- Use a non-soap cleanser, if any.
- Try to avoid tight clothing, rubbing and scratching.
- Activities such as riding a bicycle or horse may aggravate symptoms.
- If incontinent, seek medical advice and treatment.
- Apply emollients to relieve dryness and itching, and as a barrier to protect sensitive skin in genital and anal areas from contact with urine and faeces.

TOPICAL STEROID OINTMENT

Topical steroids are the main treatment for lichen sclerosus. An ultrapotent topical steroid is often prescribed, e.g. clobetasol propionate 0.05%. Lower potency topical steroids may be used in mild disease or when symptoms are controlled.

- An ointment base is less likely than cream to sting or to cause contact dermatitis.
- A thin smear should be precisely applied to the white plaques and rubbed in gently.
- Most patients will be told to apply the steroid ointment once a day. After one to three months (depending on the severity of the disease), the ointment can be used less often.
- Topical steroid may need to be continued once or twice a week to control symptoms or to prevent lichen sclerosus recurring.
- Itch often settles within a few days but it may take weeks to months for the skin to return to normal (if at all).
- One 30 g tube of topical steroid should last 3 to 6 months or longer.

The doctor should reassess the treated area after a few weeks, as response to treatment is quite variable.

Topical steroids are safe when used appropriately. However, excessive use or application to the wrong site can result in adverse effects. In anogenital areas, these include:

- red, thin skin.
- burning discomfort.
- periorificial dermatitis.
- *Candida albicans* infection.

It is most important to follow instructions carefully and to attend follow-up appointments regularly.

OTHER TOPICAL THERAPY

Other topical treatments used in patients with lichen sclerosus include the following:

- Intravaginal oestrogen cream or pessaries in postmenopausal women. These reduce symptoms due to atrophic vulvovaginitis (dry, thin, fissured and sensitive vulval and vaginal tissues due to hormonal deficiency).
- Topical calcineurin inhibitors tacrolimus ointment and pimecrolimus cream instead of or in addition to topical steroids. They tend to cause burning discomfort (at least for the first few days). Early concern that

these medications may have the potential to accelerate skin cancer growth in the presence of oncogenic human papilloma virus appears unfounded.

- Topical retinoid (e.g. tretinoin cream) is not well tolerated on genital skin but may be applied to other sites affected by lichen sclerosus. It reduces scaling and dryness.

ORAL MEDICATIONS

When lichen sclerosus is severe, acute, and not responding to topical therapy, systemic treatment may, rarely, be prescribed. Options include:

- intralesional or systemic corticosteroids.
- oral retinoids – acitretin, isotretinoin.
- methotrexate.
- ciclosporin.

SURGERY

Surgery is essential for high-grade squamous intraepithelial lesions or cancer. In males, circumcision is effective in lichen sclerosus affecting prepuce and glans of the penis. It is best done early if initial topical steroids have not controlled symptoms and signs. If the urethra is stenosed or scarred, reconstructive surgery may be necessary.

In females, release of vulval and vaginal adhesions and scarring from vulval lichen sclerosus may occasionally be performed to reduce urination difficulties and allow intercourse if dilators have not proved effective. Procedures include:

- simple perineotomy (division of adhesions).
- Fenton procedure (an incision that is repaired transversely).
- perineoplasty (excison of involved tissue and vaginal mucosal advancement).

Unfortunately, lichen sclerosus sometimes closes up the vaginal opening again after surgery has initially appeared successful. It can be repeated.

OTHER TREATMENTS

Other reported treatments for lichen sclerosus are considered experimental at this time:

- Phototherapy.
- Laser treatment.
- Photodynamic therapy.
- Fat injections.
- Stem cell and platelet-rich plasma injections.

What is the outlook for lichen sclerosus?

Lichen sclerosus is a chronic disease and usually persists for years.

- Extragenital lichen sclerosus is more likely than genital disease to clear.
- Early treatment occasionally leads to complete and long-term remission.
- Scarring is permanent.

Long-term follow-up is recommended to monitor the disease, optimise treatment and ensure early diagnosis of cancer.

3.13 Mouth ulcers

What are mouth ulcers?

Mouth ulcers are common. They are one form of stomatitis. A mouth ulcer is damaged epithelium and its underlying lamina propria. Mouth ulcers may be due to trauma, irritation, radiation, infections, drugs, inflammatory disorders and unknown causes.

The most common presentation is with painful, recurrent aphthous stomatitis, also known as aphthosis, aphthae, aphthous ulceration and canker sores.

Patients may present to doctors or to dentists with mouth ulcers for assessment and treatment. They may also have cutaneous and systemic symptoms and signs.

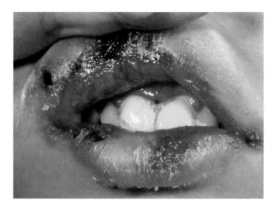

Figure 3.184. Herpes simplex infection.

Who gets mouth ulcers and how are they classified?

Males and females of all ages and races experience mouth ulcers. They may appear fairly similar, whatever the underlying cause.

ACUTE AND RECURRENT INFECTIONS

- *Candida albicans* infection: oral thrush in babies, the elderly and debilitated (see *Fig. 3.183*).
- Herpes simplex: primary (in children) or recurrent cold sores (any age); see *Fig. 3.184*.
- Enterovirus 71 infection: enteroviral vesicular stomatitis (HFM) (children or any age); see *Fig. 3.185*.
- Herpangina (children).
- Epstein–Barr virus and cytomegalovirus (adolescents).
- Varicella-zoster virus: chickenpox (children) or sometimes, shingles (any age, especially elderly); see *Fig. 3.186*.

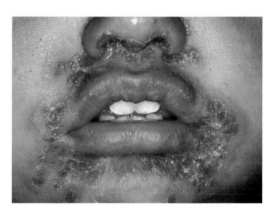

Figure 3.185. Enterovirus 71 infection.

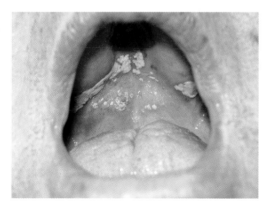

Figure 3.183. Candida albicans infection.

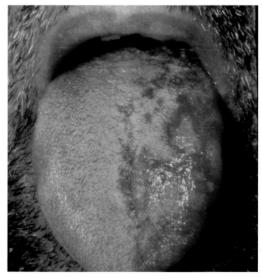

Figure 3.186. Varicella-zoster virus.

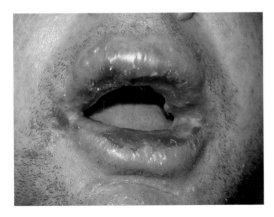

Figure 3.187. SJS/TEN.

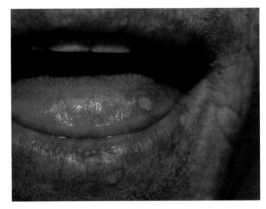

Figure 3.189. Aphthous ulceration.

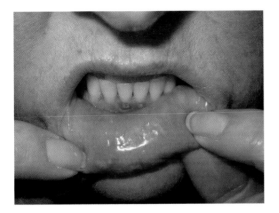

Figure 3.188. Sweet syndrome.

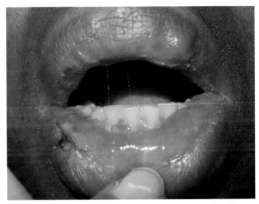

Figure 3.190. Erythema multiforme major.

- Various consequences of human immunodeficiency virus infection.
- Secondary syphilis – snail track ulcers.

ACUTE SINGLE-EPISODE ULCERATION
- Stevens–Johnson/toxic epidermal necrolysis (any age); see *Fig. 3.187*.
- Acute necrotising ulcerative gingivitis.
- Drug-induced stomatitis – e.g. to chemotherapy, low-dose methotrexate (irritant), NSAIDs (lichenoid pattern).
- Acute neutrophilic dermatosis or Sweet syndrome – with papulovesicular plaques, fever, neutrophilia (see *Fig. 3.188*).

RECURRENT/MULTIPLE ULCERS
- Aphthous ulceration (up to 20% children > older age; more common in Caucasians than other races, more common in females than in males); see *Fig. 3.189*.

- Complex aphthosis: almost constant ulcers, oral and genital aphthous ulcers (adolescents, adults).
- Behçet disease – oral and genital aphthous ulcers, ocular inflammation, skin lesions, pathergy and other symptoms and signs due to multisystem vasculitis (adults).
- Contact stomatitis – (adults) e.g. to nicotine (irritant) or rubber (allergy).
- Fixed drug eruption – to topical or oral medicine.
- Erythema multiforme major – associated with herpes simplex virus activation (adolescents, young adults); see *Fig. 3.190*.
- Oral lichen planus – may have cutaneous and mucosal lichen planus at other sites (middle-aged adults); see *Fig. 3.191*.
- Systemic lupus erythematosus (young females); see *Fig. 3.192*.
- Chronic ulcerative stomatitis (middle-aged women).

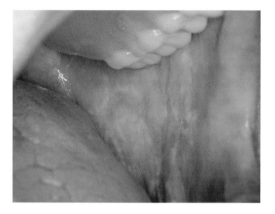

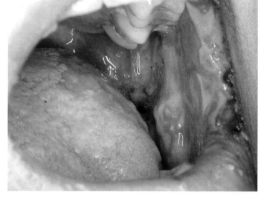

Figure 3.191. Oral lichen planus in mild and more severe form.

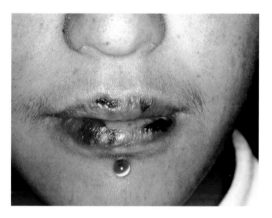

Figure 3.192. Systemic lupus erythematosus.

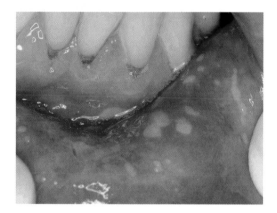

Figure 3.193. Orofacial granulomatosis.

- Orofacial granulomatosis – may have swollen lips and other orofacial features (young adults); see *Fig. 3.193*.
- Immunobullous disease: especially pemphigus, linear IgA bullous dermatosis, mucous membrane pemphigoid – vesicles

that erode/ulcerate, may have cutaneous lesions (adults); see *Fig. 3.194*.

Chronic mouth ulcer

- Trauma, e.g. due to dentures (adults) or chemical injury from aspirin, cocaine.
- Infection: tertiary syphilitic gumma, tuberculosis, aspergillus, histoplasmosis, leishmaniasis.
- Eosinophilic ulcer (children or adults).
- Membranous mucositis due to radiation therapy (see *Fig. 3.195*).
- Necrotising sialometaplasia – an ischaemic event.
- Squamous cell carcinoma: invasive and/ or *in situ* (smokers, chronic inflammatory disease); see *Fig. 3.196*.
- Non-Hodgkin lymphoma.

Differential diagnosis includes other inflammatory disorders in which there is no true ulceration, such as migratory glossitis/ geographic tongue (see *Fig. 3.197*).

What causes aphthous mouth ulcers?

The cause or causes of aphthous mouth ulcers are not well understood. Current thinking is that the immune system is disturbed by some external factor and reacts abnormally against a protein in mucosal tissue.

Although most people with aphthous stomatitis are healthy, it may relate to:

- genetic factors; a strong family history of aphthous stomatitis is common.
- other illness, lack of sleep, being "run down", psychogenic stress.
- trauma from inadvertent bite or brushing teeth.

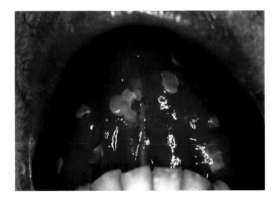

Figure 3.194. Pemphigus.

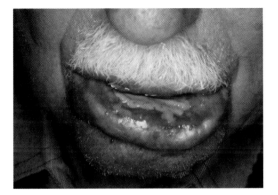

Figure 3.195. Radiation therapy.

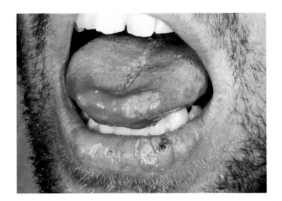

Figure 3.196. SCC.

In some patients, there are additional predisposing factors.
- Hormones: ulcers may recur according to menstrual cycle.
- Micronutritional deficiencies: iron, B12, folate.
- Gluten-sensitive enteropathy.
- Food or food-preservative allergy.
- Nicorandil (drug given for angina).

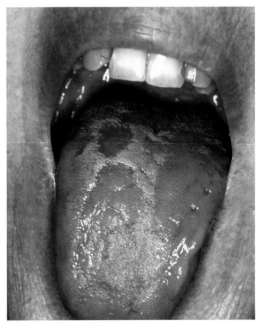

Figure 3.197. Migratory glossitis.

- Inflammatory bowel disease.
- Reiter syndrome.
- Cyclic neutropenia.

What are the clinical features of mouth ulcers?

A patient with mouth ulcers should be questioned and examined with a differential diagnosis in mind. In particular the following questions should be asked:
- Is the ulcer solitary or are there multiple ulcers?
- What part or parts of the mouth are involved?
- Is the patient feeling well or unwell?
- Is this a single episode, or have the ulcers occurred before?
- Does the patient have any underlying condition or disease?
- Does anyone else close to the patient have similar symptoms?

RECURRENT APHTHOUS ULCERATION
Recurrent aphthous ulcers are usually:
- one or many lesions scattered throughout the mouth.
- round or ovoid in shape.
- surrounded by erythematous halo.
- punched-out yellow–grey centre.
- painful, especially on eating or drinking.

Recurrent aphthous ulcers are divided into three types:

- Minor recurrent aphthous ulceration: lesions are <10 mm in diameter and heal within 10–14 days.
- Major recurrent aphthous ulceration (much less common): coalescent or large ulcers with raised margins >10 mm in diameter that take longer to heal; often associated with fever, dysphagia, malaise.
- Herpetiform recurrent aphthous ulceration: this is uncommon, and is characterised by crops of numerous grouped 1–3 mm ulcers on or under the tongue.

Complications of mouth ulcers

Most mouth ulcers heal without problem. Consider biopsy of non-healing ulcers.

- Major aphthous ulcers and Behçet mouth ulcers may heal with scarring.
- Acute ulceration can lead to secondary bacterial infection.
- Chronic ulceration due to oral lichen planus predisposes to oral squamous cell carcinoma (in ~5%).

How are mouth ulcers diagnosed?

Mouth ulcers are diagnosed by taking a careful history and examining the patient. Occasionally biopsy is performed, particularly if considering cancer. It should be taken from the indurated edge of an inflammatory ulcer or from an inflamed but non-ulcerated site.

- Aphthous ulceration has varying and non-specific features.
- Lichen planus and erythema multiforme may show a lichenoid tissue reaction.

If the patient has frequent, prolonged or large ulcers, or is unwell, the following tests may be done to assess general and gastrointestinal health:

- bacterial and viral swabs from the ulcers.
- complete blood cell count.
- iron, B12 and folate.
- coeliac antibodies.
- faecal calprotectin.

Selected patients may undergo further assessment including endoscopy if there is suspicion of inflammatory bowel disease.

If specific toothpaste or food is thought to precipitate ulcers, allergy tests including prick tests, patch tests and specific IgE testing may be performed. The results can be difficult to interpret.

What is the treatment for mouth ulcers?

GENERAL MEASURES

Symptomatic relief may be obtained from:

- avoidance of hard, spicy, salty or acid food.
- avoidance of toothpaste containing sodium lauryl/laureth sulphate.
- antiseptic, anti-inflammatory and analgesic mouthwash or spray.

PAIN RELIEF AND LOCAL TREATMENT

- Choline salicylate gel applied to ulcers (adults only).
- Nd:YAG laser or silver nitrate cautery.
- Topical corticosteroid paste, solution, spray or ointment.
- Topical calcineurin inhibitors: topical pimecrolimus or tacrolimus.

Nicotine-containing gum has been reported to be effective, but it is not recommended because it's highly addictive and has many adverse effects (see smoking, *Section 5.3*).

SYSTEMIC THERAPY

Systemic therapy is intended to reduce frequency of ulceration. A Cochrane review (2012) of systemic treatments for recurrent aphthous stomatitis was inconclusive. The following are reported to be useful in at least some patients:

- tetracycline.
- colchicine.
- dapsone.
- systemic corticosteroids.
- immunomodulatory agents such as azathioprine, methotrexate, ciclosporin.
- tumour necrosis factor (TNF) antagonists (adalimumab, etanercept, infliximab).
- thalidomide (in exceptional cases).

Mouth ulcers are not preventable in all patients. However, some people can reduce the number and severity of their ulcers by ensuring plenty of rest and avoidance of known triggers.

What is the outlook for mouth ulcers?

The outlook depends on the type of mouth ulcers and their cause, if known.

There is a gradual tendency for recurrent aphthous stomatitis to become less severe in later life.

3.14 Panniculitis

What is panniculitis?

Panniculitis refers to a group of conditions that involve inflammation of subcutaneous fat. Despite having very diverse causes, most forms of panniculitis have the same clinical appearance. The diagnosis is established by a skin biopsy as there are characteristic microscopic features depending on the type of panniculitis. The most common form of panniculitis is erythema nodosum, which arises as a reaction to an underlying illness.

Panniculitis is classified as mostly septal panniculitis or mostly lobular panniculitis, depending on the site of the most intense microscopic inflammation. Most types of panniculitis have both lobular and septal inflammation. Further classification is based on whether or not there is subcutaneous vasculitis.

Classification of panniculitis

Mostly septal panniculitis with vasculitis:
- leucocytoclastic vasculitis.
- superficial thrombophlebitis.
- cutaneous polyarteritis nodosa (*Fig. 3.198*).

Mostly septal panniculitis without vasculitis:
- necrobiosis lipoidica (*Fig. 3.199*).
- scleroderma, which may be localised (morphoea); see *Fig. 3.200*.
- subcutaneous granuloma annulare.
- rheumatoid nodule.
- necrobiotic xanthogranuloma.
- erythema nodosum (*Fig. 3.201*).

Mostly lobular panniculitis with vasculitis:
- erythema nodosum leprosum (leprosy).

- Lucio phenomenon.
- neutrophilic lobular panniculitis associated with rheumatoid arthritis.
- erythema induratum of Bazin associated with tuberculosis (*Fig. 3.202*).
- Crohn disease.
- nodular vasculitis.

Mostly lobular panniculitis without vasculitis:
- sclerosing panniculitis (lipodermatosclerosis); see *Fig. 3.203*.
- calciphylaxis (*Fig. 3.204*).
- oxalosis.
- sclerema neonatorum.
- cold panniculitis.
- lupus panniculitis.
- panniculitis in dermatomyositis.
- pancreatic panniculitis.
- alpha-1 antitrypsin deficiency.
- infective panniculitis.
- factitial panniculitis.

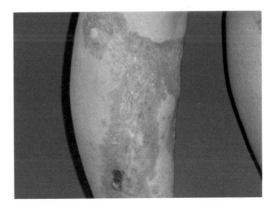

Figure 3.199. Necrobiosis lipoidica.

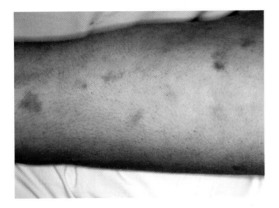

Figure 3.198. Cutaneous polyarteritis nodosa.

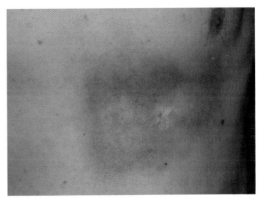

Figure 3.200. Localised scleroderma (morphoea).

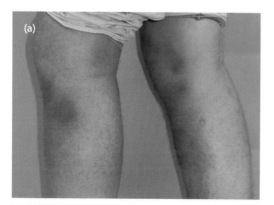

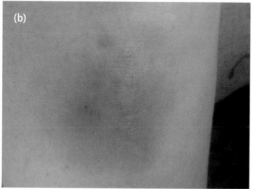

Figure 3.201. Erythema nodosum (a) and close-up of erythema nodosum nodules (b).

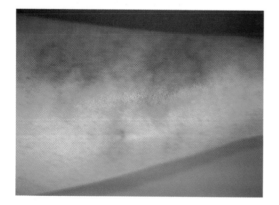

Figure 3.202. Erythema induratum of Brazin in a patient with active tuberculosis.

- subcutaneous sarcoidosis.
- traumatic panniculitis.
- lipoatrophy (Fig. 3.205).
- subcutaneous fat necrosis of the newborn.
- post-steroid panniculitis.
- gout panniculitis.
- crystal-storing panniculitis.

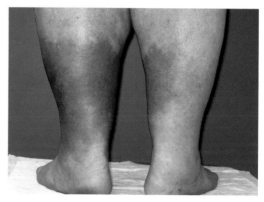

Figure 3.203. Lipodermatosclerosis.

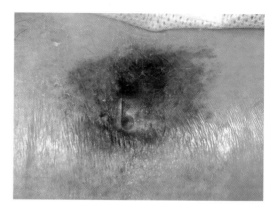

Figure 3.204. Calciphylaxis.

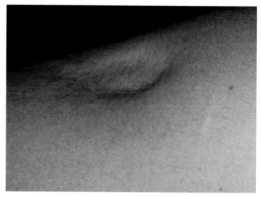

Figure 3.205. Lipoatrophy.

- cytophagic histiocytic panniculitis (Fig. 3.206).
- post-irradiation pseudosclerodermatous panniculitis.
- panniculitis associated with halogenodermas (iodides, bromides).

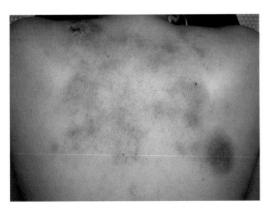

Figure 3.206. Cytophagic histiocytic panniculitis.

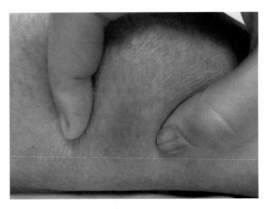

Figure 3.207. Nodules in panniculitis.

What are the clinical features of panniculitis?

Panniculitis presents typically with:
- thickened and firm nodules and plaques (see *Fig. 3.207*).
- erythematous or pigmented overlying skin.
- pain or tenderness.

Sometimes, lesions resolve to leave localised subcutaneous atrophy (lipodystrophy).

ERYTHEMA NODOSUM

Particular features of erythema nodosum (*Fig. 3.201*) are
- peak age group is 20–30 years, mainly females.
- associated in 50% with underlying infection (streptococcus, mycoplasma, tuberculosis and others), sarcoidosis (Löfgren syndrome), inflammatory bowel disease, pregnancy, drugs.
- erythematous nodules are associated with fever, myalgia, arthralgia and malaise.
- the usual duration of an episode is 6–12 weeks but it may relapse or become chronic.

How is panniculitis diagnosed?

Panniculitis is diagnosed by a combination of clinical features, biopsy findings and microbiological culture. Sometimes other investigations are necessary.

Treatment of panniculitis

Treatment of panniculitis includes:
- treat the underlying cause, if known (e.g. stop a medication, treat an infection).
- rest and elevate the affected area.
- compression hosiery (18–25 mmHg pressure) if these can be tolerated.
- pain relief using anti-inflammatory medications such as aspirin, ibuprofen or diclofenac.
- systemic steroids (oral or injected) to settle the inflammation.
- anti-inflammatory antibiotics including tetracycline or hydroxychloroquine.
- potassium iodide.
- surgical removal of persistent or ulcerated lesions.

3.15 Periorificial dermatitis

What is periorificial dermatitis?

Periorificial dermatitis is a common facial skin problem characterised by groups of itchy or tender small red papules. It is given this name because the papules occur around the eyes, the nostrils, the mouth and, occasionally, the genitals.

The more restrictive term, perioral dermatitis, is often used when the eruption is confined to the skin in the lower half of the face, particularly around the mouth. Periocular dermatitis may be used to describe the rash affecting the eyelids.

Who gets periorificial dermatitis?

Periorificial dermatitis and its variants mainly affect adult women aged 15–45 years. It is less common in men. It may affect children of any age. People with periorificial dermatitis are often using topical or inhaled corticosteroids.

What is the cause of periorificial dermatitis?

The exact cause of periorificial dermatitis is not understood. Periorificial dermatitis may be related to:
- epidermal barrier dysfunction.
- altered cutaneous microflora.
- fusiform bacteria.

Unlike seborrhoeic dermatitis, which can affect similar areas of the face, malassezia yeasts are not involved in periorificial dermatitis.

Periorificial dermatitis is thought to be a variant of rosacea, which is now known to be due to a complex activation of the innate immune system. Patients who are susceptible to periorificial dermatitis tend to have an oily face, at least in the affected areas.

Periorificial dermatitis may be induced by:

- topical steroids, whether applied deliberately to facial skin or inadvertently.
- nasal steroids, steroid inhalers, and oral steroids.
- cosmetic creams, make-up and sunscreens.
- fluorinated toothpaste.
- neglecting to wash the face.
- hormonal changes and/or oral contraceptives.

What are the clinical features of periorificial dermatitis?

The characteristics of facial periorificial dermatitis are (see *Fig. 3.208*):
- unilateral or bilateral eruption on chin, upper lip and eyelids in perioral, perinasal and periocular distribution.
- sparing of the skin bordering the lips (which then appears pale), eyelids, nostrils.
- clusters of 1–2 mm erythematous papules or papulopustules.
- dry and flaky skin surface.
- burning irritation.

In contrast to steroid-induced rosacea, periorificial dermatitis spares the cheeks and forehead.

Genital periorificial dermatitis has a similar clinical appearance. It involves the skin on and around labia majora (in females), scrotum (in males) and anus.

Complications of periorificial dermatitis

Granulomatous periorificial dermatitis is a variant of periorificial dermatitis that presents with persistent yellowish papules. It occurs mainly in young children and nearly always follows the use of a corticosteroid. There is granulomatous perifollicular infiltrate on histopathology.

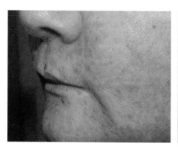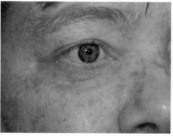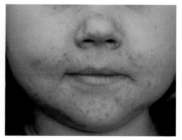

Figure 3.208. Periorificial dermatitis on chin and eyelids, but sparing the cheeks.

Steroid rosacea presents with steroid-induced large facial papules, papulopustules and telangiectasia on the mid-face, including forehead and cheeks.

Rebound flare of severe periorificial dermatitis may occur after abrupt cessation of application of potent topical corticosteroid to facial skin.

How is periorificial dermatitis diagnosed?

The presentation of periorificial dermatitis is usually typical, so clinical diagnosis is usually straightforward. There are no specific tests.

Skin biopsy shows follicular and perivascular chronic inflammation similar to rosacea.

What is the treatment for periorificial dermatitis?

Periorificial dermatitis responds well to treatment, although it may take several weeks before there is noticeable improvement.

GENERAL MEASURES
- Discontinue applying all face creams including topical steroids, cosmetics and sunscreens (zero therapy).
- Consider a slower withdrawal from topical steroid/face cream if there is a severe flare after steroid cessation. Temporarily, replace it with a less potent or less occlusive cream or apply it less and less frequently until it is no longer required.
- Wash the face with warm water alone while the rash is present. When it has cleared up, a non-soap bar or liquid cleanser can be used if desired.
- Choose a liquid or gel sunscreen.

TOPICAL THERAPY
Topical therapy is used to treat mild periorificial dermatitis. Choices include:
- erythromycin.
- clindamycin.
- metronidazole.
- pimecrolimus.
- azelaic acid.

ORAL THERAPY
In more severe cases, a course of oral antibiotics may be prescribed for 6–12 weeks.
- Most often, a tetracycline such as doxycycline is recommended. Sub-antimicrobial dose may be sufficient.
- Oral erythromycin is used during pregnancy and in pre-pubertal children.
- Oral low-dose isotretinoin may be used if antibiotics are ineffective or contraindicated.

How can periorificial dermatitis be prevented?

Periorificial dermatitis can generally be prevented by the avoidance of topical steroids and occlusive face creams. When topical steroids are necessary to treat an inflammatory facial rash, they should be applied accurately to the affected area, no more than once daily in the lowest effective potency, and discontinued as soon as the rash responds.

What is the outlook for periorificial dermatitis?

Periorificial dermatitis sometimes recurs when the antibiotics are discontinued, or at a later date. The same treatment can be used again.

3.16 Photosensitivity

What is photosensitivity?

Photosensitivity refers to various symptoms, diseases and conditions caused or aggravated by exposure to sunlight.

- A rash due to photosensitivity is a photodermatosis (plural photodermatoses).
- If the rash is eczematous, it is a photodermatitis.
- A chemical or drug that causes photosensitivity is a photosensitiser.
- A phototoxic reaction to a photosensitiser results in an exaggerated sunburn reaction and no immune reaction is involved.
- A photoallergic reaction to a photosensitiser results in photodermatitis and is due to delayed hypersensitivity reaction.
- A photoexacerbated condition describes a flare of an underlying skin disease on exposure to sunlight.

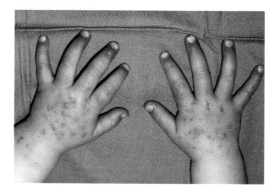

Figure 3.209. Polymorphic light eruption.

Who gets photosensitivity?

Photosensitivity occurs in males and females of all races and at all ages. Different types of photosensitivity may be prevalent at different times of life. Genetic and environmental factors are involved.

People with very white skin who don't tan on exposure to the sun (Fitzpatrick skin type 1), especially if they also have red hair and blue eyes, are often considered photosensitive, relative to people with darker skin types that tan more easily. These fair-skinned individuals do not have a photodermatosis.

Classification of photosensitivity

Photosensitivity is classified into the following groups:

PRIMARY PHOTODERMATOSES

The causes of primary or idiopathic photodermatoses have not yet been discovered. Exposure to the sun produces a clearly defined disease entity. These include:

- polymorphic light eruption (*Fig. 3.209*).
- juvenile spring eruption.
- actinic prurigo (*Fig. 3.210*).
- solar urticaria (*Fig. 3.211*).
- chronic actinic/photosensitivity dermatitis (*Fig. 3.212*).
- hydroa vacciniforme (associated with Epstein–Barr virus).
- pseudoporphyria (induced by drugs and/or renal insufficiency), see *Fig. 3.213*.

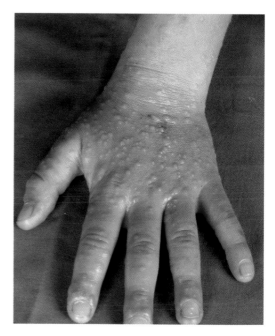

Figure 3.210. Actinic prurigo.

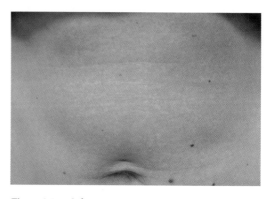

Figure 3.211. Solar urticaria.

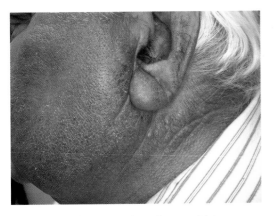

Figure 3.212. Chronic actinic or photosensitivity dermatitis.

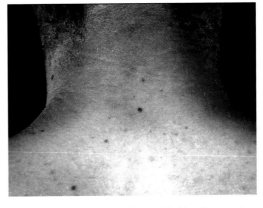

Figure 3.215. Photocontact dermatitis, showing reaction to creosote.

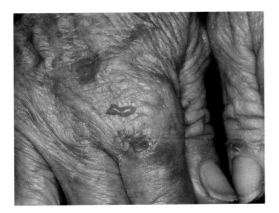

Figure 3.213. Pseudoporphyria induced by naproxen.

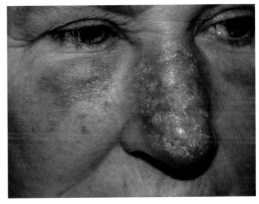

Figure 3.216. Cutaneous LE.

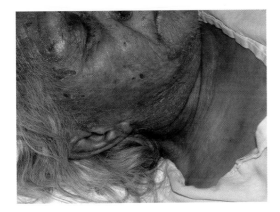

Figure 3.214. Drug-induced photosensitivity.

EXOGENOUS PHOTODERMATOSES

Exogenous photodermatoses are those in which phototoxic or photoallergic reaction is caused by an external photosensitiser. These include:

- drug-induced photosensitivity – common photosensitising drugs are thiazides, tetracyclines, non-steroidal anti-inflammatory drugs (NSAIDs), phenothiazines, voriconazole and quinine (see *Fig. 3.214*). There are many others.
- photocontact dermatitis – due to phototoxic chemicals such as psoralens in plants, vegetables, fruit; fragrances in cosmetics; sunscreen chemicals; dyes and disinfectants (see *Fig. 3.215*).

PHOTOEXACERBATED DERMATOSES

Photoexacerbated dermatoses include:
- cutaneous lupus erythematosus (*Fig. 3.216*).
- dermatomyositis.
- Darier disease.
- rosacea.
- pemphigus vulgaris.
- pemphigus foliaceus.
- atopic dermatitis (*Fig. 3.217*).
- psoriasis.

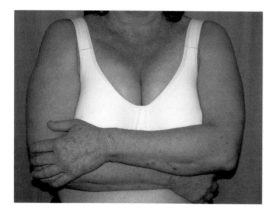

Figure 3.217. Photoaggravated atopic eczema.

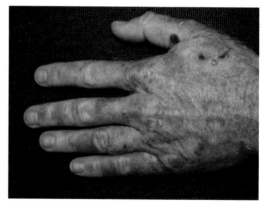

Figure 3.218. Porphyria cutanea tarda.

METABOLIC PHOTODERMATOSES

Photosensitivity can be caused by a metabolic defect. The most common disorders of this type are porphyrias, in which phototoxic porphyrins accumulate in the skin. There are genetic defects in various enzymes, and the diseases may be activated by exposure to certain medications or toxins. Clinical presentation depends on which enzyme is defective.

- Porphyria cutanea tarda (*Fig. 3.218*).
- Erythropoietic protoporphyria.
- Variegate porphyria.
- Erythropoietic porphyria (Gunther disease).

GENETIC PHOTODERMATOSES

Photosensitivity can be associated with a pre-existing genetic disorder. These are rare.

- Xeroderma pigmentosum.
- Bloom syndrome.
- Rothmund–Thomson syndrome.
- Cockayne syndrome.

What causes photosensitivity?

The electromagnetic spectrum of sunlight ranges from short invisible light rays called ultraviolet radiation (UVR), through visible light to infrared, microwaves and radiowaves. UVR has three portions:

- UVB (ultrashort wavelength rays 200–290 nm that do not reach the earth's surface).
- UVB (short wavelength rays 290–320 nm that cause sunburn and tan).
- UVA (longer wavelength rays 320–400 nm that cause tanning and also suppress immune reactions in the skin).

Patients can be sensitive to one kind of sunlight (i.e. only to UVB, UVA or visible light) or to a wider range of radiation. The most common photosensitivity is to UVA. Properties of UVA include:

- present throughout the year, but there is more UVA during summer.
- present throughout the day, but UVA is maximal around the solar noon.
- UVA is of lower energy than UVB, thus, photon for photon, less damaging to DNA in skin cells.
- UVA is, however, 100 times more prevalent at the earth's surface than UVB.
- UVA can penetrate through the epidermis into the dermis, thus damages more deeply than UVB.
- UVA can penetrate untreated and untinted glass.
- UVA is blocked by polycarbonate and densely woven fabric.

Porphyria is mainly triggered by exposure to visible light.

What are the clinical features of photosensitivity?

The clinical features depend on the specific photodermatosis. In general, photodermatoses:

- affect areas exposed to sunlight (face, neck, hands) and do not affect areas not exposed to the light (covered at least by underwear), or are less severe in covered areas.
- sometimes spare areas that are habitually exposed to the light, e.g. the face in polymorphic light eruption.
- sometimes only affect certain parts of the body, e.g. juvenile spring eruption is confined to the tops of the ears.
- may also occur following indoor exposure to artificial sources of UVR or visible radiation.

Rashes on exposed sites may be due to another cause. For example:

- facial acne.
- contact dermatitis due to make-up applied to the face.
- airborne contact dermatitis due to plant pollens.

Clues to photosensitivity include:

- summer exacerbation; note that many photodermatoses are present year round.
- sharp cut-off between affected area and skin covered by clothing or jewellery (e.g. watch strap, ring).
- sparing of folds of upper eyelids.
- sparing of deep furrows on face and neck.
- sparing of skin covered by hair.
- sparing of skin shadowed by the ears, under the nose and under the chin.
- sparing of the web spaces between the fingers.

Complications of photosensitivity

Severe photosensitivity can lead to a person being unable to go outdoors during the day unless completely covered (including face). This leads to social isolation and depression.

How is photosensitivity diagnosed?

Photosensitivity is diagnosed by the history of a skin problem arising on exposure to sunlight. The specific type is determined by examination of the skin and specific tests.

Photosensitivity is sometimes confirmed by phototests – artificial light from various different sources and at different doses is shone on small areas of the skin to see whether the rash can be reproduced, or if sunburn occurs more easily than expected. These tests can be difficult to perform and to interpret, and are only available in specialised centres.

Contact photosensitivity can be tested by photopatch tests. Adhesive patches containing known photosensitising materials are applied to the upper back, removed after two days, and light is shone on the area. The reaction is observed two days later.

Tests may include:

- full blood count.
- connective tissue antibodies including antinuclear antibodies (ANA) and extractable nuclear antigens (ENA).
- porphyrins in blood, urine and faeces.

Patients suspected of porphyria cutanea tarda may also have liver function and iron tests.

What is the treatment for photosensitivity?

Management of photosensitivity involves sun protection and treatment of the underlying disorder.

How can photosensitivity reactions be prevented?

Photosensitivity is mainly prevented by careful protection from sun exposure and avoidance of exposure to artificial sources of UVR. However, the following should be noted.

- The degree of protection needed from UVR depends on the severity of the disorder and the geographic location of the patient.
- Protection from UVR is not effective for porphyria. Affected areas must be covered when outdoors.
- Graduated exposure to small amounts of UVR may reduce sun-induced reactions in polymorphous light eruption.

PROTECTION FROM UVR

When considering sun protective measures, observe the following.

- Take note of the time of year and time of day. UVR is greater when the sun is overhead.
- Find out local ultraviolet levels from meteorological services. Smartphone apps provide geolocation and time-specific sun protection guidance. In New Zealand, Sun Alert reports from NIWA's National Climate Database indicate the hours when the UV index (UVI) is over 3 and therefore significant.
- Note that the temperature and to some extent weather conditions make little difference to environmental UV.
- Be aware of greater UVR at altitude, and when reflected by bright surfaces such as snow, concrete and sand.
- Do not rely on shade from tree, umbrella or sail. UVR is scattered by dust particles, meaning they may provide only partial protection.
- Watch out for a small amount of UVR released from some unguarded fluorescent daylight lamps.

Sunscreens are essential.

- Sunscreens often fail to completely prevent photodermatoses.
- Sunscreens are best at filtering out UVB. To be most effective, they need to be applied thickly and frequently to all exposed skin.

- Select a sunscreen with a very high Sun Protection Factor (SPF 50+), which is a water resistant and broad-spectrum product that complies with current standards.
- Sunscreens containing reflectants such as zinc may be more effective than pure chemical sunscreens, as they filter out more UVA. They can be messy to use and cosmetically unappealing.
- Contact photodermatitis to sunscreen chemicals can occur uncommonly, particularly to benzophenone or butyl methoxy dibenzoylmethane, and in the past, para-aminobenzoic acid (PABA).

Patients with photodermatoses also may need to:
- take vitamin D supplements.
- confine summer excursions out of doors to early in the morning or late in the evening.
- cover up, wearing shirts with high collar and long sleeves, trousers or a long skirt, socks and shoes, a wide-brimmed hat, and if possible gloves.
- wear opaque sun protective clothing (dark coloured and densely woven fabric is the most effective); some clothes are now labelled with UPF, the sun protection factor for fabrics – choose those with a UPF of 40+
- protect their skin indoors and when in a vehicle.
- apply UVR-absorbing film to windows at home or in the car.
- wear a clear plastic mask to protect the face.

Oral antioxidants such as polyphenols have been reported to provide limited extra protection, particularly nicotinamide, *Polypodium leucotomos* extract and carotenoids.

What is the outlook for photosensitivity?

The prognosis depends on the specific disorder, its treatment, where the patient lives, and how carefully they protect their skin from exposure to sunlight.

For the most acutely light sensitive patients, normal activities may be severely curtailed. Some find night work and sleep during the day, others put up with the rash.

3.17 Polymorphic light eruption

What is polymorphic light eruption?

Polymorphic light eruption is a common form of primary photosensitivity that mainly occurs in young adult women in temperate climates during spring and summer.

The name 'polymorphic' refers to the fact that the rash can take many forms, although in one individual it usually looks the same every time it appears.

Polymorphic light eruption is also known as polymorphous light eruption, PLE or PMLE.

Who gets polymorphic light eruption?

PLE generally affects adult females aged 20–40, although it sometimes affects children and males (25%). It is particularly common in places where sun exposure is uncommon, such as Northern Europe, where it is said to affect 10–20% of women holidaying in the Mediterranean area. It is less common in Australasia. It has also been reported to be relatively common at higher altitudes compared to sea level.

PLE can occur in all races and skin phototypes and may be more prevalent in skin of colour than in white skin. There is a genetic tendency to PLE, and it is sometimes associated with or confused with photosensitivity due to lupus erythematosus (which generally is more persistent than PLE).

Some patients experience PLE during phototherapy, which is used to treat skin conditions such as psoriasis and dermatitis.

What causes polymorphic light eruption?

Genetic factors may be important with many affected individuals reporting a family history of PLE. Native Americans have a hereditary form of PLE (actinic prurigo).

PLE is caused by a delayed hypersensitivity reaction to a compound in the skin that is altered by exposure to ultraviolet radiation (UVR). UVR leads to impaired T cell function and altered production of cytokines in affected individuals. There is a reduction in the normal UV-induced immune suppression in the skin. This has been suggested to be either due to oestrogen or deficiency of vitamin D.

The rash is usually provoked by UVA (in 90%). This means the rash can occur when the sunlight is coming through window glass, and that standard sunscreens may not prevent it. Occasionally, UVB and/or visible light provoke PLE.

What are the clinical features of polymorphic light eruption?

PLE may be a rare occurrence in the individual concerned or may occur every time the skin is exposed to sunlight. In most affected individuals, it occurs each spring, provoked by several hours outside on a sunny day. If further sun exposure is avoided, the rash settles in a few days and is gone without a trace within a couple of weeks. It may or may not recur next time the sun shines on the skin. However, if the affected area is exposed to more sun before it has cleared up, the condition tends to get more severe and extensive.

The arms, the back of the hands, the V of the neck, the chest and lower legs/feet, may be affected, but the face is usually spared (*Fig. 3.219*). A few people complain of ocular and/or lip lesions. Juvenile spring eruption is a variant of PLE that is confined to the ears of children (usually boys).

The commonest variety of PLE presents as crops of 2–5 mm pink or red papules on the arms. Other presentations include:

- erythema (red macules).
- erythematous plaques.
- dry, red patches or plaques (dermatitis).
- vesicles (blisters).
- pinpoint papules (especially in skin of colour).
- lichenoid plaques.
- target lesions (bullseye appearance).
- prurigo confined to exposed areas.

PLE persists for several days, and often longer if the affected skin is exposed to more sunlight. It resolves without scarring. PLE usually causes a burning sensation or itch. A few individuals also report fever and malaise following sun exposure.

PLE can be the first sign of lupus erythematosus, but this is not usually the case.

Complications from polymorphic light eruption

Severe PLE can lead to emotional distress, anxiety and depression.

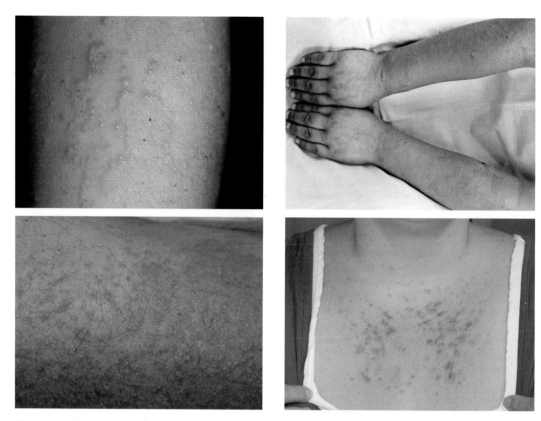

Figure 3.219. Polymorphic light eruption on arm, hands, leg and chest.

How is polymorphic light eruption diagnosed?

PLE is diagnosed clinically by its typical onset within hours of exposure to sunlight, and clearance after a few days. The rash is confined to exposed sites, and is often composed of erythematous papules and plaques.

Sometimes a skin biopsy is necessary to make a diagnosis. PLE has characteristic histopathological features, with upper dermal oedema and a dense perivascular lymphocytic infiltrate. Eczematous changes may be present. Direct immune fluorescence is negative, unless the patient has cutaneous lupus erythematosus.

It is usual to have a blood count and a check for circulating antinuclear antibodies (ANA) and extractable nuclear antigens (ENA) in case of photosensitive intermittent cutaneous lupus erythematosus.

Phototesting is not usually carried out, but provocation tests of exposure to UVA daily for 3 days to a small area of skin can confirm the diagnosis.

How can polymorphic light eruption be prevented?

It is not known how to prevent PLE altogether. However, many people can avoid developing a rash by using effective sun protection during the middle hours of the day during summer. In New Zealand, patients are advised to dress appropriately during the hours indicated by NIWA's National Climate Database regional Sun Protection Alert, when the UV index is >3. Elsewhere, local meteorological services or a smartphone app can provide geolocation and time-specific UVI reports.

- Cover affected areas with densely woven sun protective clothing. Choose UPF 40+ clothing where available.
- Apply SPF 50+ semi-opaque sunscreen frequently to all uncovered skin.
- Stay in the shade.
- Many patients find antioxidant nutritional supplements somewhat helpful. These include nicotinamide, *Polypodium leucotomos* extract, and the carotenes, beta carotene, astaxathanin and canthaxanthin.

Some people with PLE successfully manage to gradually harden their skin by slowly increasing how long they spend outdoors with uncovered skin, starting with a few minutes' exposure during spring.

What is the treatment for polymorphic light eruption?

The following treatments may reduce the severity of PLE:

- topical corticosteroid creams to relieve symptoms.
- short course of oral steroids, e.g. to cover a summer holiday.
- hydroxychloroquine.
- phototherapy – narrowband UVB, or PUVA for several weeks in early spring.

What is the outlook for polymorphic light eruption?

In most individuals, there is a hardening as the summer progresses and more sun can be tolerated without a rash appearing. This does not always occur, and some very sensitive individuals even develop PLE in the winter.

It has been noted that PLE appears to be less frequent and severe in women after the menopause.

3.18 Pruritus vulvae/vulval itch

What is the vulva?

The vulva, or external genitalia of the female, includes the mons pubis, labia majora (outer lips), labia minora (inner lips), clitoris, perineum (tissue between vagina and anus) and the external openings of the urethra and vagina.

Itching often affects the vulva. The sensation of itch in this site is also referred to as pruritus vulvae. Pruritus vulvae should be distinguished from vulval pain and from vulvodynia, which refers to chronic burning symptoms in the absence of clinical signs. Vulval itch, pain and/or burning can co-exist.

Who gets an itchy vulva?

Girls and women of any age and race can experience mild, moderate or severe vulval itch, which can be intermittent or continuous. There are a number of diseases and conditions that may be responsible.

What causes an itchy vulva?

One or more specific conditions may be the cause of vulval itch.

ITCH DUE TO INFECTIONS

Candida albicans infection (vulvovaginal thrush) is the most important microorganism to consider in a post-pubertal woman with vulval itch (*Fig. 3.220*). Candida can be a cause of napkin dermatitis in babies. Post-menopausal women are unlikely to have *Candida albicans* infection, unless they are diabetic, being treated with oestrogen or antibiotics, or the infection is secondary to an underlying skin disease.

There are several less common infections that may cause vulval itch.

- Bacterial vaginosis causes a frothy, malodorous discharge, and causes vulval itch or stinging, possibly as a result of a contact dermatitis.
- Genital viral warts are often itchy (see *Fig. 3.221*).
- Pinworms can reside in the vagina or anus and cause itch when they exit at night.
- Infections that rarely cause vulval itch include cytolytic vaginosis (associated with vaginal lactobacilli) and trichomoniasis.

ITCH DUE TO AN INFLAMMATORY SKIN CONDITION

Irritant contact dermatitis is the most common cause of an itchy vulva at all ages. It can be acute, relapsing or chronic. It may be due to diverse causes (see *Figs 3.222* and *3.223*), including:

- age-related pre-pubertal or post-menopausal lack of oestrogen (see *Fig. 3.224*).
- underlying tendency to atopic dermatitis.
- scratching for another reason.
- friction from skin folds, clothing, activity, or sexual intercourse.
- moisture due to occlusive underwear.
- urine and/or faeces.

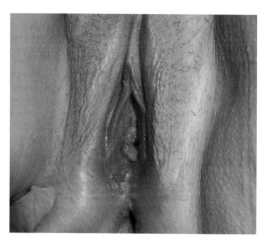

Figure 3.220. Vulval itch due to *Candida albicans* infection.

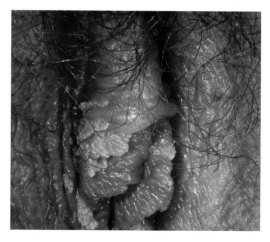

Figure 3.221. Genital viral warts.

- soap or harsh cleanser.
- frequent washing.
- inappropriate or unnecessary chemical applications, including over-the-counter or prescribed medications.
- fissuring of the posterior fourchette.
- normal, excessive or infected vaginal secretions.

Severe vulval itch may be due to:
- lichen simplex, see *Fig. 3.225.*
- lichen sclerosus, see *Fig. 3.226.*
- lichen planus, which can also be very painful when erosive, see *Fig. 3.227.*

Other common skin disorders that may cause vulval itch include:
- psoriasis (*Fig. 3.228*).
- seborrhoeic dermatitis (*Fig. 3.229*).
- allergic contact dermatitis*
- irritant or allergic contact urticaria.
- dermographism.

- folliculitis (*Fig. 3.230*).

*Potential vulval allergens include:
- methylisothiazolone, a preservative in moist wipes.
- various textile dyes in underwear (see *Fig. 3.231*).
- fragrance in a douche or antiperspirant.
- rubber in condom, menstrual cup or underwear.

Latex rubber and semen are potential causes of contact urticaria.

ITCH DUE TO NEOPLASIA

Benign and malignant neoplastic disorders of the vulva are often asymptomatic in their early stages, but they can cause itch. The most common cancerous lesions are:
- squamous intraepithelial lesions (also known as vulval intraepithelial neoplasia or VIN); see *Fig. 3.232.*

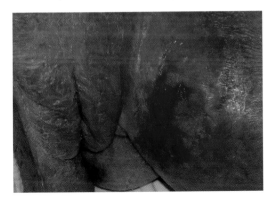

Figure 3.222. Severe irritant contact dermatitis due to chronic urinary incontinence.

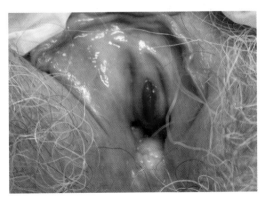

Figure 3.224. Pale vulva with urethral caruncle typical of post-menopausal lack of oestrogen.

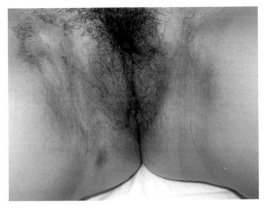

Figure 3.223. Contact irritant dermatitis due to inadequately rinsed underwear.

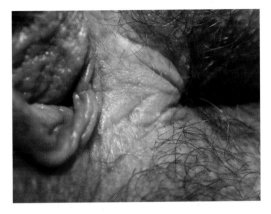

Figure 3.225. Lichen simplex.

- extramammary Paget disease (*Fig. 3.233*).
- invasive squamous cell carcinoma (*Fig. 3.234*).

ITCH DUE TO NEUROPATHY

Neuropathy should be considered if there are no signs of infection or skin disease apart from lichen simplex – which can be secondary to neuropathy – especially if vulvodynia is present. The neuropathy may be caused by injury, surgery or disease locally, within the pelvis or in the spine.

What are the clinical features of an itchy vulva?

The clinical features depend on the underlying cause of the vulval itch. There may be an obvious or subtle rash, or no signs of disease at all.

When assessing the cause, it is important to determine the precise location of the symptoms. Itch often only affects one anatomic part of the vulva:

- convex areas and thighs – irritant contact dermatitis due to urinary incontinence (symmetrical) or rarely, allergic contact dermatitis e.g. to preservative (asymmetrical).
- flexures – seborrhoeic dermatitis, non-specific/candida intertrigo irritation by underwear.
- mons pubis – seborrhoeic dermatitis, folliculitis.
- labia majora – psoriasis, atopic dermatitis, lichen simplex (unilateral or bilateral).
- labia minora – lichen sclerosus, lichen planus.
- vaginal introitus – erosive lichen planus, atrophic vulvovaginitis, vaginal discharge or infection.
- perineum – dermatitis, lichen sclerosus.
- any site – neoplasia.

The itch can also involve other adjacent skin of the abdomen, thighs and perianal area.

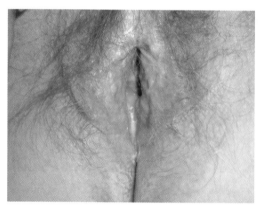

Figure 3.226. Lichen sclerosus.

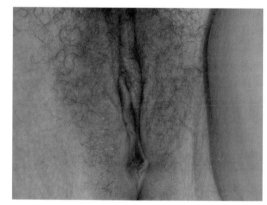

Figure 3.228. Psoriasis.

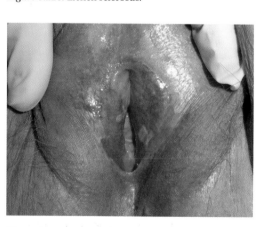

Figure 3.227. Erosive lichen planus.

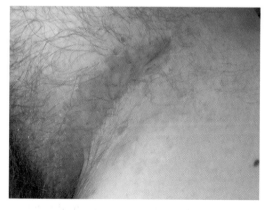

Figure 3.229. Seborrhoeic dermatitis.

Examination may reveal apparently normal skin, scratch marks (excoriations) and the specific features associated with the underlying cause of the itch.

Morphology may be modified according to the site, with minimal scale evident.

- *Candida albicans* causes thick white vaginal discharge, erythema, oedema and/or satellite red superficial papules, pustules, desquamation and erosions. See *Section 2.2.2.*
- Candida can also cause subtle fissuring and subclinical dermatitis.
- Viral warts are clustered as soft condylomata. See *Section 2.3.2.*
- Acute irritant contact dermatitis may be shiny, waxy or scald-like. See *Section 3.6.4.*
- Psoriasis has symmetrical circumscribed erythematous plaques, but they are rarely scaly. See *Section 3.19.*
- Seborrhoeic dermatitis presents with salmon-pink, poorly defined patches, sometimes with mild exfoliation. See *Section 3.6.12.*

- Allergic contact dermatitis can have varied morphology, but tends to be asymmetrical, intermittent. See *Section 3.6.4.*
- Lichen simplex presents as confluent thickened papules with broken-off hairs. See *Section 3.6.8.*
- Lichen sclerosus typically has white plaques, ecchymoses and erosions. See *Section 3.12.*
- Lichen planus may present as violaceous or hyperpigmented papules with reticulated white network (thighs). It may appear similar to lichen sclerosus, or cause tender well-defined red patches and erosions (introitus/vagina). See *Section 3.6.11.*
- Neoplasia should be considered if there is a solitary plaque with irregular shape, structure, surface and colour. Firm or hard consistency and/or ulceration and bleeding are particularly concerning.

Complications of an itchy vulva

An itchy vulva can result in a lot of psychological distress and sleeplessness. Scratching injures

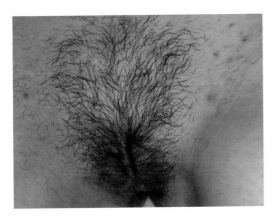

Figure 3.230. Folliculitis following waxing.

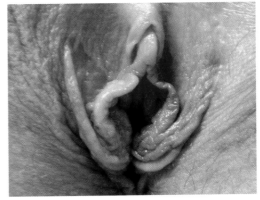

Figure 3.232. Vulval intraepithelial neoplasia (VIN).

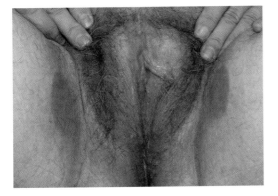

Figure 3.231. Contact allergic eczema caused by dye in underwear.

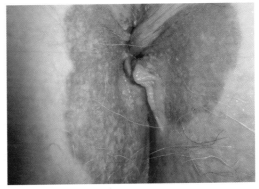

Figure 3.233. Perianal extramammary Paget disease.

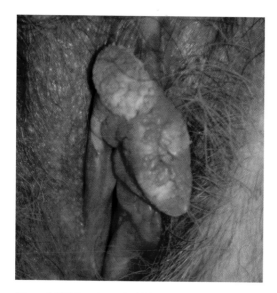

Figure 3.234. Invasive vulval SCC.

the skin, which can lead to pain and secondary bacterial infection.

Erosive lichen planus can also cause significant pain/soreness as well as itch.

How is the cause of an itchy vulva diagnosed?

The cause or causes of an itchy vulva may be diagnosed through careful history (include genitourinary and musculoskeletal systems) and examination.

A full skin examination may reveal a skin condition or disease in another site that gives a clue to why the vulva is itchy.

Swabs of the affected area and of the vagina may be taken for microbiological examination.

Skin biopsy of the area affected by itch or visible skin condition may be necessary to determine its exact nature. Sometimes several biopsies may be taken.

Patch tests are sometimes performed to see whether any contact allergy is present, such as to a fragrance, medicament or other material.

What is the treatment for pruritus vulvae?

The conditions causing an itchy vulva often require specific treatment. For example:
- antifungal, antibacterial or antiviral medications for infection.
- topical steroids or calcineurin inhibitors for inflammatory disease.
- oral antihistamines for contact urticaria.
- surgery for neoplasia.
- tricyclic antidepressants, serotonin reuptake agents, and anticonvulsants for neuropathic symptoms.

NON-SPECIFIC TREATMENT
- Minimise scratching or rubbing the affected area.
- Wear loose-fitting absorbent underwear and outer clothing.
- Avoid occlusive nylon such as tights (pantyhose).
- Select modern absorbent underwear.
- Keep cool, especially at night-time.
- Apply emollients (e.g. sorbolene, cetomacrogol cream) and barrier preparations (e.g. petroleum jelly).
- Hydrocortisone cream can be used safely and purchased without prescription.

Contact dermatitis occurs quite readily when inflamed skin affects the genital area.
- Wash once or twice daily with lukewarm water alone or use a soap-free cleanser.
- Do not use leave-on moist wipes, antiperspirants or other cosmetics in the vulva.
- Insert tampons with care or use reusable silicone menstrual cups.
- Change sanitary pads, pantiliners and/or incontinence products frequently.
- Avoid riding bicycles or horses.

Tricyclic antidepressants may be prescribed to control intractable itch, even in the absence of a defined neuropathy.

How can vulval itch be prevented?

Vulval itch cannot always be prevented, depending on its cause. However, vulval health is optimised by the non-specific measures described above.

What is the outlook for vulval itch?

Vulval itch is usually a minor, short-lived nuisance. However, some women may suffer from vulval itch for years, and may only receive temporary relief from treatment.

3.19 Psoriasis

3.19.1 Psoriasis – general

What is psoriasis?

Psoriasis is a chronic inflammatory skin condition characterised by well-circumscribed, erythematous and scaly plaques. It is classified into several subtypes and by severity.

Who gets psoriasis?

Psoriasis affects 2–4% of males and females. It can start at any age, with bimodal peaks of onset at 15–25 years and 50–60 years. It tends to persist lifelong, fluctuating in extent and severity. It is particularly common in Caucasians, but may affect people of any race. About one third of patients with psoriasis have family members with psoriasis.

What causes psoriasis?

Psoriasis is multifactorial. It is classified as an immune-mediated inflammatory disease.

Genetic factors are important; at least 36 psoriasis susceptibility loci have been identified in Caucasians. An individual's genetic profile influences the phenotypic features of their psoriasis and its response to treatment.

Genome-wide association studies report that HLA-Cw6 is associated with early onset psoriasis and guttate psoriasis. This major histocompatibility complex is not associated with arthritis, nail dystrophy or late onset psoriasis.

Theories of pathogenesis need to explain vascularity, inflammation and keratinocyte proliferation. It is clear that immune factors and inflammatory cytokines such is IL1β and TNF-α are responsible for the clinical features of psoriasis. Current theories are exploring the TH17 pathway and release of the cytokine IL17A.

What are the clinical features of psoriasis?

Psoriasis usually presents with symmetrically distributed, red, scaly plaques with well-defined edges (*Fig. 3.235*). The scale is typically silvery white, except in skin folds where the plaques often appear shiny and they may have a moist peeling surface. The most common sites are scalp, elbows and knees, but any part of the skin can be involved. The plaques are usually very persistent without treatment.

Itch is mostly mild but may be severe in some patients, leading to excoriations, eczematisation (oozing, crusting), and lichenification (thickened leathery skin with increased skin markings). Painful fissuring may occur.

When psoriatic plaques resolve, post-inflammatory hypopigmentation or hyperpigmentation may be noted. These can be expected to fade over several months.

How is psoriasis classified?

Certain features of psoriasis can be categorised (see *Table 3.2*) to help determine appropriate investigations and treatment pathways. Overlap may occur.

TYPES OF PSORIASIS

Typical patterns of psoriasis are shown in *Table 3.3*.

Generalised pustulosis and localised palmoplantar pustulosis are no longer classified within the psoriasis spectrum.

AGGRAVATING FACTORS

- Streptococcal tonsillitis and other infections.
- Injuries such as cuts, abrasions, sunburn (Koebner psoriasis).
- Sun exposure in 10% (sun exposure is more often beneficial).
- Obesity.
- Smoking.
- Excessive alcohol.
- Stressful event.
- Medications such as lithium, beta-blockers, anti-malarials, non-steroidal anti-inflammatories.
- Stopping oral or strong topical corticosteroids.

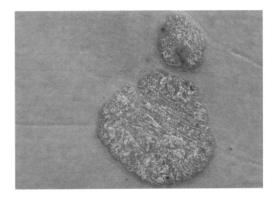

Figure 3.235. Psoriasis.

Comorbidities associated with psoriasis

- Inflammatory arthritis, "psoriatic arthritis" and spondyloarthropathy (in up to 40% of patients with early onset chronic plaque psoriasis).
- Inflammatory bowel disease (Crohn disease and ulcerative colitis).

Table 3.2. Features used to classify psoriasis.

Early age of onset <35 years (75%)	Late age of onset >50 years
Acute, e.g. guttate psoriasis	Chronic plaque psoriasis
Localised, e.g. scalp, palmoplantar	Generalised
Small plaques <3 cm	Large plaques >3 cm
Thin plaques	Thick plaques
Nail involvement	No nail involvement

- Uveitis.
- Metabolic syndrome: obesity, hypertension, hyperlipidaemia, gout, cardiovascular disease, type 2 diabetes (most often affecting patients with early onset, large plaque, generalised psoriasis).

How is psoriasis diagnosed?

Psoriasis is diagnosed by its clinical features. If necessary, diagnosis is supported by typical biopsy findings.

Assessment of psoriasis

Medical assessment entails a careful history, examination, questioning about effect of psoriasis on daily life, and evaluation of comorbid factors. Psoriasis is mild in 60%, moderate in 30% and severe in 10% of patients.

Validated tools that are used to evaluate psoriasis are listed in *Table 3.4*.

Table 3.3. Typical patterns of psoriasis.

Post-streptococcal acute guttate psoriasis (*Fig. 3.236*)	- Widespread small plaques - Often resolves after several months
Small plaque psoriasis (*Fig. 3.237*)	- Often late age of onset
Chronic plaque psoriasis (*Fig. 3.238*)	- Persistent and treatment-resistant - Most often affects elbows, knees and lower back - Ranges from mild to very extensive disease
Unstable plaque psoriasis (*Fig. 3.239*)	- Rapid extension of existing or new plaques - Koebnerisation: new plaques at sites of skin injury - Induced by infection, stress, drugs or drug withdrawal
Flexural psoriasis (*Fig. 3.240*)	- Affects body folds - Smooth, well-defined patches - Colonised by candida
Scalp psoriasis (*Fig. 3.241*)	- Often the first or only site of psoriasis
Sebopsoriasis (*Fig. 3.242*)	- Overlap of seborrhoeic dermatitis and psoriasis - Affects scalp, face, ears and chest - Colonised by malassezia
Palmoplantar psoriasis (*Fig. 3.243*)	- Palms and/or soles - Keratoderma - Painful fissuring
Nail psoriasis (*Fig. 3.244*)	- Pitting, onycholysis, yellowing and ridging - Associated with inflammatory arthritis
Erythrodermic psoriasis (rare), see *Fig. 3.245*	- May or may not be preceded by another form of psoriasis - Acute and chronic forms - May result in systemic illness with temperature dysregulation, electrolyte imbalance, cardiac failure

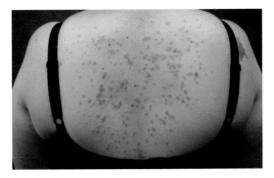

Figure 3.236. Post-streptococcal acute guttate psoriasis.

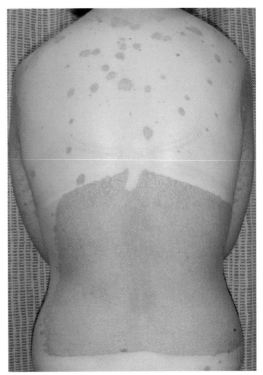

Figure 3.239. Koebner psoriasis after sunburn.

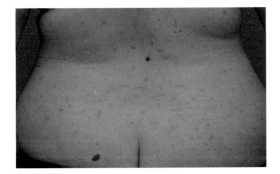

Figure 3.237. Small plaque psoriasis.

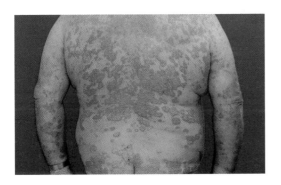

Figure 3.238. Chronic large plaque psoriasis.

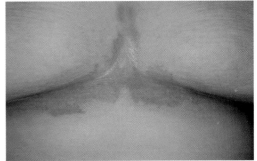

Figure 3.240. Flexural psoriasis.

- Mild psoriasis: PASI ≤10 and DLQI ≤10 or <5% BSA.
- Moderate psoriasis: (5–10% BSA) to severe psoriasis (>10% BSA): PASI >10 and DLQI >10; involvement of visible areas such as face, palms, soles and/or genitals; severe pruritus and significant nail disease.

Treatment of psoriasis

GENERAL ADVICE

- Education: emphasising chronicity of psoriasis and that it is not contagious.

- Explain purpose, expected efficacy, and use of treatments.
- Lifestyle advice: benefits of not smoking, avoiding excessive alcohol and maintaining optimal weight.
- Review effects of treatment regularly.

TOPICAL THERAPY

Mild psoriasis is generally treated with topical agents alone. Which treatment is selected may depend on body site, choice of vehicle, extent and severity of the psoriasis; see *Table 3.5.*

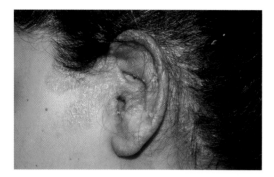

Figure 3.241. Scalp psoriasis.

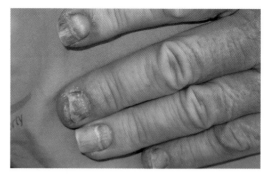

Figure 3.244. Nail psoriasis.

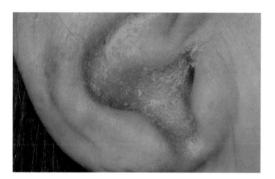

Figure 3.242. Sebopsoriasis.

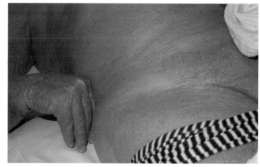

Figure 3.245. Erythrodermic psoriasis.

- Risks of phototherapy include erythema and burning, premature ageing of the skin, and possible increase in skin cancer.
- Phototherapy is contraindicated in patients with known photosensitivity, particularly lupus erythematosus or xeroderma pigmentosum.

SYSTEMIC THERAPY

Moderate to severe psoriasis warrants referral for a systemic agent and/or phototherapy.

- Systemic corticosteroids are best avoided due to risk of severe withdrawal flare of psoriasis and adverse effects.
- Methotrexate given as a single weekly oral or subcutaneous dose (range 10–30 mg) is effective for at least 60% of psoriasis patients. It is contraindicated in pregnancy and lactation, in patients with cirrhosis or renal impairment, and in patients with significant anaemia, leucopenia or thrombocytopenia. Patients require ongoing monitoring to reduce the risk of haematological toxicity and hepatotoxicity developing.

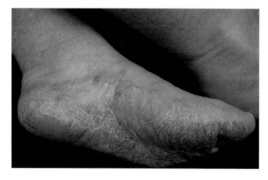

Figure 3.243. Palmoplantar psoriasis.

PHOTOTHERAPY

- Most psoriasis treatment centres offer narrowband UVB as monotherapy or in combination with topical or systemic agents.
- Dosage of UVB starts low and is slowly increased according to tolerance.
- Administered 2–3 times per week for up to 3 months or longer.
- Most effective for acute guttate psoriasis or generalised small plaque psoriasis.

Table 3.4. Tools for evaluation of psoriasis.

Extent and severity of psoriasis	PASI	▪ Psoriasis Area and Severity Index ▪ Score 0–72 ▪ Assess erythema, thickness, scaling in 4 body regions ▪ Use online tool or smartphone app to score
	PGA	▪ Physicians/Patients Global Assessment ▪ Clear, nearly clear, mild, moderate, severe, very severe
	BSA	▪ Body Surface Area as percentage of total ▪ Palm of patient's hand is 1%
Functional impairment	DLQI	▪ Dermatology Life Quality Index ▪ 10 questions about symptoms, activities, feelings and treatment
	SKINDEX-16	▪ Single page survey ▪ Cognitive, social and psychological effects and physical limitations
Arthritis	PASE	▪ Psoriatic Arthritis Screening Evaluation ▪ Joint involvement, severity of symptoms and functional impairment
	PEST	▪ Psoriasis Epidemiology Screening Tool ▪ Questions on symptoms ▪ Check affected joints on mannequin
Cardiovascular system	BMI BP HbA1c/glucose Lipid profile	▪ Identify comorbidities ▪ Complete medical history and examination

Table 3.5. Topical treatments of psoriasis.

Topical treatment	Features
Emollient	▪ Helps to lift scale and reduce fissuring ▪ Use as a soap substitute
Coal tar	▪ Limited use because of poor patient acceptance due to cosmetic issues such as smell, staining of skin and clothes, and mess of application ▪ Most often used for scalp psoriasis
Dithranol	▪ Effective on large, thick plaques as "short-contact therapy" rinsed off with water after 10–30 minutes ▪ Often irritant to surrounding normal skin and may stain skin and clothing
Salicylic acid	▪ Keratolytic agent that reduces scaling to allow other topical treatments to penetrate
Vitamin D analogue (calcipotriol)	▪ Initially apply twice daily and reduce to once daily as condition improves ▪ Ointment base is better absorbed than cream base ▪ Can irritate facial and flexural skin ▪ To avoid risk of hypercalcaemia, do not use with calcium or vitamin D supplements ▪ Total dose should not exceed 5 mg/week (i.e. 100 g of 50 mcg/g ointment or cream) ▪ Often used in combination with corticosteroid agent as it has a corticosteroid-sparing effect
Corticosteroid	▪ Suitable for most patients, especially those with limited disease. Easy to use and causes no irritation ▪ Use mild to moderate potency corticosteroid once or twice daily on the face, intertriginous areas, areas with thin skin, and in infants (for a maximum of 2 weeks). If response unsatisfactory consider using a topical calcineurin inhibitor

Table 3.5. *(continued)*	
Topical treatment	**Features**
	▪ Moderate to high potency corticosteroids can be used in other areas of the body (trunk, limbs and scalp). Apply once daily for up to 4 weeks. Avoid for a further 4 weeks ▪ Thick chronic plaques and plaques on hands and feet may require very high potency agents (class I steroids) for 2–4 weeks. Do not exceed 50 g/week ▪ Potential side-effects that limit use include local skin atrophy, telangiectasia, striae, acne and folliculitis. Systemic effects include adrenal suppression, increased intraocular pressure, glaucoma and cataracts ▪ Tachyphylaxis may occur with long-term use and results in decreased efficacy, and sometimes acute flare-up when treatment is stopped ▪ Minimise side-effects and tachyphylaxis by gradual reduction in frequency, or change to less potent formulation following clinical response. Another strategy is to have corticosteroid-free times
Calcineurin inhibitor (tacrolimus, pimecrolimus)	▪ Suitable for psoriasis on face, genitals and flexures to reduce need for potent topical steroids ▪ Apply twice daily ▪ Most common side-effect is burning and itching that generally reduces with ongoing usage

- Ciclosporin produces a rapid response, particularly for thin plaques. Useful in crisis management when rapid or short-term disease control is required, e.g. psoriasis flare. Patients must be monitored for nephrotoxicity and hypertension.
- Acitretin is particularly useful for erythrodermic psoriasis. It is a known teratogen so is contraindicated in pregnancy.
- The phosphodiesterase 4 inhibitor, apremilast, is a new oral agent for moderately severe psoriasis.

BIOLOGICS
- Biologics are reserved for conventional treatment-resistant severe psoriasis, mainly because of expense, as side-effects compare favourably with other systemic agents.
- Anti-tumour necrosis factor alpha (anti-TNF-α) biologics infliximab, adalimumab and etanercept, and IL-12/23 antagonist ustekinumab are effective for 50–80% of patients but efficacy reduces in time for a proportion of patients.
- IL-17 antagonists such as secukinumab and ixekizumab may be more effective than anti-TNF-α drugs.

3.19.2 Nail psoriasis

What is nail psoriasis?

Nail psoriasis is nail disease associated with psoriasis. It is also known as psoriatic nail dystrophy.

Who gets nail psoriasis?

Only 5% of patients present with typical nail psoriasis as an isolated disorder; most patients have plaque psoriasis. About 50–80% have psoriatic arthritis, particularly arthritis mutilans.

Patients with nail psoriasis may be of any age or race. Nail dystrophy is often precipitated or aggravated by trauma.

What causes nail psoriasis?

Nail psoriasis arises within the nail matrix. The specific pathogenesis of nail psoriasis is unknown.

What are the clinical features of nail psoriasis?

Nail psoriasis can affect any part of one or more nails. There are often scaly plaques on the dorsum of the hands and fingers due to associated plaque psoriasis (*Fig. 3.246*). Signs depend on the part of the nail affected. Its severity may or may not reflect the severity of the skin or joint psoriasis (*Fig. 3.247*).

- Psoriasis can enhance speed of nail growth and thickness of the nail plate.
- Pitting is a sign of loss of cells from the surface of nail plate. It is due to psoriasis in the proximal nail matrix (see *Fig. 3.248*).
- Leuconychia (areas of white nail plate) is due to parakeratosis within the body of the nail plate and is due to psoriasis in the mid-matrix.
- Onycholysis describes separation of the nail plate from the underlying nail bed and hyponychium. The affected distal nail plate appears white or yellow.
- Oil drop or salmon patch is a translucent yellow–red discoloration in the nail bed proximal to onycholysis. It reflects inflammation and can be tender.
- Subungual hyperkeratosis is scaling under the nail due to excessive proliferation of keratinocytes in the nail bed and hyponychium.
- Transverse lines and ridges are due to intermittent inflammation causing growth arrest followed by hyperproliferation in the proximal nail matrix. The lines and ridges move out distally as the nail grows.
- Psoriatic inflammation can also lead to nail plate crumbling, splinter haemorrhages, and a spotted lunula.
- Acrodermatitis continua of Hallopeau is a rare pustular eruption that affects nail bed, nail matrix and tips of digits (*Fig. 3.249*).

Complications of nail psoriasis

Nail psoriasis is unsightly. It can also lead to:
- pain and tenderness.
- functional disability.
- psychological distress.
- secondary bacterial infection (acute paronychia) or fungal infection (chronic paronychia, onychomycosis).

How is nail psoriasis diagnosed?

Psoriatic nail disease is readily recognised in a patient with current or prior plaque psoriasis. It is frequently confused with fungal nail infection.

If in doubt, or antifungal treatment is planned, nail clippings and scrapings of

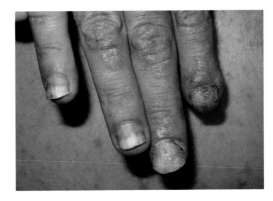

Figure 3.246. Nail psoriasis with associated plaque psoriasis on digits.

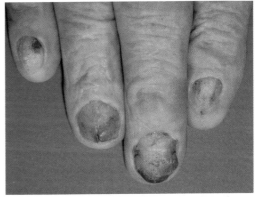

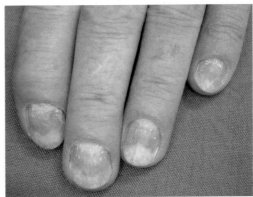

Figure 3.247. Nail psoriasis.

subungual debris should be sent for potassium hydroxide microscopy and fungal culture.

A nail biopsy is occasionally needed to confirm the diagnosis of nail psoriasis, particularly if dystrophy affects a single nail and

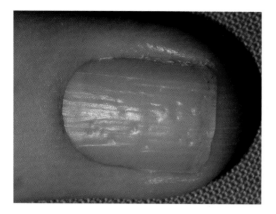

Figure 3.248. Pitting.

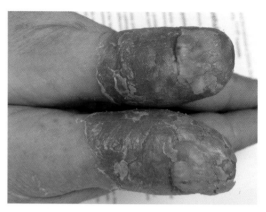

Figure 3.249. Acrodermatitis continua of Hallopeau.

a tumour is a possible explanation. The biopsy can lead to permanent nail deformity.

What is the treatment for nail psoriasis?

It is difficult to treat nail psoriasis effectively. Topical treatment must be applied to the nail matrix and hyponychium for months or years, and its effects are often disappointing. Options include:

- calcipotriol solution twice daily.
- topical high-potency corticosteroid solution or ointment as weekend pulses under occlusion at night.
- triamcinolone acetonide injected into proximal nail folds.
- fluorouracil cream twice daily.
- phototherapy with UVB or photochemotherapy (PUVA).
- systemic treatment with methotrexate, acitretin, ciclosporin or biologics.

Note: acitretin thins the nail plate and reduces its speed of growth, which can be helpful or not, depending on the type of nail psoriasis.

Antibiotic or antifungal treatment may be prescribed if secondary infection is present.

Chemical or surgical avulsion therapy, i.e. complete removal of the nail, is occasionally recommended. A risk is that the regrowing nail may be as badly or more severely affected than prior to the procedure.

How can nail psoriasis be prevented?

At this time, we do not know how to prevent nail psoriasis. Avoidance of trauma is essential.

What is the outlook for nail psoriasis?

Nail psoriasis varies in severity over time. In some patients, it resolves completely spontaneously or as a response to systemic treatment. In others, it persists long term.

3.20 Rosacea

What is rosacea?

Rosacea is a common condition involving the central face characterised by flushing, papules, pustules and telangiectasia.

Although once known as "acne rosacea", this is a misnomer, as rosacea is unrelated to acne.

Who gets rosacea?

Rosacea is very common in males and females aged 30 to 60.
- It can affect younger people including children.
- The phymatous subtype is more common in males than in females.
- Rosacea is common in people with fair skin and uncommon in people with dark skin.
- It fluctuates in severity.
- Rosacea may be aggravated by facial creams or oils, and especially by topical steroids.

What causes rosacea?

There are several theories regarding the cause of rosacea, which involves genetic, environmental, vascular and inflammatory factors. These include:
- skin damage due to chronic exposure to ultraviolet radiation.
- activation of the innate immune response to microbes.
- nitric acid may be involved.
- inflammation can lead to lymphatic obstruction and swelling.

High concentrations of antimicrobial peptides such as cathelicidins have been observed in rosacea.
- Cathelicidins promote infiltration of neutrophils in the dermis and dilation of blood vessels.
- Neutrophils release nitric acid also promoting vasodilation.
- Fluid leaks out of these dilated blood vessels causing swelling (oedema); and proinflammatory cytokines leak into the dermis, increasing the inflammation.

In wounds, matrix metalloproteinases (MMPs) such as collagenase and elastase, remodel tissue and cause new blood vessels to grow (angiogenesis).

- They are in high concentration in rosacea and may contribute to cutaneous inflammation and thickened, hardened skin.
- MMPs may also activate cathelicidins.

Other theories try to explain an increased prevalence in rosacea of:
- hair follicle mites, *Demodex folliculorum*.
- stomach bacteria, *Helicobacter pylori*.

Typically, rosacea flares from time to time. Triggers include:
- hot, cold or windy weather.
- sun exposure.
- emotional stress.
- exercise or hot shower.
- hot or spicy food and drink.
- alcohol.
- vasodilator drugs.

What are the clinical features of rosacea?

Rosacea is classified into several types, which may overlap.

Erythemato-telangiectatic rosacea
- Frequent blushing or flushing (*Fig. 3.250*).
- Persistent redness of central face.
- Inflamed, swollen cheeks.
- Prominent blood vessels – telangiectasia.
- Sensitive skin, e.g. stinging from various normally innocuous face creams.
- Dryness and flaky scale due to concomitant seborrhoeic dermatitis.

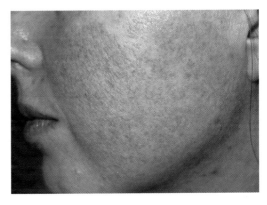

Figure 3.250. Erythemato-telangiectatic rosacea.

PAPULOPUSTULAR ROSACEA

- Lesions on mid face: nose, forehead, cheeks and chin (*Fig. 3.251*).
- These may spread to scalp, neck, upper trunk.
- Dome-shaped erythematous papules.
- Tiny pustules.
- Absence of comedones (blackheads, whiteheads).

OCULAR ROSACEA

- Red, sore or gritty eyelid margins (posterior blepharitis); see *Fig. 3.252*.
- Sore or tired eyes (conjunctivitis, keratitis, episcleritis).
- Papules and pustules centred on eyelashes and meibomian glands.

PHYMATOUS ROSACEA

- Enlarged nose with prominent pores (sebaceous hyperplasia).
- Fibrous thickening – rhinophyma (*Fig. 3.253*).
- Firm swelling of eyelids – blepharophyma.
- Persistent redness and swelling or solid oedema of the upper face – Morbihan disease.

GRANULOMATOUS ROSACEA

- Uncommon variant usually diagnosed histologically.
- Most often affects upper face around eyes and nose.
- Firm yellowish red papules.

How is rosacea diagnosed?

In most cases, no investigations are required and the diagnosis of rosacea is made clinically.

Occasionally a skin biopsy is performed, which shows chronic follicular inflammation and vascular changes. Granulomatous rosacea is characterised by caseating and non-caseating granulomas.

Complications of rosacea

Severe untreated rosacea is unsightly and can lead to social withdrawal.

Application of topical steroids to rosacea can result in periorificial dermatitis (see *Section 3.15*) or steroid rosacea (asymmetric papulopustular rosacea with telangiectasia).

Ocular rosacea can cause keratitis and keratoconjunctivitis sicca.

Rosacea fulminans (also called pyoderma faciale) is an acute form of rosacea with nodules and abscesses and sinus tracts. The patients may also have fever and elevated white cell count (neutrophil leucocytosis); see *Fig. 3.254*.

What is the treatment for rosacea?

Rosacea generally responds to treatment reasonably well.

GENERAL MEASURES

Where possible:

- minimise factors causing facial flushing.
- never apply a topical steroid to rosacea.
- protect from sun exposure – when outdoors apply broad-spectrum, high protection, non-greasy sunscreen to the face.

TOPICAL TREATMENT OF ROSACEA

Intermittent or continuous topical anti-inflammatory therapy is often sufficient for mild rosacea.

- Metronidazole cream or gel.
- Azelaic acid cream or lotion.
- Ivermectin cream.

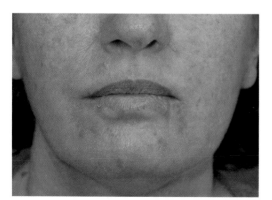

Figure 3.251. Papulopustular rosacea.

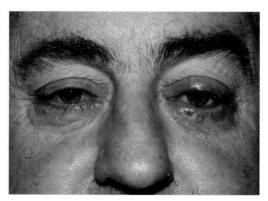

Figure 3.252. Ocular rosacea.

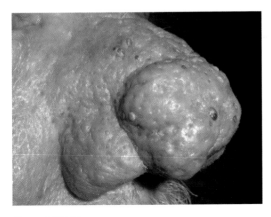

Figure 3.253. Phymatous rosacea.

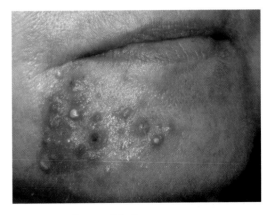

Figure 3.254. Rosacea fulminans.

Brimonidine gel is used to treat facial redness. It results in short-term vasoconstriction (12 hours duration) but has no effect on telangiectasia.

Calcineurin inhibitors such as tacrolimus ointment and pimecrolimus cream are reported to reduce redness in some patients with rosacea. Anti-acne products are also of some benefit.

ORAL TREATMENT OF INFLAMMATORY ROSACEA

Moderate or severe rosacea is often treated with tetracycline antibiotics such as doxycycline or minocycline (black ▼ in UK).
- To reduce risk of bacterial resistance, use subantibiotic dose of under 50 mg daily.
- They are usually prescribed as 6 to 12-week courses, taken as needed.
- Other options include erythromycin and derivatives, cotrimoxazole and metronidazole, dapsone.

Antibiotics have anti-inflammatory effects; they inhibit MMP function and in turn reduce cathelicidins and inflammation.

Low-dose oral isotretinoin is an effective non-antibiotic option. It has important side-effects and is not suitable for everyone.

MEDICATIONS TO REDUCE FLUSHING

There are several oral options that target flushing and facial redness.
- Nutraceuticals.
- Clonidine (an alpha2-receptor agonist).

- Carvedilol (a non-selective beta-blocker with some alpha-blocking activity).
- Selective serotonin reuptake inhibitors.

Side-effects may include low blood pressure, gastrointestinal symptoms, dry eyes, blurred vision and low heart rate.

VASCULAR LASER

Persistent telangiectasia can be successfully improved with vascular laser or intense pulsed light treatment. Where these are unavailable, cautery, diathermy (electrosurgery) or sclerotherapy (strong saline injections) may be helpful.

SURGERY FOR RHINOPHYMA

Rhinophyma can be treated successfully by reshaping the nose surgically or by laser.

How can rosacea be prevented?

Flares can be reduced by avoiding trigger factors (see above).

What is the outlook for rosacea?

Rosacea is often a chronic, relapsing disorder.

3.21 Transient acantholytic dermatosis

What is transient acantholytic dermatosis?

Transient acantholytic dermatosis causes a truncal rash characterised by acantholysis on histopathology. It can be transient, as the name suggests, in contrast to the rare and persistent inherited acantholytic dermatoses, Darier disease and benign familial pemphigus (Hailey–Hailey disease).

Transient acantholytic dermatosis is also known as Grover disease.

Who gets transient acantholytic dermatosis?

Transient acantholytic dermatosis most often affects men over 50. It is less common in women or younger people. It is common in those who are unwell in some way, but can arise in healthy people as well.

What causes transient acantholytic dermatosis?

The cause of transient acantholytic dermatosis is unknown. Sometimes, it follows sweating or some unexpected heat stress, so there has been suspicion that it may relate to sweat or sweat ducts. But it also may arise in dry skin. Many affected individuals are sun damaged.

What are the clinical features of transient acantholytic dermatosis?

Transient acantholytic dermatosis often starts quite suddenly. It is more common in winter than in summer. The following characteristics have been noted:

- The most common sites are central back, mid chest, see *Fig. 3.255*.
- Lesions are small red, crusted or eroded papules, see *Fig. 3.256*.
- There may be vesicles and non-follicular pustules.
- Lesions may bleed.

Although frequently itchy, transient acantholytic dermatosis may cause no symptoms.

Complications of transient acantholytic dermatosis

Transient acantholytic dermatosis may be complicated by the development of dermatitis, usually in a discoid pattern, i.e. with round or oval, dry or crusted plaques.

The plaques start on the chest and back, and may spread to affect other areas of the body.

How is transient acantholytic dermatosis diagnosed?

Transient acantholytic dermatosis is usually diagnosed clinically, but a skin biopsy may be necessary.

The pathology of transient acantholytic dermatosis is characteristic, with acantholysis (separated skin cells) with or without dyskeratosis (abnormal rounded skin cells). Spongiotic dermatitis may also be noted.

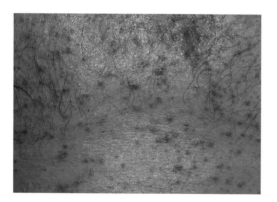

Figure 3.255. Transient acantholytic dermatosis.

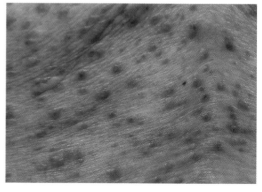

Figure 3.256. Papules in transient acantholytic dermatosis.

What is the treatment for transient acantholytic dermatosis?

There is no curative treatment for transient acantholytic dermatosis, but the following suggestions may be helpful:

- Remain cool, as sweating may induce more itchy spots.
- Apply a mild topical steroid such as hydrocortisone, if possible as a lotion. It can be applied frequently to the affected areas to relieve itching.
- Moisturising creams or antipruritic lotions containing menthol and camphor may also help.
- Calcipotriol cream has been reported to be of benefit.
- A course of tetracycline or an oral antifungal medication such as itraconazole helps some patients.
- Phototherapy can be helpful, but may also provoke the disease.
- Experimentally, oral retinoids such as acitretin or isotretinoin have been reported to be helpful. However, they have important side-effects and are not necessary for mild cases.
- Dermatitis, if present, responds to topical and systemic steroids.

How can transient acantholytic dermatosis be prevented?

Keep cool. Wear garments designed to prevent sweat rash.

What is the outlook for transient acantholytic dermatosis?

The duration of transient acantholytic dermatosis is variable – from days to decades. It can come and go, often with a seasonal variation. It may also become chronic/persistent.

NSAIDS, penicillin, ACEI, Thiazides, codeine

3.22 Urticaria

What is urticaria?

Urticaria is characterised by weals (hives) or angioedema (swellings, in 10%) or both (in 40%). There are several types of urticaria.

A weal (or wheal) is a superficial skin-coloured or pale skin swelling, usually surrounded by erythema (redness) that lasts anything from a few minutes to 24 hours. Usually very itchy, it may have a burning sensation.

Angioedema is deeper swelling within the skin or mucous membranes, and can be skin-coloured or red. It resolves within 72 hours. Angioedema may be itchy or painful but is often asymptomatic.

Classification of urticaria

Urticaria is classified according to its duration.

1. Acute urticaria (<6 weeks' duration, and often gone within hours to days).
2. Chronic urticaria (daily or episodic weals, >6 weeks' duration).

Chronic urticaria may be spontaneous or inducible. Both types may co-exist.

Inducible urticaria includes:
- symptomatic dermographism.
- cold urticaria.
- cholinergic urticaria.
- contact urticaria.
- delayed pressure urticaria.
- solar urticaria.
- heat urticaria.
- vibratory urticaria.
- aquagenic urticaria.

Who gets urticaria?

One in five children or adults has an episode of acute urticaria during their lifetime. It is more common in atopics. It affects all races.

Chronic spontaneous urticaria affects 0.5–2% of the population; two-thirds are women. Inducible urticaria is more common. There are genetic and autoimmune associations.

What are the clinical features of urticaria?

Urticarial weals can be a few millimetres or several centimetres in diameter, coloured white or red, with or without a red flare. Each weal may last a few minutes or several hours, and may change shape. Weals may be round, or form rings, a map-like pattern or giant patches (see *Fig. 3.257*).

Urticaria can affect any site of the body and tends to be distributed widely.

Angioedema is more often localised. It commonly affects the face (especially eyelids and perioral sites, see *Fig. 3.258*), hands, feet and genitalia. It may involve tongue, uvula, soft palate, or larynx.

In chronic inducible urticaria, weals appear about 5 minutes after the stimulus and last a few minutes or up to one hour. Characteristically, weals are:
- linear in symptomatic dermographism (see *Fig. 3.259*).
- tiny in cholinergic urticaria (see *Fig. 3.260*).
- confined to contact areas in contact urticaria (see *Fig. 3.261*).
- diffuse in cold urticaria – if large areas of skin are affected, they can lead to fainting

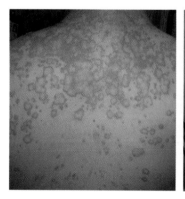
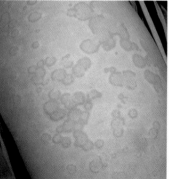
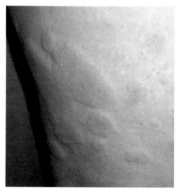

Figure 3.257. Urticaria.

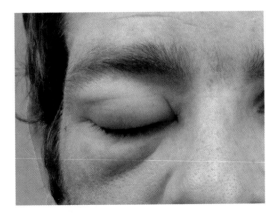

Figure 3.258. Angioedema of eyelids.

(potentially dangerous if swimming in cold water); see *Fig. 3.262.*

The weals are more persistent in chronic spontaneous urticaria, but each has gone or has altered in shape within 24 hours. They may occur at certain times of day.

The activity of chronic spontaneous urticaria can be assessed using the UAS7 scoring system. The daily weal/itch scores are added up for 7 days; the maximum score is 42.

Score	Weals/24 hours	Itch
0	None	None
1	<20	Mild
2	20–50	Moderate
3	>50	Intense

The emotional impact of urticaria and its effect on quality of life should also be assessed. The Dermatology Life Quality Index (DLQI) and CU-Q2oL, a specific questionnaire for chronic urticaria, have been validated for chronic urticaria, where sleep disruption is a particular problem.

What causes urticaria?

Weals are due to release of chemical mediators from tissue mast cells and circulating basophils. These chemical mediators include histamine, platelet-activating factor and cytokines. The mediators activate sensory nerves and cause dilation of blood vessels and leakage of fluid into surrounding tissues. Bradykinin release causes angioedema.

Several hypotheses have been proposed to explain the pathogenesis of urticaria. The immune, arachidonic acid and coagulation systems are involved, and genetic mutations are under investigation.

ACUTE URTICARIA
Acute urticaria can be induced by the following factors but the cause is not always identified:
- Acute viral infection – upper respiratory infection, hepatitis, mononucleosis, mycoplasma.
- Acute bacterial infection – dental abscess, sinusitis.
- Food allergy (IgE-mediated) – usually milk, egg, peanut, shellfish.
- Drug allergy (IgE-mediated) – often an antibiotic.
- Drug pseudoallergy – aspirin, non-selective non-steroidal anti-inflammatory drugs, opiates, radiocontrast media cause urticaria without immune activation.
- Vaccination.
- Arthropod stings – bees, wasps.
- Widespread reaction to contact with an allergen – e.g. rubber latex.

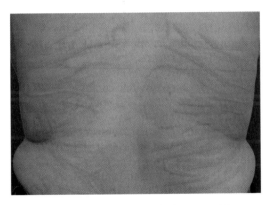

Figure 3.259. Weals in symptomatic dermographism.

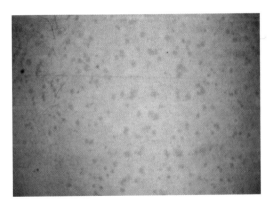

Figure 3.260. Weals in cholinergic urticaria.

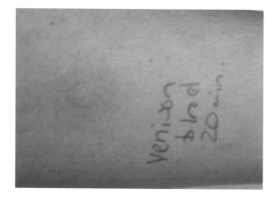

Figure 3.261. A weal in contact urticaria.

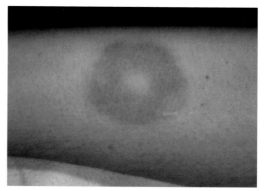

Figure 3.262. Ice block test used to confirm a weal in cold urticaria.

Severe allergic urticaria may lead to anaphylactic shock (bronchospasm, collapse).

Immune complexes due to blood transfusion and certain drugs cause serum sickness, when urticaria is associated with fever, lymphadenopathy, arthralgia and nausea.

A single episode or recurrent episodes of angioedema without urticaria can be due to angiotensin-converting enzyme (ACE) inhibitor drugs.

CHRONIC URTICARIA

Chronic spontaneous urticaria is mainly idiopathic. An autoimmune cause is likely. About half of investigated patients carry functional IgG autoantibodies to immunoglobulin IgE or high-affinity receptor FcεRIα.

Chronic spontaneous urticaria has also been associated with:
- chronic underlying infection, e.g. *Helicobacter pylori*, bowel parasites.
- chronic autoimmune disease, e.g. systemic lupus erythematosus, thyroid disease, coeliac disease, vitiligo and others.

Weals in chronic spontaneous urticaria may be aggravated by:
- heat.
- viral infection.
- tight clothing.
- drug pseudoallergy – aspirin, non-steroidal anti-inflammatory drugs, opiates.
- food pseudoallergy – salicylates, azo dye food colouring agents, benzoate preservatives.

Inducible urticaria is a response to a physical stimulus; see *Table 3.6.*

Recurrent angioedema without urticaria can be due to inherited or acquired complement C1 esterase deficiency.

How is urticaria diagnosed?

Urticaria is diagnosed in people with a history of weals that last less than 24 hours with or without angioedema. A thorough physical examination should be undertaken to evaluate the cause.

Skin prick testing and radioallergosorbent tests (RAST) or CAP fluoroimmunoassay may be requested if a drug or food allergy is suspected in acute urticaria.

There are no routine diagnostic tests in chronic spontaneous urticaria apart from blood count (CBC/FBC) and C-reactive protein (CRP), but investigations may be undertaken if an underlying disorder is suspected.

The autologous serum skin test is sometimes carried out in chronic spontaneous urticaria, but its value is uncertain. It is positive if an injection of the patient's serum under the skin causes a red weal.

Inducible urticaria is often confirmed by inducing the reaction, e.g. scratching the skin in dermographism or applying an ice cube in suspected cold urticaria.

A family history should be elicited. Investigations for a systemic condition or autoinflammatory disease should be undertaken in urticaria patients with fever, joint or bone pain, and malaise. Patients with angioedema without weals should be asked if they take ACE inhibitor drugs and tested for complement C4; C1-INH levels, function and antibodies; and C1q.

Biopsy of urticaria can be non-specific and difficult to interpret. The pathology shows

Table 3.6. Types of inducible urticaria and stimuli.

Type of inducible urticaria	Examples of stimuli inducing wealing
Symptomatic dermographism	Stroking or scratching the skin Tight clothing Towel drying after hot shower
Cold urticaria	Cold air on exposed skin Cold water Ice block Cryotherapy
Cholinergic urticaria	Sweat induced by exercise Sweat induced by emotional upset Hot shower
Contact urticaria	Eliciting substance absorbed through skin or mucous membrane Allergens (IgE-mediated): white flour, cosmetics, textiles, latex, saliva, meat, fish, vegetables Pseudoallergens: stinging nettle, hairy caterpillar, medicines
Delayed pressure urticaria	Pressure on affected skin several hours earlier Carrying heavy bag Pressure from seat belt Standing on ladder rung Sitting on a horse
Solar urticaria	Sun exposure to non-habituated body sites Often spares face, neck, hands May involve long wavelength UV or visible light
Heat urticaria	Hot water bottle Hot drink
Vibratory urticaria	Pneumatic drill (jack hammer)
Aquagenic urticaria	Hot or cold water Fresh, salt or chlorinated water

oedema in the dermis and dilated blood vessels, with variable mixed inflammatory infiltrate. Vessel-wall damage indicates urticarial vasculitis.

What is the treatment for urticaria?

The main treatment of all forms of urticaria in adults and in children is with an oral second-generation antihistamine chosen from the list below. If the standard dose is not effective, the dose can be increased up to fourfold. They are best taken continuously rather than on demand. They are stopped when the acute urticaria has settled down. There is not thought to be any benefit from adding a second antihistamine.

- Cetirizine.
- Loratidine.
- Fexofenadine.
- Desloratadine.
- Levocetirizine.
- Rupatadine.
- Bilastine.

Terfenadine and astemizole should not be used, as they are cardiotoxic in combination with ketoconazole or erythromycin.

Although systemic treatment is best avoided during pregnancy and breastfeeding, there have been no reports that second-generation antihistamines cause birth defects. If treatment is required, loratidine and cetirizine are currently preferred.

Conventional first-generation antihistamines such as promethazine or chlorpheniramine are no longer recommended for urticaria.

- They are short-lasting.
- They have sedative and anticholinergic side-effects.
- They impair sleep, learning and performance.
- They cause drowsiness in nursing infants if taken by the mother.
- They interact with alcohol and other medications.
- Lethal overdoses are reported.

AVOIDANCE OF TRIGGER FACTORS

In addition to antihistamines, the cause of urticaria should be eliminated if known (e.g. drug or food allergy). Avoidance of relevant type 1 (IgE-mediated) allergens clears urticaria within 48 hours.

In addition to antihistamines, the triggers for urticaria should be avoided where possible. For example:

- treat identified chronic infections such as *H. pylori*.

- avoid aspirin, opiates and NSAIDs.
- minimise dietary pseudoallergens for a trial of at least 3 weeks.
- avoid known allergens that have been confirmed by positive specific IgE/skin prick tests if these have clinical relevance for urticaria.
- cool the affected area with a fan, cold flannel, ice pack or soothing moisturising lotion.

The physical triggers for inducible urticaria should be minimised; see examples below. However, symptoms often persist.

- Symptomatic dermographism: reduce friction, e.g. avoid tight clothing.
- Cold urticaria: dress up carefully in cold or windy conditions and avoid swimming in cold water.
- Delayed pressure urticaria: broaden the contact area of a heavy bag.
- Solar urticaria: wear covering clothing and apply broad-spectrum sunscreens.

Some patients benefit from daily induction of symptoms to induce tolerance. Phototherapy may be helpful for symptomatic dermographism.

TREATMENT OF REFRACTORY ACUTE URTICARIA

If non-sedating antihistamines are not effective, a 4 to 5-day course of oral prednis(ol)one may be warranted in severe acute urticaria.

Intramuscular injection of adrenaline (epinephrine) is reserved for life-threatening anaphylaxis or swelling of the throat.

TREATMENT OF REFRACTORY CHRONIC URTICARIA

Patients with chronic urticaria that has failed to respond to maximum-dose second generation oral antihistamines taken for 4 weeks should be referred to a dermatologist or immunologist/allergy specialist.

There is good evidence to support treatment with omalizumab or ciclosporin, which each have a 65% response rate in antihistamine-resistant patients.

- Omalizumab is a monoclonal antibody directed against IgE, with low toxicity.
- Ciclosporin is a calcineurin inhibitor, with potential serious side-effects (e.g. may increase blood pressure and reduce renal function).

Other treatments that are sometimes used in chronic urticaria include:

- montelukast.
- tricyclic antidepressants.
- methotrexate.
- dapsone.
- phototherapy.
- anti-TNF alpha agents, e.g. infliximab, adalimumab.
- intravenous immunoglobulins.

Long-term systemic corticosteroids are not recommended, as high doses are required to reduce symptoms of urticaria and they have inevitable adverse effects that can be serious.

Differential diagnosis of urticaria

SCOMBROID FISH POISONING

Histamine release from decomposing scombroid fish causes erythema without weals, tachycardia, abdominal pain and diarrhoea and diaphoresis.

PAPULAR URTICARIA

Insect bites are localised, often clustered in groups of 3–5 lesions, and they appear in crops. Bites persist for days. Close inspection reveals a central punctum. Chronic hypersensitivity to insect bites is often called papular urticaria.

MASTOCYTOSIS

The most common form of mastocytosis, maculopapular cutaneous mastocytosis, is also called urticaria pigmentosa. Itchy brown patches or freckles on the skin are due to abnormal collections of mast cells.

URTICARIAL VASCULITIS

Urticarial vasculitis causes persistent urticaria-like plaques that last more than 24 hours and resolve with bruising. Biopsy reveals leucocytoclastic vasculitis.

AUTOINFLAMMATORY SYNDROMES

Urticarial rashes are rarely due to autoinflammatory syndromes, which are mediated by interleukin (IL) 1. These include:

- hereditary periodic fever and cryopyrin-associated syndromes.
- Schnitzler syndrome (onset in adult life).
- adult-onset Still disease and juvenile idiopathic arthritis.

Urticarial rashes in autoinflammatory syndromes differ from urticaria:

- patches are flat.
- lesions persist longer.
- distribution is symmetrical.
- systemic symptoms.
- elevated inflammatory markers such as C-reactive protein (CRP).
- biopsy of skin lesion shows dense neutrophilic infiltrate.
- lack of response to antihistamines.

What is the outlook for chronic urticaria?

Although chronic urticaria clears up in most cases, 15% continue to have wealing at least twice weekly after 2 years.

3.23 Vasculitis: cutaneous

What is cutaneous vasculitis?

Cutaneous vasculitis is a group of disorders in which there are inflamed blood vessels in the skin. These may include capillaries, venules, arterioles and lymphatics.

- Cutaneous vasculitis has several different causes.
- There are a wide variety of clinical presentations.
- It is associated with systemic vasculitis in a minority of patients.

In most cases an underlying cause is not found and the disease is self-limiting.

Classification of cutaneous vasculitis

CAPILLARITIS

- Progressive pigmented purpura (*Fig. 3.263*).
- Itching purpura.
- Pigmented purpuric lichenoid dermatosis.
- Purpura annularis telangiectodes.
- Contact allergy.
- Lichen aureus (*Fig. 3.264*).

SMALL VESSEL VASCULITIS

- Idiopathic cutaneous small vessel vasculitis (*Fig. 3.265*).
- Drug- or infection-induced hypersensitivity vasculitis (*Fig. 3.266*).
- Henoch–Schönlein purpura (*Fig. 3.267*).
- Acute haemorrhagic oedema of infancy (*Fig. 3.268*).
- Urticarial vasculitis (*Fig. 3.269*).
- Exercise-induced vasculitis (*Fig. 3.270*).
- Livedo vasculitis (strictly speaking an occlusive vasculopathy; *Fig. 3.271*).
- Erythema elevatum diutinum.
- Malignant atrophic papulosis (Degos).
- Cryoglobulinaemia.
- ANCA-associated vasculitis:
  - ☐ Microscopic polyangiitis
  - ☐ Eosinophilic granulomatosis with polyangiitis (Churg–Strauss)
  - ☐ Granulomatosis with polyangiitis (Wegener) (*Fig. 3.272*)
  - ☐ Lymphomatoid granulomatosis.

MEDIUM VESSEL VASCULITIS

- Cutaneous polyarteritis nodosa (*Fig. 3.273*).
- Kawasaki disease (*Fig. 3.274*).
- Nodular vasculitis (*Fig. 3.275*).

LARGE VESSEL VASCULITIS

- Temporal arteritis.
- Takayasu disease.

Who gets cutaneous vasculitis?

Cutaneous vasculitis can affect people of all ages and races. Some types of vasculitis have a predilection for certain age groups.

- Acute haemorrhagic oedema affects infants.
- Henoch–Schönlein purpura affects children.
- Hypersensitivity vasculitis affects adults.

What causes vasculitis?

Many different insults may cause an identical inflammatory response within the blood vessel wall. Three main mechanisms are proposed:

1. Direct injury to the vessel wall by bacteria or viruses.
2. Indirect injury by activation of antibodies.

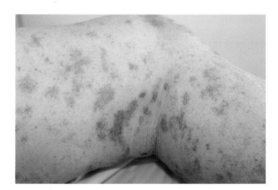

Figure 3.263. Pigmented purpura of capillaritis.

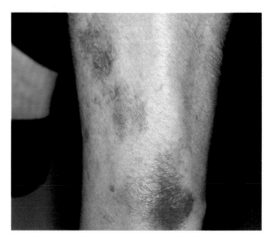

Figure 3.264. Lichen aureus.

3. Indirect injury through activation of complement, a group of proteins in the blood and tissue fluids that attack infection and foreign bodies.

Vasculitis can be triggered by one or more factors. In the past, it was frequently seen with administration of antisera (serum sickness), but is now more often due to drugs, infections and disease. In most cases an underlying cause is not found.

DRUGS

Drugs are frequently responsible for cutaneous small vessel vasculitis, particularly in association with infection, malignancy or autoimmune disorders. Onset of vasculitis is often 7–10 days after introduction of a new medicine, such as:
- Antibiotics.
- Thiazide diuretics.
- Phenytoin.
- Allopurinol.

- Oral anticoagulants such as warfarin and coumarin.
- NSAIDs.

Foods and food additives, e.g. tartrazine, are rare causes of vasculitis.

INFECTION

Examples of infections associated with cutaneous small vessel vasculitis include:
- Bacterial infection, e.g. *Streptococcus pyogenes*, bacterial endocarditis.
- Viral infection, e.g. hepatitis B, hepatitis C (by causing cryoglobulinaemia), human immunodeficiency virus (HIV), and haemorrhagic fever.

DISEASES

Cancer is found in fewer than 5% of patients with cutaneous vasculitis. It is thought that malignancy leads to more circulating antibodies and viscous proteins that may sludge within small blood vessels.

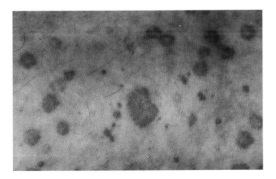

Figure 3.265. Idiopathic cutaneous small vessel vasculitis.

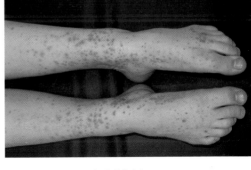

Figure 3.267. Henoch–Schönlein purpura.

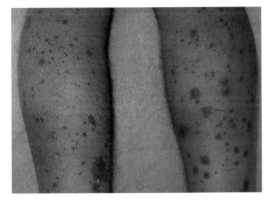

Figure 3.266. Hypersensitivity vasculitis.

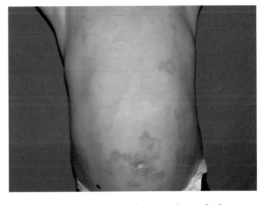

Figure 3.268. Acute haemorrhagic oedema of infancy.

Autoimmune disorders such as systemic lupus erythematosus (SLE), dermatomyositis, and rheumatoid arthritis are characterised by circulating antibodies that target the individual's own tissues. Some of these antibodies can target blood vessels, resulting in vasculitis.

What are the clinical features of vasculitis?

Clinical presentation of cutaneous vasculitis mainly depends on the size of the inflamed blood vessel.

CAPILLARITIS

Capillaritis presents as pigmented purpura (*Fig. 3.276*), most often on the lower legs, characterised by:
- Initial pin-point red or purple petechiae.
- Subsequent golden-brown haemosiderin deposition.

Capillaritis is often chronic or relapsing.

SMALL VESSEL VASCULITIS

Small vessel vasculitis presents acutely as palpable purpura (purple, non-blanching papules and plaques) (*Fig. 3.277*).
- Prominent involvement of lower legs with fewer lesions on proximal sites.
- Sometimes, petechiae and ecchymoses.
- Often, non-purpuric erythematous weals, macules and papules.
- Haemorrhagic bullae, necrosis and superficial ulceration may occur.
- Local pruritus, burning pain and swelling.
- Variable systemic symptoms with fever, joint pains, lymphadenopathy and gastrointestinal upset.

The initial acute rash of small vessel vasculitis usually subsides within 2–3 weeks, but crops of lesions may recur over weeks to several months. If the cause is not removed, hypersensitivity vasculitis (see *Fig. 3.266*) may rarely become relapsing or chronic.

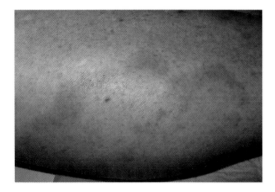

Figure 3.269. Urticarial vasculitis.

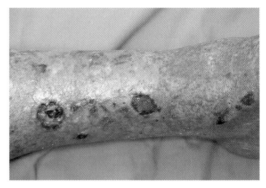

Figure 3.271. Livedo vasculopathy.

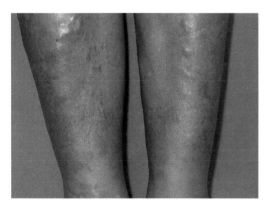

Figure 3.270. Exercise-induced vasculitis.

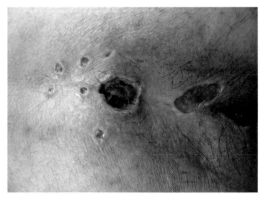

Figure 3.272. Granulomatosis with polyangiitis.

MEDIUM VESSEL VASCULITIS

Medium vessel cutaneous vasculitis is associated with nodules, deep and persistent ulceration (*Fig. 3.278*). It may be accompanied by livedo reticularis. Medium vessel vasculitis tends to persist.

LARGE VESSEL VASCULITIS

Large vessel vasculitis infrequently results in cutaneous features.

How is vasculitis diagnosed?

In many cases the diagnosis of capillaritis or small vessel vasculitis can be made on the basis of its appearance without requiring any further tests.

Cutaneous small vessel vasculitis is confirmed by 4mm punch biopsy of an early purpuric papule, ideally present for 24–48 hours. Medium vessel vasculitis requires a larger, deeper biopsy to involve panniculus.

Histopathology of hypersensitivity vasculitis reveals neutrophils around arterioles and venules, and fibrinoid necrosis (fibrin within

or inside the vessel wall). There may be extravasated red cells, leukocytoclasis (broken-up neutrophils within the vessel wall) and/or signs of an underlying disease.

Other forms of vasculitis may have lymphocytic and granulomatous inflammation.

Direct immunofluorescence of a vasculitic lesion less than 24 hours old often reveals immunoglobulins and complement.

- Perivascular IgA confirms Henoch–Schönlein purpura.
- Perivascular IgM suggests cryoglobulinaemia or rheumatoid arthritis.
- It is often negative in cutaneous polyarteritis nodosa and ANCA-positive vasculitis.

Screening tests are requested to identify any underlying cause and to determine the extent of involvement of internal organs. These may be suggested by the history and symptoms. Patients should have:

- Urinalysis, looking for protein, blood and glomerular casts.
- Full blood count, liver and kidney function.

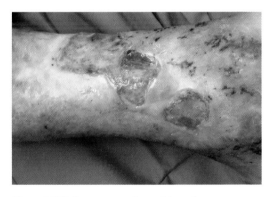

Figure 3.273. Cutaneous polyarteritis nodosa.

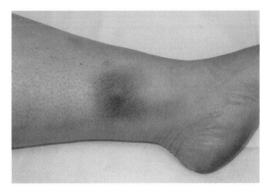

Figure 3.275. Nodular vasculitis.

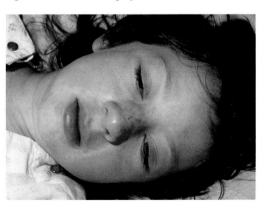

Figure 3.274. Kawasaki disease.

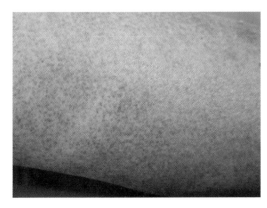

Figure 3.276. Capillaritis.

Additional tests may include:
- Anti-nuclear antibodies (ANA), extractable nuclear antigen profile (ENA).
- Anti-streptococcal antibodies, HIV, hepatitis B and C serology.
- Serum complement levels.
- Protein and immunoglobulin electrophoresis.
- Cryoglobulins.
- Anti-neutrophil cytoplasmic antibody (ANCA).
- Chest X-ray if symptoms suggest lung disease.

If an initial screen indicates an abnormality, or there is clinical suspicion of a more widespread vasculitic process, further investigations will be required. The majority of patients presenting with palpable purpura have primary cutaneous small vessel vasculitis and no underlying cause is found in spite of extensive investigations.

What is the treatment for vasculitis?

Treatment depends on the severity of the disease and may include general measures, systemic corticosteroids, and immune modulating agents.
- If an underlying cause is found, remove the trigger (e.g. stop the drug) and treat associated diseases.
- Rest – exercise often induces new lesions (see *Fig. 3.270*).
- Compress and/or elevate the affected limb(s).

- Use simple analgesics and NSAIDs for pain.
- Protect fragile skin from injury.
- Apply emollients to relieve dryness and itch.
- Dress ulcers.
- Treat secondary infection.

Medications used to control cutaneous vasculitis have not been subjected to randomised trials. They are recommended in acute vasculitis when ulcerated, and in symptomatic relapsing or chronic disease. They include:
- Corticosteroids, e.g. prednis(ol)one 0.5 mg/kg/day for 1–2 weeks, tapered over 3–6 weeks.
- Colchicine 0.5 or 0.6 mg bd.
- Dapsone 50–100 mg daily.
- Other immune modulators.

If cutaneous vasculitis is a manifestation of systemic vasculitis then treatment of the systemic disorder is required.

What is the outlook for vasculitis?

Vasculitis limited to the skin has a good prognosis, with most cases resolving within a period of weeks to months. The vasculitis may recur at variable intervals after the initial episode.

The prognosis of systemic vasculitis is dependent upon the severity of involvement of other organs. If vasculitis affects the kidneys, lungs or brain it can be life-threatening.

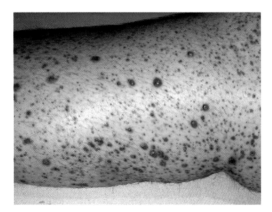

Figure 3.277. Purpura in small vessel vasculitis.

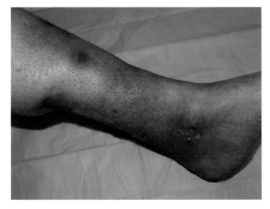

Figure 3.278. Medium vessel vasculitis (cutaneous polyarteritis nodosa).

Chapter 4

Non-inflammatory conditions

4.1 Alopecia areata

What is alopecia areata?

The term alopecia means hair loss. In alopecia areata, one or more round bald patches appear suddenly, most often on the scalp. Alopecia areata is the most common form of autoimmune alopecia.

Who gets alopecia areata?

Alopecia areata can affect males and females at any age. It starts in childhood in about 50%, and before the age of 40 years in 80%. Lifetime risk is 1–2% and is independent of ethnicity.

- A family history of alopecia areata and/or of other autoimmune conditions is present in 10–25% of patients.
- At least eight susceptibility genes have been detected.
- Patients with alopecia areata have higher than expected rates of thyroid disease, vitiligo and atopic eczema.
- There is increased prevalence in patients with chromosomal disorders such as Down syndrome.
- It is possibly drug-induced when arising in patients on biologic medicines.

What causes alopecia areata?

Alopecia areata is classified as an autoimmune disorder. It is histologically characterised by T lymphocytes around the hair follicles. These CD8(+)NK group 2D-positive (NKG2D(+)) T cells release pro-inflammatory cytokines and chemokines that reject the hair. The exact mechanism is not yet understood.

The onset or recurrence of hair loss is sometimes triggered by:

- viral infection.
- trauma.
- hormonal change.
- emotional/physical stressors.

What are the clinical features of alopecia areata?

Several clinical patterns are described below. More severe disease is associated with young age, concurrent atopic eczema, and chromosomal abnormalities.

Most patients have no symptoms, and a bald patch or thinning hair is noted incidentally, often discovered by a hairdresser. Other patients describe a burning, prickly discomfort in the affected areas – this is known as trichodynia.

Patchy alopecia areata

Any hair-bearing area can be affected, most often the scalp, eyebrows, eyelashes and beard (see *Fig. 4.1*).

Patchy alopecia areata has three stages.

1. Sudden loss of hair.
2. Enlargement of bald patch or patches.
3. Regrowth of hair.

The bald areas may have a smooth surface, completely devoid of hair or with scattered "exclamation mark" hairs (see *Fig. 4.2*).

- Exclamation mark hairs are 2–3 mm in length, broken or tapered, with a club-shaped root. Microscopy shows a thin proximal shaft and normal calibre distal shaft.

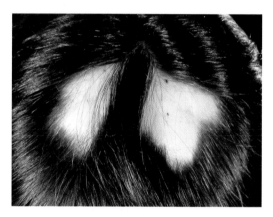

Figure 4.1. Patchy alopecia areata.

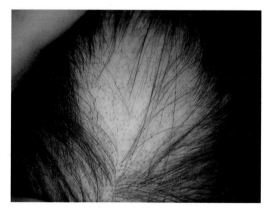

Figure 4.2. "Exclamation mark" hairs.

- Regrowing hairs are often initially coloured white or grey; they may be curly when previously straight.
- It may take months and sometimes years to regrow all the hair.
- One patch can be falling out while another is regrowing.

ALOPECIA TOTALIS
- Affects up to 5% of patients with autoimmune hair loss.
- All or nearly all scalp hair is lost (*Fig. 4.3*).

ALOPECIA UNIVERSALIS
- Affects less than 1% of cases.
- All hair or nearly all hair on the entire body is lost.

OPHIASIS
- Pattern of alopecia areata affecting occipital scalp.
- Bald area can encircle scalp (see *Fig. 4.4*).

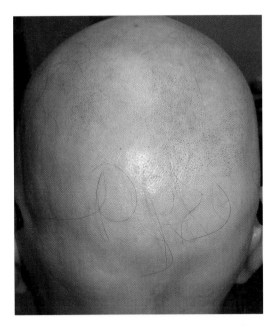

Figure 4.3. Alopecia totalis.

DIFFUSE ALOPECIA AREATA
- Sometimes called alopecia areata incognito.
- Presents with sudden diffuse thinning of scalp hair (see *Fig. 4.5*).
- Persisting hair tends to grey, hence descriptions of "turning white overnight".
- Positive hair pull test.
- May be confused with telogen effluvium or hair loss due to medications.

ALOPECIA AREATA OF THE NAILS
- Affects 10–50% of those with alopecia areata.
- Regular pitting and ridging are the most common findings (see *Fig. 4.6*).
- May also cause koilonychia, trachyonychia, Beau lines, onychorrhexis, onychomadesis, onycholysis and haemorrhagic spotting of the lunula.

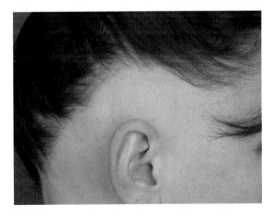

Figure 4.4. Ophiasis.

Complications of alopecia areata

Alopecia areata patients are at risk for psychosocial consequences of their disease, such as depression and anxiety.

They should be assessed for atopy, vitiligo, thyroid disease and other autoimmune conditions.

How is alopecia areata diagnosed?

Alopecia areata is diagnosed clinically. Although usually straightforward,

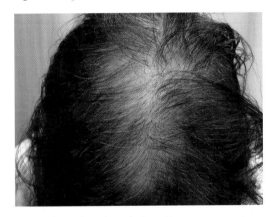

Figure 4.5. Diffuse alopecia areata.

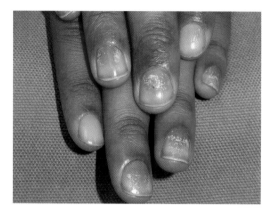

Figure 4.6. Alopecia areata of the nails.

additional tests are sometimes needed
to confirm the diagnosis:
- trichoscopy (use of a dermatoscope
  to examine hair and scalp).
- skin biopsy (histopathology).

What is the treatment for alopecia areata?

There is not yet any reliable cure for alopecia
areata and other forms of autoimmune hair loss.
Because spontaneous regrowth is common in
alopecia areata, and research has often been
of poor quality, the effectiveness of reported
treatments is mostly unknown.

TOPICAL TREATMENTS
Several topical treatments used for alopecia
areata are reported to result in temporary
improvement in some people. The hair falls out
when they are stopped. These include:
- potent or ultrapotent topical steroids.
- minoxidil solution or foam.
- dithranol (anthralin) ointment.

INTRALESIONAL CORTICOSTEROID INJECTION
Injecting triamcinolone acetonide 2.5–10 mg/ml
into patchy scalp, beard or eyebrow alopecia
areata may speed up regrowth of hair. Its effect is
temporary. If bald patches reappear, they can be
reinjected.

SYSTEMIC CORTICOSTEROIDS
Oral and pulse intravenous steroids in high dose
can lead to temporary regrowth of hair. Most
physicians agree that long-term systemic steroid
treatment is not justified because of potential
and actual adverse effects.

IMMUNOTHERAPY
The sensitising agents diphenylcyclopropenone
and dinitrochlorobenzene provoke contact
allergic dermatitis in treated areas. These
sensitisers can be reapplied once weekly to bald
areas on the scalp. The resultant dermatitis
is irritating and may be unsightly. It is often
accompanied by a swollen lymph gland.

OTHER TREATMENTS
A combination of the lipid-lowering agents
simvastatin and ezetimibe (which have
immunomodulating effects) has been reported
to be effective.

There is no convincing data to support the use
of methotrexate, sulfasalazine, azathioprine,
ciclosporin or phototherapy.

JAK INHIBITORS
Several patients with severe alopecia areata
have had improvement when treated with oral
tofacitinib and oral ruxolitinib, which are Janus
kinase (JAK) inhibitors. It is thought they may act
by blocking interleukin (IL)-15 signalling.

What else should be considered for alopecia areata?

COUNSELLING
Some people with alopecia areata seek and
benefit from professional counselling to come
to terms with the disorder and regain self-
confidence.

CAMOUFLAGING HAIR LOSS – SCALP
A hairpiece is often the best solution to
disguise the presence of hair loss. These cover
the whole scalp or only a portion of the scalp,
using human or synthetic fibres tied or woven
to a fabric base.
- A full wig is a cap that fits over the whole
  head.
- A partial wig must be clipped or glued to
  existing hair.
- A hair integration system is a custom-made
  hair net that provides artificial hair where
  required, normal hair being pulled through
  the net.
- Hair additions are fibres glued to existing
  hair and removed after 8 weeks.

Styling products include gels, mousses and sprays to keep hair in place and add volume. They are reapplied after washing or styling the hair.

CAMOUFLAGING HAIR LOSS – EYELASHES

Artificial eyelashes come as singlets, demilashes and complete sets. They can be trimmed if necessary. The lashes can irritate the eye and eyelids. They are stuck on with methacrylate glue, which can also irritate and sometimes causes contact allergic dermatitis.

Eyeliner tattooing is permanent and should be undertaken by a professional cosmetic tattooist. The colour eventually fades and may move slightly from the original site. It is extremely difficult to remove the pigment, should the result turn out to be unsatisfactory.

CAMOUFLAGING HAIR LOSS – EYEBROWS

Artificial eyebrows are manufactured from synthetic or natural human hair on a net that is glued in place.

Eyebrow pencil can be obtained in a variety of colours made from inorganic pigments.

Tattooing can also be undertaken to disguise the loss of eyebrows, but tends to look rather unnatural because of the shine of hairless skin.

How can alopecia areata be prevented?

We do not yet know how to prevent the onset of alopecia areata.

What is the outlook for alopecia areata?

In 80% of patients with a single bald patch, spontaneous regrowth occurs within a year. Even in the most severe cases of alopecia totalis and alopecia universalis, recovery may occur at some future date.

Poor prognostic factors include:
- extensive disease.
- bald patches persisting for more than 1 year.
- ophiasis pattern of hair loss.
- alopecia areata of the nails.
- onset of alopecia areata before puberty.
- family members with alopecia areata.
- personal or family history of other autoimmune diseases.
- Trisomy 21.

New treatments with monoclonal antibody biologic agents targeting cytokine pathways hold promise for the future.

4.2 Dry skin

What is dry skin?

Dry skin refers to skin that feels dry to touch. Dry skin is lacking moisture in the outer horny cell layer (stratum corneum) and this results in cracks in the skin surface. Dry skin is also called xerosis, xeroderma or asteatosis (lack of fat).

Who gets dry skin?

Dry skin can affect males and females of all ages. There is some racial variability in water and lipid content of the skin.

- Dry skin that starts in early childhood may be one of about 20 types of ichthyosis (fish-scale skin; see *Fig. 4.7*). There is often a family history of dry skin.
- Dry skin is commonly seen in people with atopic dermatitis (see *Fig. 4.8*).
- Nearly everyone older than 60 years has dry skin.

Dry skin that begins later may be seen in people with certain diseases and conditions:

- post-menopausal females.
- hypothyroidism (see *Fig. 4.9*).
- chronic renal disease.
- malnutrition and weight loss.
- subclinical dermatitis.

- treatment with certain drugs such as oral retinoids (see *Fig. 4.10*), diuretics and epidermal growth factor receptor inhibitors.

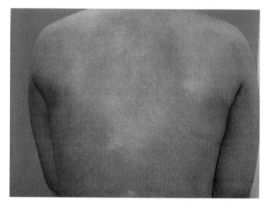

Figure 4.8. Dry skin in atopic dermatitis.

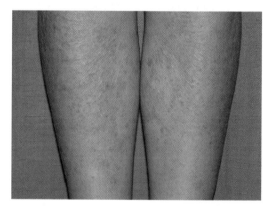

Figure 4.9. Dry skin in hypothyroidism.

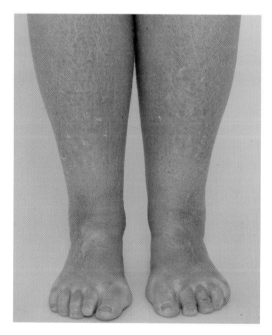

Figure 4.7. Ichthyosis vulgaris.

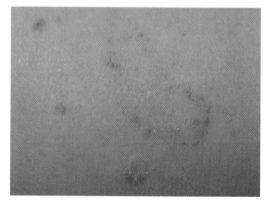

Figure 4.10. Dry skin and dermatitis due to isotretinoin.

People exposed to a dry environment may experience dry skin.

- Low humidity: in desert climates or cool, windy conditions.
- Excessive air conditioning.
- Direct heat from a fire or fan heater.
- Excessive bathing.
- Contact with soap, detergents and solvents.
- Inappropriate topical agents such as alcohol.
- Frictional irritation from rough clothing or abrasives.

What causes dry skin?

Dry skin is due to abnormalities in the integrity of the barrier function of the stratum corneum, which is made up of corneocytes.

- There is an overall reduction in the lipids in the stratum corneum.
- Ratio of ceramides, cholesterol and free fatty acids may be normal or altered.
- There may be a reduction in proliferation of keratinocytes.
- Keratinocyte subtypes change in dry skin with decrease in K1, K10 and increase in K5, K14.
- Involucrin (a protein) may be expressed early, increasing cell stiffness.
- The result is retention of corneocytes and reduced water-holding capacity.

The inherited forms of ichthyosis are due to loss of function mutations in various genes (listed in parentheses below); see www.DermNetNZ.org for details.

- Ichthyosis vulgaris (*FLG*); see *Fig. 4.7* above.
- Recessive X-linked ichthyosis (*STS*); see *Fig. 4.11*.
- Autosomal recessive congenital ichthyosis (*ABCA12, TGM1, ALOXE3*); see *Fig. 4.12*.

- Keratinopathic ichthyoses (*KRT1, KRT10, KRT2*); see *Fig. 4.13*.

Acquired ichthyosis may be due to:

- metabolic factors: thyroid deficiency.
- illness: lymphoma, internal malignancy, sarcoidosis, HIV infection.
- drugs: nicotinic acid, kava, protein kinase inhibitors, hydroxyurea.

What are the clinical features of dry skin?

Dry skin has a dull surface with a rough, scaly quality. The skin is less pliable and cracked. When dryness is severe, the skin may become inflamed and fissured.

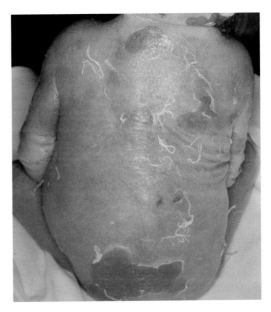

Figure 4.12. Epidermolytic ichthyosis.

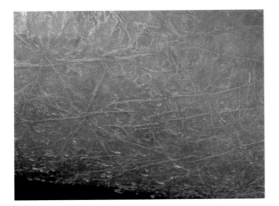

Figure 4.11. Recessive X-linked ichthyosis.

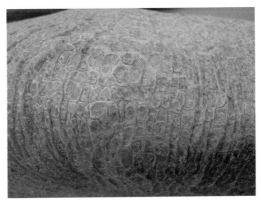

Figure 4.13. Keratinopathic ichthyosis.

Although any body site can be dry, dry skin tends to affect the shins more than any other site.

The clinical features of ichthyosis depend on the specific type of ichthyosis.

Complications of dry skin

Dry areas of skin may become itchy, indicating a form of eczema/dermatitis has developed.

- Atopic eczema – especially in people with ichthyosis vulgaris (see *Fig. 4.7* above).
- Eczema craquelé – especially in elderly people; also called asteatotic eczema.
- A dry form of nummular dermatitis/discoid eczema – especially in people who wash their skin excessively (see *Fig. 4.14*).

When the dry skin of an elderly person is itchy without a visible rash, it is sometimes called winter itch, seventh age itch, senile pruritus or chronic pruritus of the elderly.

Other complications of dry skin may include:

- skin infection, when bacteria or viruses penetrate a break in the skin surface.
- overheating, especially in some forms of ichthyosis.
- food allergy, e.g. to peanuts, has been associated with filaggrin mutations.
- contact allergy, e.g. to nickel, has also been correlated with barrier function defects.

How is the type of dry skin diagnosed?

The type of dry skin is diagnosed by careful history and examination.

In children:

- family history.
- age of onset.
- appearance at birth, if known.
- distribution of dry skin.
- other features, e.g. eczema, abnormal nails, hair, dentition, sight, hearing.

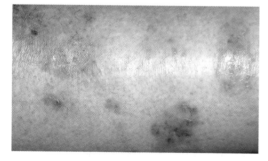

Figure 4.14. Dry form of nummular dermatitis/discoid eczema.

In adults:

- medical history.
- medications and topical preparations.
- bathing frequency and use of soap.
- evaluation of environmental factors that may contribute to dry skin.

Sometimes, skin biopsy may be requested. There may be additional tests requested to diagnose some types of ichthyosis.

What is the treatment for dry skin?

The mainstay of treatment of dry skin and ichthyosis is moisturisers/emollients. They should be applied liberally and often enough to:

- reduce itch.
- improve barrier function.
- prevent entry of irritants, bacteria.
- reduce transepidermal water loss.

When considering which emollient is most suitable, consider:

- severity of the dryness.
- tolerance.
- personal preference.
- cost.

Emollients generally work best if applied to damp skin, if pH is below 7 (acidic), and if containing humectants such as urea.

Additional treatments include topical corticosteroid if itchy or there is dermatitis – choose an emollient base.

How can dry skin be prevented?

Eliminate aggravating factors.

- Reduce frequency of bathing.
- Humidifier in winter and air conditioner in summer.
- Compare having a short shower with a prolonged soak in a bath.
- Use lukewarm, not hot, water.
- Replace standard soap with a substitute such as a synthetic detergent cleanser, water-miscible emollient, bath oil, anti-pruritic tar oil, colloidal oatmeal, etc.
- Apply an emollient liberally and often, particularly shortly after bathing, and when itchy. The drier the skin, the thicker this should be, especially on the hands.

What is the outlook for dry skin?

A tendency to dry skin may persist life-long, or it may improve once contributing factors are controlled.

4.3 Excessive hair

Excessive hair comprises two entities:
- hirsutism (also known as hirsutes).
- hypertrichosis.

What is hirsutism?

Hirsutism (*Fig. 4.15*) is a male pattern of secondary or post-pubertal hair growth occurring in women. It arises in the moustache and beard areas at puberty when hair also appears in non-hirsute women in the underarm and pubic areas. Hirsute women may also develop thicker, longer hair than is usual on their limbs and trunk.

What is hypertrichosis?

Hypertrichosis is non-hirsute excessive hair growth over and above the normal for the age, sex and race of a male or female (*Fig. 4.16*). It can refer to unpigmented vellus hair or darker, longer, terminal hair, and can be generalised or localised.

Who gets hirsutism?

Which women are considered hirsute varies according to culture and ethnicity, as the normal range of secondary hair growth varies with race. It should also be noted that women spend a great deal of time and energy removing unwanted hair, resulting in an unnaturally hair-free norm in today's society.
- A hirsute pattern of hair growth is usually genetically determined, confirmed by male and female family members also having more hair than average.
- Late onset hirsutism may be due to hyperandrogenism, i.e. an increase in circulating androgens including testosterone.

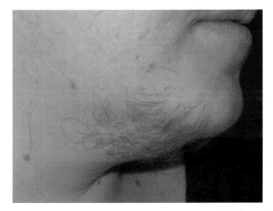

Figure 4.15. Hirsutism.

Hyperandrogenism is often associated with polycystic ovaries, insulin resistance and obesity. Rare causes include:
- Cushing syndrome.
- congenital adrenal hyperplasia.
- androgenic medications.
- tumour of adrenal gland or ovary.

Who gets hypertrichosis?

Normal hair growth is genetically determined and highly variable. Hypertrichosis may be a subjective complaint of healthy individuals. Pathological hypertrichosis can be congenital or acquired.

CONGENITAL HYPERTRICHOSIS

- Congenital hypertrichosis lanuginosa, also known as hypertrichosis universalis, and congenital hypertrichosis terminalis are very rare syndromes with autosomal dominant inheritance.
- Naevoid hypertrichosis is a solitary circumscribed area of terminal hair growth. A faun-tail on the lower back may be associated with underlying spina bifida.
- Localised hypertrichosis may also be a feature of congenital melanocytic naevus, vascular malformation, Becker naevus and less frequently, other birthmarks.

ACQUIRED HYPERTRICHOSIS

Generalised acquired hypertrichosis may be associated with:
- porphyria cutanea tarda.
- malnutrition, e.g. anorexia nervosa.
- malignancy.
- drugs, e.g. ciclosporin, phenytoin, androgenic steroids, minoxidil.

Localised acquired hypertrichosis may be associated with:
- increased vascularity.
- repetitive rubbing or scratching (lichen simplex).
- application of plaster cast (temporary).
- repeated application of minoxidil, corticosteroid, iodine, psoralens.
- trichomegaly (long eyelashes) can arise from local bimatoprost or systemic erlotinib.

What causes hirsutism?

Different genes expressed in individual hair follicles vary in their response to androgens.

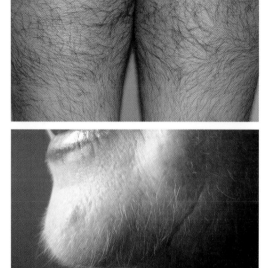
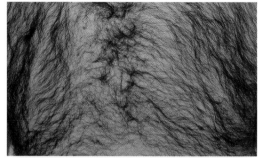
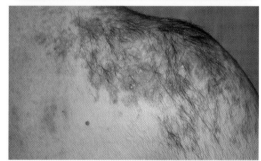
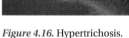

Figure 4.16. Hypertrichosis.

- Hair follicles in the secondary hair growth sites are more sensitive to androgens than those in other areas.
- Androgens alter mesenchyme-epithelial cell interactions, changing the duration of hair growth, dermal papilla size and dermal papilla cell, keratinocyte and melanocyte activity.
- Small vellus follicles producing tiny, virtually invisible hairs become larger intermediate and terminal follicles making bigger, pigmented hairs.

What causes hypertrichosis?

Hypertrichosis is due to non-hormonal alteration in hair growth driven by genes and cytokines. Precise causes in an individual are often unknown.

What are the clinical features of hirsutism and hypertrichosis?

Hirsutism is usually first noted in late teenage years and tends to gradually get more severe as the woman gets older. Hypertrichosis can be present at birth or appear at any time later on. Affected areas vary.

Hirsutism is usually isolated. It can involve a single site or multiple sites.
- Facial hair: moustache, beard, eyebrows.
- Abdomen: diamond shape of pubic hair extending to umbilicus.
- Chest: around nipples or more extensive growth.
- Upper back.
- Inner thighs.

Severity is assessed using a modified version of the Ferriman–Gallwey visual scale, which assesses nine areas of the body. The score varies from 0 (no hair) to 4 (extensive hair growth) in each area.
- Total score <8: normal hair growth.
- Total score 8–14: mild hirsutes.
- Total score ≥15: moderate to severe hirsutes.

General examination may reveal clues as to the cause of hirsutism.
- Acanthosis nigricans suggests insulin resistance.
- Galactorrhoea suggests hyperprolactinaemia.
- Purple striae, thin skin, bruising and facial plethora suggest Cushing syndrome.
- Virilisation suggests hyperandrogenism. Signs include:
  - deepening voice
  - balding
  - acne
  - decrease in breast size
  - enlargement of the clitoris
  - increased muscle bulk.

Complications of hirsutism and hypertrichosis

People affected by excessive hair may suffer from great embarrassment with consequent psychosocial effects. They may go to considerable lengths and expense to remove the hair.

Other complications can arise from underlying disease, if any.

How are hirsutism and hypertrichosis diagnosed?

Hirsutism and hypertrichosis are diagnosed clinically. Investigations are not usually necessary, unless the hirsutism has a Ferriman–Gallwey score of >15, when blood tests are done to evaluate male hormone levels and underlying diseases.

Free androgen index is total testosterone concentration divided by sex hormone binding globulin concentration and multiplied by 100. If elevated, check:
- dihydroxyepiandrosterone sulphate (elevated if androgen is of adrenal origin).
- androstenedione (elevated if androgen is of ovarian origin).

If early onset of hirsutism, premature adrenarche, and/or family history of congenital adrenal hyperplasia:
- 17-hydroxyprogesterone.

If Cushingoid features:
- urinary and serum cortisol or overnight dexamethasone test.

If menstrual disorder:
- luteinising hormone (LH) and follicle-stimulating hormone (FSH).
- prolactin.

General health:
- thyroid function.
- glucose.
- lipids (cholesterol and triglyceride).
- imaging, according to any symptoms.

A pelvic examination and abdominal/transvaginal ultrasound examination of the ovaries may be performed, as polycystic ovaries are a common cause of hirsutism.

Diagnostic features for polycystic ovary syndrome are:
1. Oligo-/anovulation.
2. Clinical/biochemical signs of hyperandrogenism.
3. Presence of ≥12 follicles in each ovary, measuring 2–9 mm in diameter and/or increased ovarian volume (>10 ml) on pelvic/transvaginal ultrasound (optional).

If skin fragility and blisters in sun exposed sites:
- check urinary and faecal porphyrins.

Image the lower spine to evaluate the significance of a faun tail.

What is the treatment for hirsutism and hypertrichosis?

Bleaching makes the excessive hair less obvious. Hair can be physically removed.

PHYSICAL METHODS OF HAIR REMOVAL
Hair removal needs to be repeated regularly as hair continues to grow back. Methods include:
- shaving.
- depilatory creams.
- waxing.
- electric hair removers.
- electrolysis and thermolysis.
- laser hair removal.

MEDICAL TREATMENT
Some women with hirsutism may be treated medically with variable response. Eflornithine is a topical option. Oral anti-androgen therapy is not effective in hypertrichosis. Drugs to consider include:
- low-dose glucocorticoids.
- oral contraceptives.
- spironolactone.
- flutamide.
- finasteride.
- cyproterone acetate.
- metformin.
- rosiglitazone.

How can hirsutism and hypertrichosis be prevented?

It is not possible to prevent genetically predetermined excessive hair growth. Insulin resistance associated with obesity can be reduced by weight loss and dietary control.

What is the outlook for hirsutism and hypertrichosis?

Prognosis depends on the cause. The most common types of excessive hair growth persist life-long. Hirsutism has a tendency to be more pronounced with age.

4.4 Hair loss

What is hair loss?

The medical term for hair loss is alopecia.

- Alopecia may be localised or diffuse.
- It can affect the scalp or other parts of the body.
- It may be due to hair shedding, poor quality hair, or hair thinning.
- There may be areas of skin that are completely bald.
- There may be associated skin disease or scarring.

Unfortunately, hair loss may not be easy to remedy.

Who gets hair loss?

As all our hair follicles are formed during fetal growth, it is inevitable that we will notice hair loss of some kind in later life.

Hair loss occurs in:

- males and females.
- children and adults.
- people with any colour or type of hair.

Hair loss can be an isolated problem, or associated with another disease or condition. It can be temporary or permanent, depending on the cause.

How does hair grow?

Hair grows on most parts of the skin surface, except palms, soles, lips and eyelids. Hair thickness and length varies according to site.

- Vellus hair is fine, light in colour, and short in length.
- Terminal or androgenic hair is thicker and longer.

A hair shaft grows within a follicle at a rate of about 1 cm per month. It is due to cell division within the hair bulb at the base of the follicle. The cells produce the three layers of the hair shaft (medulla, cortex, cuticle), which are mainly made of the protein keratin (which is also the main structure of skin and nails).

Hair growth follows a cycle. However, these phases are not synchronised and any hair may be at a particular phase at random.

The three main phases of the hair cycle are:

1. Anagen: actively growing hair, most of them.
2. Catagen: in-between phase of 2–3 weeks when growth stops and the follicle shrinks, 1–3% of hairs.
3. Telogen: resting phase for 1–4 months, up to 10% of hairs in a normal scalp.

Hair length depends on the duration of anagen. Short hairs (eyelashes, eyebrows, hair on arms and legs) have a short anagen phase of around one month. Anagen lasts up to 6 years or longer in scalp hair.

What causes hair loss?

Hair loss can be due to:

- decreased growth of the hair – anagen hair loss.
- increased shedding of the hair – telogen hair loss (see *Fig. 4.20*).
- conversion of thick terminal hairs to thin vellus hairs – pattern hair loss.
- congenital or acquired hair shaft abnormalities.
- infection, trauma or inflammatory skin disease that damages or destroys the hair bulb.

What are the clinical features of hair loss?

The features of hair loss depend on the cause. Actual symptoms such as itch and soreness are generally absent, unless caused by accompanying inflammatory skin disease. However, a burning, prickly discomfort known as trichodynia may accompany hair shedding.

ANAGEN HAIR LOSS

Anagen hair is tapered or broken off. Anagen hair loss is known as anagen effluvium and has sudden onset.

Anagen effluvium is caused by:

- autoimmune disease, e.g. severe diffuse alopecia areata (see *Section 4.1* and *Fig. 4.17*).
- medications, e.g. cytotoxic/chemotherapy drugs (see *Fig. 4.18*).

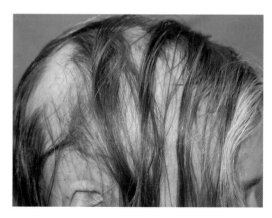

Figure 4.17. Anagen effluvium caused by diffuse form of alopecia areata.

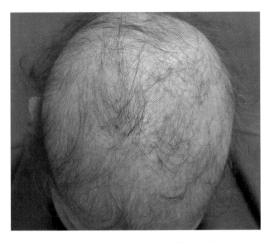

Figure 4.18. Anagen effluvium caused by medication.

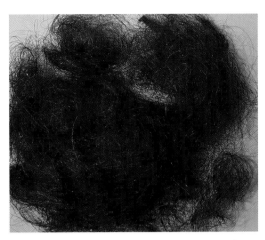

Figure 4.20. Telogen hair loss.

■ inherited/congenital condition, e.g. loose anagen syndrome (*Fig. 4.19*).

Short broken hairs and empty follicles may be observed. If caused by a drug or toxin, hair growth can return to normal within 3–6 months of its withdrawal.

TELOGEN HAIR LOSS

Telogen hair has a bulb at the end (club hair). Excessive shedding (see *Fig. 4.20*) is known as telogen effluvium (*Fig. 4.21*). It occurs 2–6 months after an event that stops active hair growth.

Telogen effluvium is caused by:
■ child-bearing.
■ fever.
■ weight loss.
■ haemorrhage.
■ surgical operation, illness or psychological stress.
■ medications, e.g. contraceptives, statins, imiquimod.

Sometimes there appears to be no recognisable cause for telogen effluvium, and shedding can continue for years (chronic telogen effluvium). Scalp hair continues to grow, but has a shorter natural length than normal.

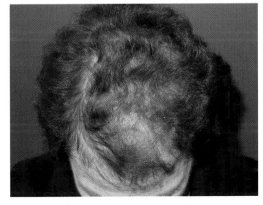

Figure 4.21. Telogen effluvium associated with systemic reaction to imiquimod cream used to treat superficial skin cancer.

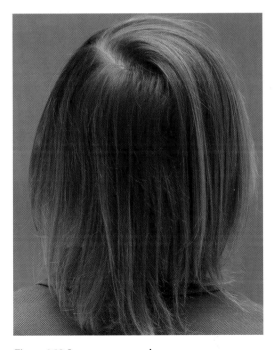

Figure 4.19. Loose anagen syndrome.

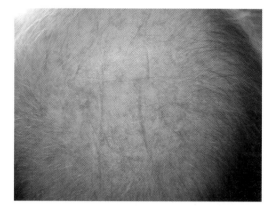

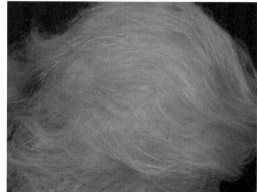

Figure 4.22. Male (left) and female (right) pattern alopecia.

Pattern hair loss

Pattern hair loss is due to genetic programming or hormonal influences. It is also called androgenetic alopecia because it is influenced by androgens.

Pattern alopecia is apparent in about 50% of individuals by the age of 50 years.

- Male pattern alopecia affects vertex and temporal scalp, see *Fig. 4.22*.
- Female pattern alopecia is less pronounced and affects the anterior scalp, see *Fig. 4.22*.

Hair shaft abnormalities

Hair shaft defects can be inherited and congenital, or acquired due to disease or injury (e.g. excessive brushing, hair pulling (trichotillomania, see *Fig. 4.23*), hair dryer heat, relaxing chemicals, bleach). They are diagnosed by microscopic examination of the hair, and sometimes by scanning electron microscopy. They include:

- fractures: trichorrhexis nodosa (see *Fig. 4.24*), trichoschisis, trichoclasis (trichothiodystrophy).
- irregularities: trichorrhexis invaginata (seen with ichthyosis in Netherton's syndrome), Marie-Unna hypotrichosis (uncombable hair), pili bifurcati, pili annulati, pseudopili annulati, monilethrix (beaded hair), pseudomonilethrix.
- coiling and twisting: pili torti (twisted hair), woolly hair, trichonodosis (knotted hair).

Dermatological disease

Conditions resulting in reversible patchy hair thinning, poor hair quality and bald patches include:

- localised alopecia areata (see *Fig. 4.1*).
- localised infection, such as tinea capitis (*Fig. 4.25*).

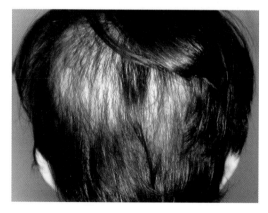

Figure 4.23. Trichotillomania.

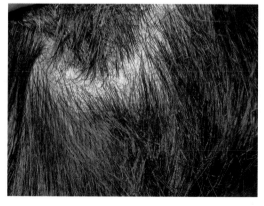

Figure 4.24. Trichorrhexis nodosa.

- severe local skin disease, such as psoriasis (*Fig. 4.26*), eczema, pityriasis rubra pilaris, cutaneous T-cell lymphoma (see *Fig. 4.27*).
- generalised skin disease (erythroderma).

SYSTEMIC DISEASE

Systemic diseases resulting in reversible patchy hair thinning, poor hair quality and bald patches include:

- iron deficiency.
- thyroid hormone deficiency.
- systemic lupus erythematosus (see *Fig. 4.28*).
- syphilis.
- severe acute or chronic illness.

DESTRUCTIVE INFLAMMATORY SKIN DISEASES

Inflammation in the dermis or subcutaneous tissue may injure the hair follicle, resulting in localised bald patches in which there are no visible follicles; this is called scarring alopecia or cicatricial alopecia. Examples include:

- trauma: surgery (see *Fig. 4.29*), radiation, traction (see *Fig. 4.30*), central centrifugal cicatricial alopecia.
- infections: boils and abscesses (*Staphylococcus aureus*, see *Section 2.1.3*), kerion (inflammatory tinea capitis, see *Fig. 4.31, Section 2.2.3*), shingles (herpes zoster see *Section 2.3.5*).
- inflammatory skin diseases: folliculitis decalvans (*Fig. 4.32*), dissecting cellulitis (*Fig. 4.33*), lichen planopilaris (*Fig. 4.34*), frontal fibrosing alopecia (*Fig. 4.35*), alopecia mucinosa (*Fig. 4.36*), discoid lupus erythematosus (*Fig. 4.37*, see *Section 3.4*), localised scleroderma.

Pseudopelade of Brocq (see *Fig. 4.38*) is a condition in which there are localised areas of the scalp in which hair follicles have disappeared without visible inflammation.

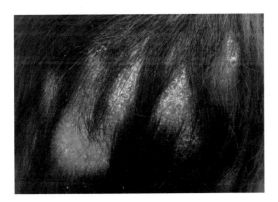

Figure 4.25. Hair loss due to tinea capitis.

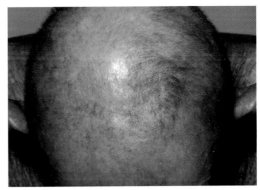

Figure 4.27. Hair loss due to cutaneous T-cell lymphoma: Sézary syndrome.

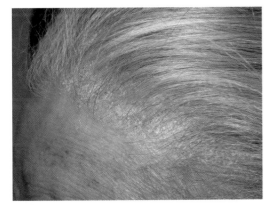

Figure 4.26. Hair thinning due to psoriasis.

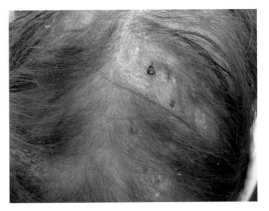

Figure 4.28. Hair loss due to SLE.

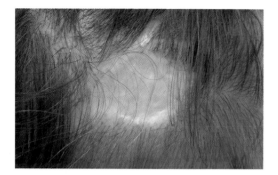

Figure 4.29. Hair loss due to skin graft.

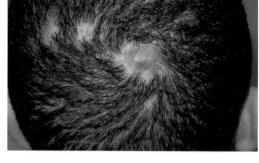

Figure 4.33. Hair loss due to dissecting cellulitis.

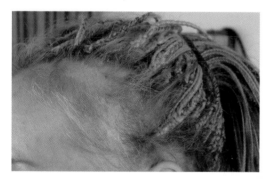

Figure 4.30. Hair loss due to tight braiding.

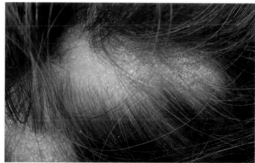

Figure 4.34. Hair loss due to lichen planopilaris.

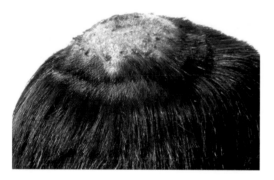

Figure 4.31. Hair loss due to kerion.

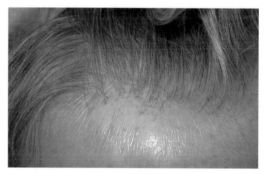

Figure 4.35. Frontal fibrosing alopecia.

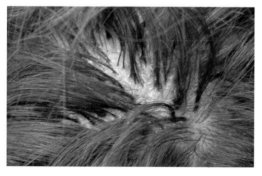

Figure 4.32. Hair loss due to folliculitis decalvans.

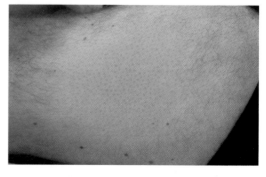

Figure 4.36. Alopecia mucinosa.

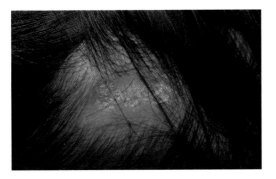

Figure 4.37. Hair loss in discoid lupus erythematosus.

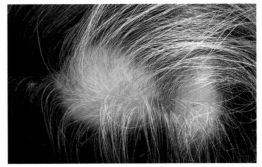

Figure 4.39. Alopecia areata showing bald patches and white regrowing hair.

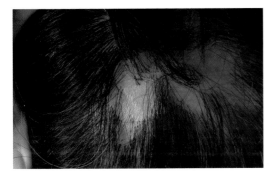

Figure 4.38. Pseudopelade of Brocq.

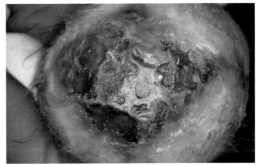

Figure 4.40. Aplasia cutis.

Differential diagnosis of hair loss

SCALP: LOCALISED HAIR LOSS WITHOUT SCARRING
- Treated bacterial or fungal infection.
- Alopecia areata (see *Section 4.1*).
  - round bald patches (see *Fig. 4.1*)
  - exclamation hairs (see *Fig. 4.2*)
  - regrowing hair is often white (*Fig. 4.39*)
  - diffuse, totalis and universalis variants

SCALP: LOCALISED HAIR LOSS WITH SCARRING
- Aplasia cutis (*Fig. 4.40*).
  - eroded or thin skin at birth
- Central centrifugal cicatricial alopecia (CCCA, see *Fig. 4.41*).
  - African ancestry
  - hair style that pulls on the hair
- Ectodermal dysplasia.
  - various syndromes
- Pseudopelade (see *Fig. 4.38*).
  - "footprints in the snow"
- Sebaceous naevus (*Fig. 4.42*).
  - yellowish–orange–pink plaque at birth
  - thickens at puberty
- Trauma or surgery.

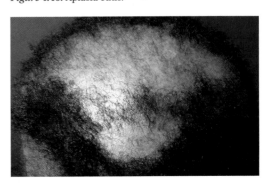

Figure 4.41. CCCA. Photo courtesy Dr Stavonnie Patterson.

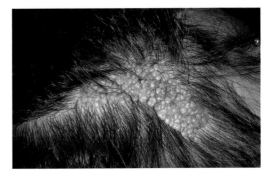

Figure 4.42. Sebaceous naevus.

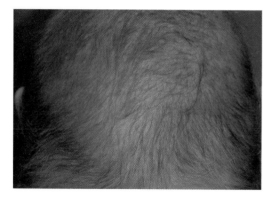

Figure 4.43. Drug-induced hair loss.

SCALP: DIFFUSE HAIR LOSS WITHOUT SCARRING

- Ageing (see *Fig. 4.22*).
- Drug-induced hair loss (*Fig. 4.43*).
  - chemotherapy, retinoids, warfarin, statins
  - diffuse hair loss
  - entire scalp bald
- Pattern balding: slow onset with reduced hair shaft diameter and minimal shedding.
  - males: vertex, anterior scalp (*Fig. 4.44*)
  - females: frontal scalp (*Fig. 4.44*)
- Systemic disease.
  - patchy hair thinning
  - moth-eaten appearance in systemic lupus erythematosus (see *Fig. 4.28*), syphilis
  - suggestive clinical features and investigations
- Telogen effluvium.
  - diffuse shedding (*Fig. 4.45*)
  - hair pull reveals telogen hairs
  - no bald areas
- Alopecia areata (see *Section 4.1*).
  - alopecia totalis/universalis
  - hair pull reveals anagen hairs (see *Fig. 4.46*).

Complications of hair loss

Whatever the type of hair loss, it may be extremely distressing and embarrassing. Loss of normal scalp hair increases the risk of:
- sunburn.
- injury.

How is hair loss diagnosed?

A careful history and full skin examination can generally result in the correct diagnosis. Additional tests may include:
- hair pull test to determine relative proportion of anagen and telogen hairs.
- Wood light examination.
- swabs of pustules for bacterial and/or viral culture.
- skin scrapings and hair clippings for mycology.
- blood tests for haematology, thyroid function, serology.

What is the treatment for hair loss?

Treatment depends on the diagnosis.
- Infections should be treated.
- Deficiencies should be remedied.
- Causative drugs may be discontinued.
- Inflammation can be suppressed.
- Treatment may be available for specific conditions.

How can hair loss be prevented?

Most types of hair loss cannot be actively prevented. However, it is prudent to avoid injury to the hair shaft.
- Dry hair naturally or with hair dryer on a cool setting.
- Minimise chemical treatments or use them infrequently.
- Use loose hair styles to avoid traction injury.

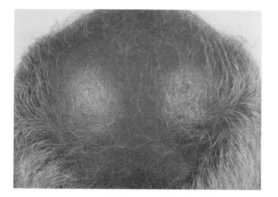

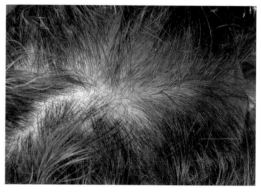

Figure 4.44. Male (left) and female (right) pattern baldness.

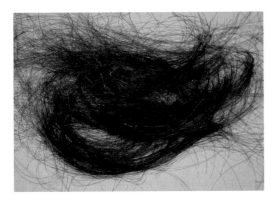

Figure 4.45. Diffuse shedding in telogen effluvium.

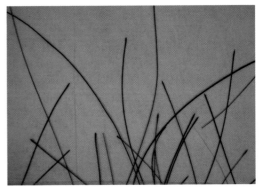

Figure 4.46. Anagen hairs.

What is the outlook for hair loss?

The outlook for hair loss depends on the diagnosis. Scarring alopecia is permanent.

- Anagen and telogen shedding generally stops in time.
- Early treatment of pattern alopecia may reduce the speed of thinning.

- Treatment of inflammatory disease may be successful.
- Hair loss can be disguised or covered.
- Hair replacement techniques include wigs, hair pieces and surgery.

4.5 Hyperhidrosis

What is hyperhidrosis?

Hyperhidrosis is the name given to excessive and uncontrollable sweating.

Sweat is a weak salt solution produced by the eccrine sweat glands. These are distributed over the entire body but are most numerous on the palms and soles.

What are the clinical features of hyperhidrosis?

Hyperhidrosis can be localised or generalised:
- localised hyperhidrosis affects armpits, palms (*Fig. 4.47*), soles (*Fig. 4.48*), face or other sites.
- generalised hyperhidrosis affects most or all of the body.

Primary hyperhidrosis:
- starts in childhood or adolescence.
- may persist lifelong, or improve with age.
- may have a family history.
- tends to involve axillae, palms and or soles symmetrically.
- usually shows reduced sweating at night and disappears during sleep.

Secondary hyperhidrosis:
- is less common than primary hyperhidrosis.
- is more likely to be unilateral and asymmetrical, or generalised.
- can occur at night or during sleep.
- is due to endocrine or neurological conditions.

What is the impact of excessive sweating?

Hyperhidrosis is embarrassing and interferes with many daily activities.

Axillary hyperhidrosis:
- clothing becomes damp, stained and must be changed several times a day.
- wet skin folds are prone to chafing, irritant dermatitis (*Fig. 4.49*) and infection.

Palmar hyperhidrosis:
- difficulty in writing neatly.
- malfunction of electronic equipment such as keypads and trackpads.
- prone to vesicular hand dermatitis (pompholyx, see *Fig. 4.50*).

Plantar hyperhidrosis:
- unpleasant smell.
- ruined footwear.
- prone to vesicular dermatitis (pedopompholyx) and to secondary infection (tinea pedis, pitted keratolysis).

What causes hyperhidrosis?

Primary hyperhidrosis appears to be due to overactivity of the hypothalamic thermoregulatory centre and is transmitted via the sympathetic nervous system to the eccrine sweat gland.

Triggers to attacks of sweating include:
- hot weather.
- exercise.
- fever.
- anxiety.
- spicy food.

Causes of secondary localised hyperhidrosis:
- stroke.
- spinal nerve damage.
- peripheral nerve damage.

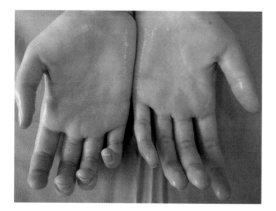

Figure 4.47. Palmar hyperhidrosis.

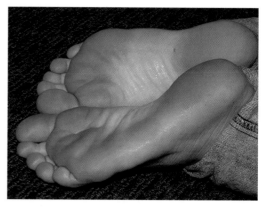

Figure 4.48. Hyperhidrosis on feet.

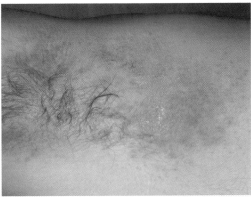

Figure 4.49. Irritant contact dermatitis with hyperhidrosis.

- surgical sympathectomy.
- neuropathy.
- brain tumour.
- chronic anxiety disorder.

Causes of secondary generalised hyperhidrosis:
- obesity.
- diabetes.
- menopause.
- overactive thyroid.
- cardiovascular disorders.
- respiratory failure.
- other endocrine tumours.
- Parkinson disease.
- drugs: caffeine, corticosteroids, cholinesterase inhibitors, tricyclic antidepressants, selective serotonin reuptake inhibitors, nicotinamide and opioids.

What tests are necessary in hyperhidrosis?

Tests relate to the potential underlying cause of hyperhidrosis and are rarely necessary in primary hyperhidrosis.

Screening tests in secondary generalised hyperhidrosis depend on other clinical features but should include as a minimum:
- blood sugar/glycosylated haemoglobin.
- thyroid function.

What is the treatment for hyperhidrosis?

GENERAL MEASURES
- Wear loose-fitting, stain-resistant, sweat-proof garments.
- Change clothing and footwear when damp.
- Socks containing silver or copper reduce infection and odour.
- Use absorbent insoles in shoes and replace them frequently.
- Use a non-soap cleanser.
- Apply talcum powder or corn starch powder after bathing, or try dusting powder containing the anticholinergic diphemanil 2%, if available.
- Avoid caffeinated food and drink.
- Discontinue any drug that may be causing hyperhidrosis.
- Apply antiperspirant.

TOPICAL ANTIPERSPIRANTS
- Antiperspirants which contain 10–25% aluminium salts reduce sweating.
- Deodorants are fragrances or antiseptics to disguise unpleasant smells.
- Available as cream, aerosol spray, stick, roll-on, wipe or paint.

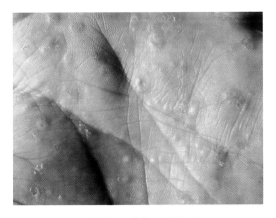

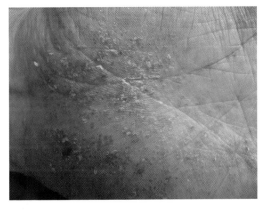

Figure 4.50. Pompholyx with hyperhidrosis.

- Applied when skin is dry, after a cool shower just before bed.
- Wash off in the morning.
- Use from once or twice weekly to daily if necessary.
- If irritating, apply hydrocortisone cream.

Iontophoresis
- For hyperhidrosis of palms, soles and armpits.
- Mains and battery-powered units are available.
- Affected area is immersed in water, an electrolyte solution or glycopyrronium solution.
- Gentle electrical current is passed across the skin surface for 10–20 minutes.
- Repeated daily for several weeks then less frequently as required.
- May cause irritation or dermatitis.
- Not always effective.

Oral medications
Anticholinergic drugs:
- propantheline, oxybutynin, glycopyrrolate (off licence).
- can also cause blurred vision, dry mouth, constipation, dizziness, palpitations and other side effects.
- should not be taken by those with glaucoma or urinary retention.

Beta blockers:
- block the physical effects of anxiety.
- unsuitable for people with asthma or peripheral vascular disease.

Calcium channel blockers, NSAIDs and anxiolytics may also be useful for some patients.

Botulinum toxin injections
- stop sweating for 3–6 months.
- approved for axillary hyperhidrosis.
- used off-licence for localised hyperhidrosis in other sites.

Surgical removal of axillary sweat glands
Overactive sweat glands in the armpits may be removed by several methods, usually under local anaesthetic:
- tumescent liposuction (sucking them out).
- subcutaneous curettage (scraping them out).
- microwave thermolysis.
- excision with primary or complex closure.

Sympathectomy
Division of the spinal sympathetic nerves by chemical or surgical endoscopic thoracic sympathectomy (ETS) may reduce sweating of face (T2 ganglion) or armpit and hand (T3 ganglion), but is reserved for the most severely affected individuals due to potential risks and complications.
- Hyperhidrosis may recur in up to 15% of cases.
- Often accompanied by undesirable skin warmth and dryness.
- New-onset hyperhidrosis of other sites in 50% of patients, severe in 2%.
- Serious complications include Horner syndrome, pneumothorax (in up to 10%), pneumonia and persistent pain (in fewer than 2%).

Lumbar sympathectomy is not recommended for hyperhidrosis affecting the feet because it can interfere with sexual function.

What is the outlook for hyperhidrosis?
Localised primary hyperhidrosis tends to improve with age. The outlook for secondary localised or generalised hyperhidrosis depends on the cause.

4.6 Keratosis pilaris

What is keratosis pilaris?

Keratosis pilaris is a very common form of dry skin characterised by hair follicles plugged by scale.

Who gets keratosis pilaris?

Keratosis pilaris affects up to half of normal children and up to three quarters of children with ichthyosis vulgaris (a dry skin condition due to filaggrin gene mutations). It is also common in children with atopic eczema.

Although most prominent during teenage years, and least common in the elderly, keratosis pilaris may occur in children and adults of all ages.

What causes keratosis pilaris?

Keratosis pilaris is due to abnormal keratinisation of the lining of the upper portion of the hair follicle (the follicular infundibulum). Scale fills the follicle instead of exfoliating.

The tendency to keratosis pilaris has genetic origins, with autosomal dominant inheritance. This means that up to half of the children of an affected individual may display signs of keratosis pilaris to a variable degree.

Keratosis pilaris-like lesions can arise as a side effect of targeted cancer therapies.

What are the clinical features of keratosis pilaris?

Keratosis pilaris (*Fig. 4.51*) most often affects the outer aspect of both upper arms. It may also occur on the thighs, buttocks and sides of the cheeks, and less often on the forearms and upper back. The distribution is symmetrical.

The scaly spots may appear skin coloured, red (keratosis pilaris rubra; see *Fig. 4.52*) or brown (hyperpigmented keratosis pilaris; see *Fig. 4.53*). They are not itchy or sore.

Keratosis pilaris tends to be more prominent at times of low humidity, such as in the winter months.

KERATOSIS PILARIS ATROPHICANS

Keratosis pilaris atrophicans refers to uncommon forms of keratosis pilaris in which

Figure 4.51. Keratosis pilaris.

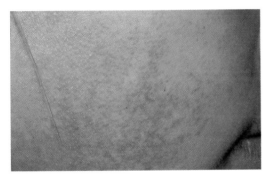

Figure 4.52. Keratosis pilaris rubra.

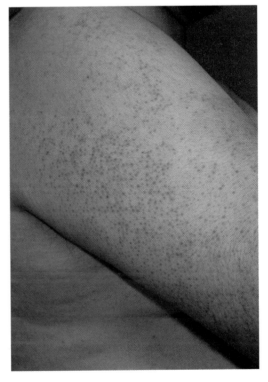

Figure 4.53. Hyperpigmented keratosis pilaris.

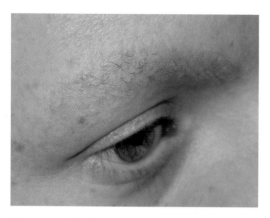

Figure 4.54. Ulerythema ophryogenes.

there are scar-like follicular depressions and loss of hair. These include:

- keratosis pilaris atrophicans faciei (face; see *Fig. 4.52*).
- erythromelanosis follicularis faciei et colli (face and neck).
- ulerythema ophryogenes (eyebrows; see *Fig. 4.54*).
- keratosis follicularis spinulosa decalvans (scalp).
- atrophoderma vermiculata/folliculitis ulerythematosa reticulata (pitted scarring of cheeks).

How is keratosis pilaris diagnosed?

Keratosis pilaris is a clinical diagnosis.
Biopsy reveals:
- epidermal hyperkeratosis.
- hypergranulosis.
- plugged hair follicles.
- mild superficial perivascular lymphocytic inflammation.

What is the treatment for keratosis pilaris?

No cure is available for keratosis pilaris. The following may be useful:
- non-soap cleansers (soap may exacerbate dryness).
- rubbing with a pumice stone or exfoliating sponge to remove scale.
- moisturising creams containing urea, salicylic acid or alpha hydroxy acids.
- topical retinoids.
- pulse dye laser treatment or intense pulsed light (IPL)—this may reduce the redness (at least temporarily), but not the roughness.
- laser assisted hair removal.

What is the outlook for keratosis pilaris?

Keratosis pilaris may become less obvious in time. Atrophy or scarring with hair loss is permanent.

4.7 Melasma

What is melasma?

Melasma is a chronic skin disorder that results in symmetrical, blotchy, brownish facial pigmentation (see *Fig. 4.55*). It can lead to considerable embarrassment and distress.

This form of facial pigmentation is sometimes called *chloasma*, but as this means green skin, the term "melasma" is preferred.

Who gets melasma?

Melasma is more common in women than in men; only 5–25% affected individuals are male, depending on the population studied.

It generally starts between the age of 20 and 40 years, but it can begin in childhood or not until middle age.

Melasma is more common in people who tan well or have naturally brown skin (Fitzpatrick skin types 3 and 4) compared with those who have fair skin (skin types 1 and 2) or black skin (skin types 5 or 6).

What causes melasma?

The cause of melasma is complex. The pigmentation is due to overproduction of melanin by the pigment cells, melanocytes, which is taken up by the keratinocytes (epidermal melanosis) and/or deposited in the dermis (dermal melanosis). There is a genetic predisposition to melasma, with at least one-third of patients reporting other family members to be affected. In most people melasma is a chronic disorder.

Known triggers for melasma include:
- sun exposure – this is the most important avoidable risk factor.
- pregnancy – when this is the cause, the pigment often fades a few months after delivery.
- hormone treatments – oral contraceptive pills containing oestrogen and/or progesterone, hormone replacement, intrauterine devices and implants, are a factor in about a quarter of affected women.

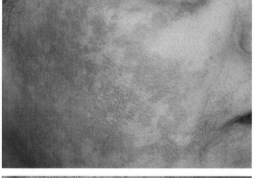
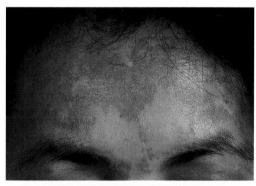
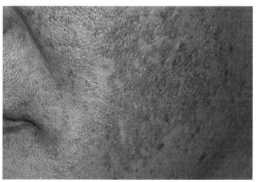
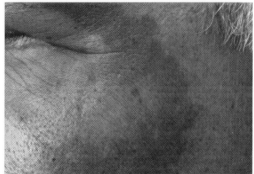

Figure 4.55. Melasma.

- certain medications, scented or deodorant soaps, toiletries and cosmetics – these may cause a phototoxic reaction that triggers melasma, which may then persist long term.
- hypothyroidism.

Melasma commonly arises in healthy, non-pregnant adults and persists for decades. Exposure to ultraviolet radiation (UVR) deepens the pigmentation because it activates the melanocytes to produce more melanin.

Research is attempting to pinpoint the roles of stem cell, neural, vascular and local hormonal factors in promoting melanocyte activation.

What are the clinical features of melasma?

Melasma presents as bilateral and symmetrical pigmented macules and patches with an irregular border. There are several distinct patterns:

- centrofacial pattern – forehead, cheeks, nose and upper lips.
- malar pattern – cheeks and nose.
- lateral cheek pattern.
- mandibular pattern – jawline.
- reddened or inflamed forms of melasma (also called erythrosis pigmentosa faciei).
- poikiloderma of Civatte – reddened, photoaging changes seen on the sides of the neck, mostly affecting patients older than 50 years.
- brachial type of melasma affecting shoulders and upper arms (also called acquired brachial cutaneous dyschromatosis).

Melasma is sometimes separated into epidermal (skin surface), dermal (deeper) and mixed types.

Type of melasma	Clinical features
Epidermal	■ Well-defined border ■ Dark brown colour ■ Appears more obvious under black light ■ Responds well to treatment
Dermal	■ The most common type ■ Ill-defined border ■ Light brown or bluish in colour ■ Unchanged under black light ■ Responds poorly to treatment
Mixed	■ Combination of bluish, light and dark brown patches ■ Mixed pattern seen under black light ■ Partial improvement with treatment

A Wood lamp that emits black light (UVA1) may be used to identify the depth of the pigment.

How is melasma diagnosed?

The characteristic appearance of melasma means diagnosis is usually straightforward and made clinically.

Occasionally, skin biopsy may be performed to make or confirm the diagnosis of melasma. Histology varies with the type of melasma. But some degree of each of the following features is usually found:

- melanin deposited in basal and suprabasal keratinocytes.
- highly dendritic (branched) deeply pigmented melanocytes.
- melanin in the dermis within melanophages.
- solar elastosis and elastic fibre fragmentation.

The extent and severity of melasma can be described using the Melasma Area and Severity Index (MASI).

What is the treatment of melasma?

Melasma can be very slow to respond to treatment. Treatment may result in irritant contact dermatitis in patients with sensitive skin, and this can result in post-inflammatory pigmentation.

Generally a combination of the following measures is helpful.

GENERAL MEASURES

- Discontinue hormonal contraception.
- Year-round sun protection. Use broad-spectrum very high protection factor (SPF 50+) sunscreen applied to the whole face every day. It should be reapplied every 2 hours if outdoors during the summer months. Wear a broad-brimmed hat.
- Use a mild cleanser, and if the skin is dry, a light moisturiser.
- Cosmetic camouflage (make-up) is invaluable to disguise the pigment.

TOPICAL THERAPY

Tyrosinase inhibitors are the mainstay of treatment. The aim is to prevent new pigment formation by inhibiting formation of melanin by the melanocytes.

- Hydroquinone 2–4% as cream or lotion, applied accurately to pigmented areas at night for 2–4 months. This may cause contact dermatitis in 25% of patients. It should not be used in higher concentration or for prolonged courses, as it has been associated with ochronosis (a bluish grey discoloration similar to that seen in alkaptonuria).

- Azelaic acid cream, lotion or gel can be used long term, and is safe in pregnancy. This may also sting.
- Kojic acid is often included in formulations, as it binds with copper, required by L-dopa (a cofactor of tyrosinase). Kojic acid can cause irritant contact dermatitis and less commonly, allergic contact dermatitis.
- Ascorbic acid (vitamin C) also acts through copper to inhibit pigment production. It is well tolerated but highly unstable, so is usually combined with other agents.
- A variety of other agents thought to reduce pigmentation are under investigation.

Other active compounds used for melasma include:

- Topical corticosteroids such as hydrocortisone. These work quickly to fade the colour and reduce the likelihood of contact dermatitis caused by other agents. Potent topical steroids are best avoided due to their potential to cause adverse effects.
- Soybean extract, which is thought to reduce the transfer of pigment from melanocytes to skin cells (keratinocytes) and to inhibit receptors.
- Tranexamic acid, a lysine analogue that inhibits plasmin and is usually used orally to stop bleeding. It reduces production of prostaglandins, the precursors of tyrosine.

Superficial or epidermal pigment can be peeled off. Peeling can also allow tyrosinase inhibitors to penetrate more effectively. These must be done carefully as peels may also induce post-inflammatory pigmentation.

- Topical alpha hydroxyacids including glycolic acid and lactic acid, as creams or as repeated superficial chemical peels, remove the surface skin and their low pH inhibits the activity of tyrosinase.

- Tretinoin is a prescription medicine. It may irritate or cause contact dermatitis in patients with sensitive skin. Do not use during pregnancy.
- Salicylic acid, a common peeling ingredient in skin creams, can also be used for chemical peels, but it is not very effective in melasma.

The most successful formulation has been a combination of hydroquinone, tretinoin, and moderate potency topical steroid. This has been found to result in improvement or clearance in up to 60–80% of those treated. Many other combinations of topical agents are in common use. However, these products are often expensive.

Devices used to treat melasma

Machines can be used to remove epidermal pigmentation but with caution – over-treatment may cause post-inflammatory pigmentation. Patients should be pretreated with a tyrosinase inhibitor (see above).

Fractional lasers, Q-switched Nd:YAG lasers and intense pulsed light (IPL) are the most suitable options.

Conventional carbon dioxide or erbium:YAG resurfacing lasers, pigment lasers (Q-switched ruby and Alexandrite devices) and mechanical dermabrasion and microdermabrasion should be used with caution in the treatment of melasma.

What is the outcome of treatment of melasma?

Results take time and the above measures are rarely completely successful.

Unfortunately, even in those who get a good result from treatment, pigmentation may reappear on exposure to summer sun and/or because of hormonal factors.

4.8 Pigmentation disorders

Introduction

Pigmentation of the skin normally varies according to racial/genetic origin and the amount of sun exposure.

The melanocytes at the base of the epidermis produce the protein melanin, which is carried by keratinocytes to the skin surface. The melanocytes of dark-skinned people produce more melanin than those of people with light skin. More melanin is produced when the skin is injured, for example following exposure to ultraviolet radiation (UVR). The facultative melanisation process in dark skin is protective against sun damage, but melanisation in white skin after sun exposure is much less protective.

Diseases and conditions may result in generalised or localised hyperpigmentation (increased skin colour), hypopigmentation (reduced skin colour), or achromia (absent skin colour).

Generalised hyperpigmentation

Generalised hyperpigmentation may rarely arise from excessive circulating melanocyte-stimulating hormone (MSH), when it often has a bronze hue. It occurs:

- in 95% of patients with Addison disease, when it is more prominent on pressure areas, in skin folds, on scars and within the mouth.
- in 90% of patients with haemochromatosis, when it is more prominent on the genitals, in skin folds and on sun-exposed sites.
- rarely in metastatic melanoma, when it is known as diffuse melanosis.
- in people treated with afamelanotide.

Localised hyperpigmentation

Localised hyperpigmentation may be due to melanin, haemosiderin or exogenous pigment.

If dark patches are observed, the main diagnoses to consider are:

- benign and malignant pigmented skin lesions, such as melanocytic naevi (*Section 5.10*), seborrhoeic keratosis (*Section 5.11*), lentigines (*Section 5.8*), melanoma (*Section 5.9*), and pigmented basal cell carcinoma (*Section 5.4*).
- idiopathic epidermal (*Fig. 4.56*) or dermal (*Fig. 4.57*) melanosis.

- pigmentation due to current or previous inflammatory skin disease, especially in normally dark-skinned individuals, see post-inflammatory pigmentation (*Section 4.9; Fig. 4.58*).
- current or previous superficial skin infection, particularly pityriasis versicolor (*Section 2.3.8, Fig. 4.59*) and erythrasma (*Fig. 4.60*).
- chronic pigmentary disorders, particularly melasma (*Section 4.7, see Fig. 4.55*).
- keratinised or thickened skin, e.g. ichthyosis, acanthosis nigricans (*Fig. 4.61*).
- pigmented purpura due to haemosiderin deposition, e.g. capillaritis (*Section 3.23, Fig. 4.62*) and bruises.

Generalised hypopigmentation

Generalised reduction in pigmentation at birth (congenital) may be racial in origin or due to albinism. Pituitary failure resulting in lack of melanocyte-stimulating hormone (MSH) rarely

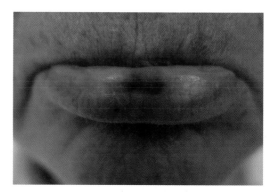

Figure 4.56. Idiopathic epidermal melanosis.

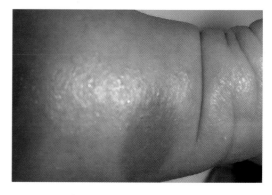

Figure 4.57. Idiopathic dermal melanosis.

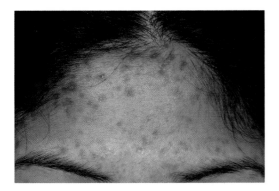

Figure 4.58. Post-inflammatory pigmentation.

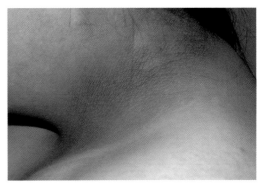

Figure 4.61. Acanthosis nigricans.

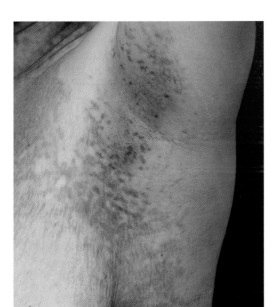

Figure 4.59. Pityriasis versicolor.

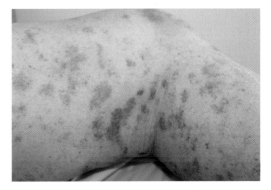

Figure 4.62. Capillaritis.

results in acquired hypomelanosis. Pallor is much more frequently due to blood loss or anaemia.

Localised hypopigmentation

Localised hypopigmentation may be due to partial or complete loss of melanin (achromia or leukoderma).

If single or multiple pale or white patches are observed, the main diagnoses to consider are:

- pityriasis alba (*Section 3.6.10*; *Fig. 4.63*).
- pityriasis versicolor (*Section 2.2.5*; *Fig. 4.64*).
- vitiligo (*Section 4.10*; *Fig. 4.65*).
- lichen sclerosus (*Section 3.12*; *Fig. 4.66*).
- guttate hypomelanosis (ageing-related pale macules on forearms, shins, sometimes elsewhere, see *Fig. 4.67*).
- post-inflammatory hypopigmentation (often surrounded by post-inflammatory hyperpigmentation) (*Fig. 4.68*).
- scarring (*Fig. 4.69*).
- leprosy.

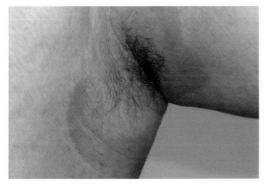

Figure 4.60. Erythrasma.

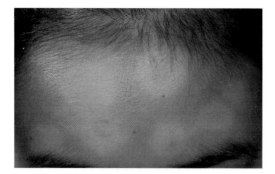

Figure 4.63. Pityriasis alba.

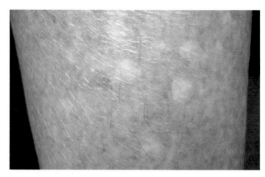

Figure 4.67. Guttate hypomelanosis.

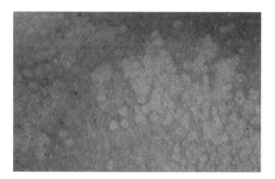

Figure 4.64. Pityriasis versicolor.

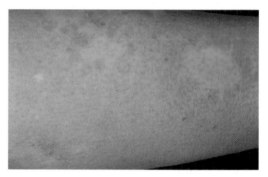

Figure 4.68. Post-inflammatory hypopigmentation (psoriasis).

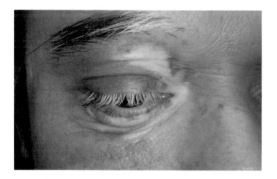

Figure 4.65. Vitiligo.

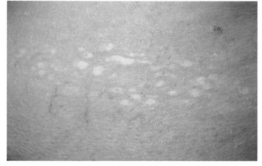

Figure 4.69. Scarring due to herpes zoster.

Treatment and outcome for pigmentation disorders

Both of these depend on what is causing the pigmentation problem.

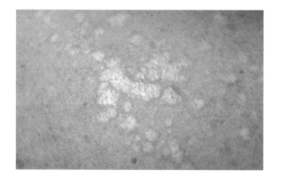

Figure 4.66. Lichen sclerosus.

4.9 Post-inflammatory pigmentation

What is post-inflammatory pigmentation?

Post-inflammatory pigmentation is temporary pigmentation that follows injury (e.g. thermal burn) or inflammatory disorder of the skin (e.g. dermatitis, infection, acne; see *Fig. 4.58*). It is mostly observed in darker skin types. Post-inflammatory pigmentation is also called acquired melanosis.

Some conditions (e.g. psoriasis; *Fig. 4.68*) and more severe injury result in post-inflammatory hypopigmentation or scarring (*Fig. 4.69*).

Who gets post-inflammatory pigmentation?

Post-inflammatory pigmentation can occur in anyone, but is more common in darker-skinned individuals, in whom the colour tends to be more intense and persist for a longer period than in lighter skin colours. Pigmentation tends to be more pronounced in sun-induced skin conditions such as phytophotodermatitis

(*Fig. 4.70*) and lichenoid dermatoses (skin conditions with a lichen planus-like pattern of inflammation, such as erythema dyschromicum perstans; see *Fig. 4.71*).

Fixed drug eruption typically causes post-inflammatory pigmentation (*Fig. 4.72*). Pigmentation is also a feature of reactions to antimalarial drugs, clofazimine, tetracycline (*Fig. 4.73*), anticancer drugs such as bleomycin (*Fig. 4.74*), doxorubicin, fluorouracil and busulfan.

What causes post-inflammatory pigmentation?

Post-inflammatory pigmentation follows damage to the epidermis with deposition of melanin within the keratinocytes and/or dermis.

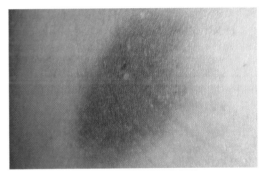

Figure 4.72. Post-inflammatory pigmentation as a result of fixed drug eruption.

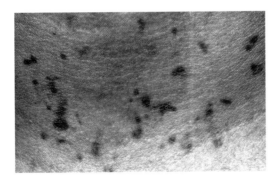

Figure 4.70. Phytophotodermatitis.

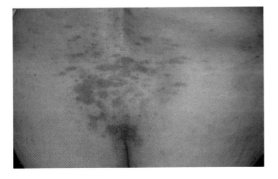

Figure 4.71. Erythema dyschromicum perstans.

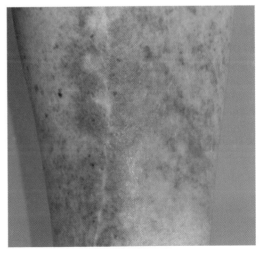

Figure 4.73. Post-inflammatory pigmentation around a scar as a result of tetracycline.

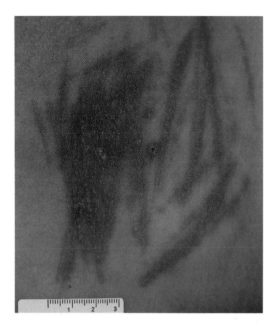

Figure 4.74. Post-inflammatory flagellate pigmentation as a result of bleomycin.

Inflammation in the epidermis stimulates melanocytes to increase melanin synthesis and to transfer the pigment to surrounding keratinocytes (epidermal melanosis). If the basal layer is injured (e.g. lichen planus), melanin pigment is released and subsequently trapped by macrophages in the papillary dermis (dermal melanosis or pigment incontinence). Dermal pigment tends to be a grey brown.

Post-inflammatory hypopigmentation is due to reduced function or destruction of melanocytes by injury to the melanocytes.

What are the clinical features of post-inflammatory pigmentation?

Post-inflammatory hyperpigmented macules or patches are located at the site of the original disease after it has healed. The lesions range from light brown to black in colour. The patches may become darker if exposed to sunlight (UV rays).

Sometimes the most severely affected areas are pale (post-inflammatory hypopigmentation).

What is the treatment for post-inflammatory pigmentation?

If pigmentation affects an exposed site, daily application of SPF 50+ broad-spectrum sunscreen is important to minimise darkening caused by UVR. Cosmetic camouflage can be used.

The following agents can be used to lighten epidermal melanosis, alone or, more effectively, in combination:

- hydroquinone.
- tretinoin.
- moderately potent topical corticosteroid.
- azelaic acid, glycolic acid, lactic acid, kojic acid and salicylic acid.
- L-Ascorbic acid (vitamin C).

These treatments do not benefit dermal pigmentation or hypopigmentation, for which there is no specific treatment.

Resurfacing using chemical peels, laser, intense pulsed light (IPL) or dermabrasion may be effective but unfortunately risks further damage to the epidermis and formation of more pigment.

Can post-inflammatory pigmentation be prevented?

Active use of treatments that treat post-inflammatory pigmentation, particularly hydroquinone, may prevent predictable pigmentation from a cosmetic procedure, such as laser treatment in skin of colour.

What is the outcome for post-inflammatory pigmentation?

Post-inflammatory pigmentation gradually lessens in time. Post-inflammatory hypopigmentation is often more persistent or permanent.

4.10 Vitiligo

What is vitiligo?

Vitiligo is an acquired depigmenting disorder of the skin, in which pigment cells (melanocytes) are lost. It presents with well-defined white patches. Vitiligo can be cosmetically very disabling, particularly in people with dark skin.

Who gets vitiligo?

Vitiligo affects 0.5–1% of the population, and occurs in all races. In 50%, pigment loss begins before the age of 20. In 20%, other family members also have vitiligo. Males and females are equally affected.

Even though most people with vitiligo are in good general health, they face a greater risk of having autoimmune diseases such as diabetes, thyroid disease, pernicious anaemia, Addison disease, systemic lupus erythematosus, rheumatoid arthritis, psoriasis, and alopecia areata.

What causes vitiligo?

Vitiligo is due to loss or destruction of melanocytes, which are the cells that produce melanin. Melanin determines the colour of skin, hair, and eyes. If melanocytes cannot form melanin or if their number decreases, skin colour becomes progressively lighter.

Although it is thought to be a systemic autoimmune disorder, this has been disputed for segmental vitiligo. There is a genetic susceptibility and vitiligo is a component of some rare syndromes.

There are three theories on the cause of vitiligo:
- The pigment cells are injured by abnormally functioning nerve cells.
- There may be an autoimmune reaction against the pigment cells.
- Autotoxic theory – the pigment cells self-destruct.

Current investigations are evaluating the pattern of cytokines and the role of the hair follicle in repigmentation.

What are the clinical features of vitiligo?

Vitiligo can affect any part of the body (see *Fig. 4.75*). Complete loss of pigment can affect a single patch of skin or it may affect multiple patches. Small patches or macules are sometimes described as *confetti*-like.
- Common sites are exposed areas (face, neck, eyelids, nostrils, fingertips and toes), body folds (armpits, groin), nipples, navel, lips and genitalia.
- Vitiligo also favours sites of injury (cuts, scrapes, thermal burns and sunburn). This is called the Koebner phenomenon.
- New-onset vitiligo also sometimes follows emotional stress.
- Vitiligo may occasionally start as multiple halo naevi, see *Fig. 4.76*.
- Loss of colour may also affect the hair on the scalp, eyebrows, eyelashes and body. White hair is called 'leukotrichia' or 'poliosis', see *Fig. 4.65*.
- The retina at the back of the eye may also be affected. However, the colour of the iris does not change.

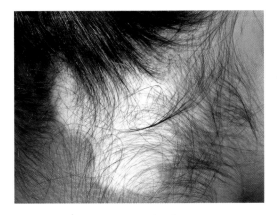

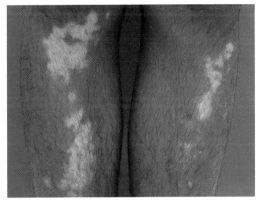

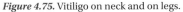

Figure 4.75. Vitiligo on neck and on legs.

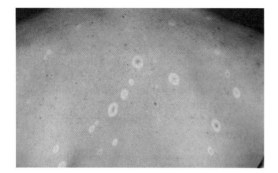

Figure 4.76. Multiple halo naevi.

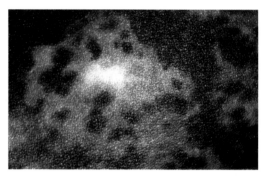

Figure 4.77. Four shades of pigment.

The colour of the edge of the white patch can vary.
- It is usually the colour of unaffected skin, but sometimes it is hyperpigmented or hypopigmented.
- The term *trichrome vitiligo* is used to describe three shades of skin colour. Very rarely, there are four shades of pigment (white, pale brown, dark brown and normal skin; see *Fig. 4.77*).
- Occasionally, each patch of vitiligo has an inflamed red border.

The severity of vitiligo differs with each individual. There is no way to predict how much pigment an individual will lose or how fast it will be lost.
- Vitiligo appears more obvious in patients with naturally dark skin.
- Extension of vitiligo can occur over a few months, then it stabilises.

- Some spontaneous repigmentation may occur. Brown spots arise from the hair follicles and the overall size of white patch may reduce.
- At some time in the future, the vitiligo begins to extend again.
- Cycles of pigment loss followed by periods of stability may continue indefinitely.
- Light-skinned people usually notice the pigment loss during the summer as the contrast between the affected skin and suntanned skin becomes more distinct.
- Pigment has occasionally been reported to be lost from the entire skin surface.

How is vitiligo classified?

The Vitiligo European Taskforce consensus classification of vitiligo (2007) has four main categories and subtypes:

Classification	Subtype	Comments
Nonsegmental vitiligo	<ul><li>Focal</li><li>Mucosal</li><li>Acrofacial</li><li>Generalised</li><li>Universal</li></ul>	<ul><li>Tends to be bilateral and symmetrical in distribution</li><li>Stable or unstable</li></ul>
Segmental vitiligo	<ul><li>Focal</li><li>Mucosal</li><li>Unisegmental, bi- or multisegmental</li></ul>	<ul><li>Single white patch in 90%</li><li>Border often irregular</li><li>Young people</li><li>Stable after first year</li><li>Cutaneous mosaicism (Blaschko, dermatomal, phylloid, checkerboard patterns)</li></ul>
Mixed vitiligo	<ul><li>Nonsegmental combined with segmental vitiligo</li></ul>	<ul><li>Rare</li></ul>
Unclassified vitiligo	<ul><li>Focal at onset</li><li>Multifocal, asymmetrical, nonsegmental</li><li>Unifocal mucosal</li></ul>	<ul><li>Early disease</li></ul>

How is the severity of vitiligo assessed?

In most cases the severity of vitiligo is not formally assessed. However, clinical photographs may be taken to monitor the condition.

At least two scoring systems for vitiligo are used in clinical trials:
- Vitiligo Area Scoring Index (VASI).
- Vitiligo European Task Force (VETF) system.

How is vitiligo diagnosed?

Vitiligo is normally a clinical diagnosis, and no tests are necessary to make the diagnosis. The white patches may be seen more easily under Wood lamp examination (black light).

Occasionally skin biopsy may be recommended, particularly in early or inflammatory vitiligo, when a lymphocytic infiltration may be observed. Melanocytes and epidermal pigment are absent in established vitiligo patches.

Blood tests to assess other potential autoimmune diseases or polyglandular syndromes may be arranged, such as thyroid function, B12 levels and autoantibody screen.

Clinical photographs are useful to document the extent of vitiligo for monitoring. Serial digital images may be arranged on follow-up. The extent of vitiligo may be scored according to the body surface area affected by depigmentation.

How is vitiligo treated?

Treatment of vitiligo is currently unsatisfactory. Repigmentation treatment is most successful on face and trunk; hands, feet and areas with white hair respond poorly. Compared to long-standing patches, new ones are more likely to respond to medical therapy.

When successful repigmentation occurs, melanocyte stem cells in the bulb at the base of the hair follicle are activated and migrate to the skin surface. They appear as perifollicular brown macules.

GENERAL MEASURES

Minimise skin injury: wear protective clothing.
- A cut, a graze, a scratch may lead to a new patch of vitiligo.

Sun protection: stay indoors when sunlight is at its peak, cover up and apply SPF 50+ sunscreen to exposed skin.

- White skin can only burn on exposure to ultraviolet radiation (UVR); it cannot tan.
- Sunburn may cause vitiligo to spread.
- Tanning of normal skin makes vitiligo patches appear more obvious.

Cosmetic camouflage can disguise vitiligo. Options include:
- make-up, dyes and stains.
- waterproof products.
- dihydroxyacetone-containing products "tan without sun".
- micropigmentation or tattooing for stable vitiligo.

TOPICAL THERAPY

Topical treatments for vitiligo include:
- Corticosteroid creams. These can be used for vitiligo on trunk and limbs for up to 3 months. Potent steroids should be avoided on thin-skinned areas of face (especially eyelids), neck, armpits and groin.
- Calcineurin inhibitors (pimecrolimus cream and tacrolimus ointment). These can be used for vitiligo affecting eyelids, face, neck, armpits and groin.

PHOTOTHERAPY

Phototherapy refers to treatment with ultraviolet (UV) radiation. Options include:
- whole-body or localised broadband or narrowband (311 nm) UVB.
- targeted UVB or excimer laser UVB (308 nm) for small areas of vitiligo.
- oral, topical, or bathwater photochemotherapy (PUVA).

Phototherapy probably works in vitiligo by two mechanisms:
- immune suppression – preventing destruction of the melanocytes.
- stimulation of cytokines (growth factors).

Treatment is usually given twice weekly for a trial period of 3–4 months. If repigmentation is observed, treatment is continued until repigmentation is complete or for a maximum of 1–2 years.
- Phototherapy is unsuitable for very fair-skinned people.
- If repigmentation is observed, treatment is continued until repigmentation is complete or for a maximum of 1–2 years.

- Treatment times are generally brief. The aim is to cause the treated skin to appear very slightly pink the following day.
- It is important to avoid burning (red, blistered, peeling, itchy or painful skin), as this could cause the vitiligo to get worse.

SYSTEMIC THERAPY

Systemic treatments for vitiligo include:
- mini-pulses of oral steroids for 3–6 months.
- subcutaneous afamelanotide.

It is anticipated that monoclonal antibody biologic agents will be developed to treat vitiligo.

SURGICAL TREATMENT OF STABLE VITILIGO

Surgical treatment for stable and segmental vitiligo requires removal of the top layer of vitiligo skin (by shaving, dermabrasion, sandpapering or laser) and replacement with pigmented skin removed from another site.
  Techniques include:
- non-cultured melanocyte-keratinocyte cell suspension transplantation.
- punch grafting.
- blister grafts, formed by suction or cryotherapy.
- split skin grafting.
- cultured autografts of melanocytes grown in tissue culture.

DEPIGMENTATION THERAPY

Depigmentation, using monobenzyl ether of hydroquinone, may be considered in severely affected, dark-skinned individuals.
  Cryotherapy and laser treatment (e.g. 755 nm Q-switched alexandrite or 694 nm Q-switched ruby) have also been used successfully to depigment small areas of vitiligo.

Psychosocial effects of vitiligo

Vitiligo results in reduced quality of life and psychological difficulties in many patients, especially in adolescents and in females. The psychosocial effects of vitiligo tend to be more severe in some countries, cultures and religions than in others. Family support, counselling and cognitive behavioural treatment can be of benefit.

Chapter 5

Skin lesions

5.1 Actinic cheilitis

What is actinic cheilitis?

Actinic cheilitis presents as diffuse or patchy dryness and variable thickening of the vermilion of the lower lip (see *Figs 5.1–5.3*). The common form of actinic cheilitis is due to chronic sun exposure. It is also called actinic cheilosis, solar cheilitis, and sometimes, actinic cheilitis with histological atypia.

Actinic cheilitis also describes lip involvement in actinic prurigo, a rare form of photosensitive dermatitis (see photosensitivity, *Section 3.16*).

Who gets actinic cheilitis?

Actinic cheilitis mainly affects adults with fair skin who live in tropical or subtropical areas, especially outdoor workers. They often recall having sunburned lips in earlier years. They may also have actinic keratoses on other sun-exposed sites of the scalp, ears, face and hands.

Actinic cheilitis is three times more common in males than in females.

What causes actinic cheilitis?

Actinic cheilitis results from chronic exposure of the lower lip to solar ultraviolet radiation. It is more vulnerable than surrounding skin because mucosal epithelium is thinner and less pigmented than the epidermis.

What are the clinical features of actinic cheilitis?

Actinic cheilitis most commonly affects the lower lip (90%), and causes:

- dry lips.
- thinned, fragile, skin.
- scaly patches (see *Fig. 5.2*).

Less common features of actinic cheilitis include:
- swelling.
- redness.
- fissuring, focal ulceration and crusting (see *Figs 5.1* and *5.3*).
- loss of demarcation between the vermilion border of the lip and adjacent skin.
- white thickened patches (called leukokeratosis or leukoplakia).
- discoloured skin with pale or yellow areas.
- prominent folds and lip lines.
- difficulty applying lipstick, which tends to "bleed" into the surrounding lines.

What are the complications of actinic cheilitis?

Actinic cheilitis is a pre-malignant condition. It predisposes to:
- intraepidermal carcinoma (Bowen disease or squamous cell carcinoma *in situ*).
- invasive squamous cell carcinoma.

Cancer of the lip is more common in smokers than in non-smokers. Other factors include human papillomavirus, alcohol abuse and immune suppression.

Squamous cell carcinoma should be suspected if the lip is focally tender, or a persistent ulcer or enlarging nodule develops.

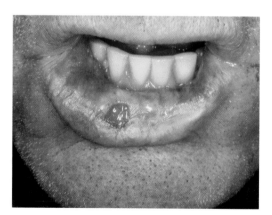
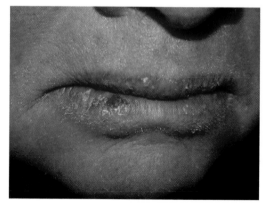

Figure 5.1. Actinic cheilitis: eroded and dry.

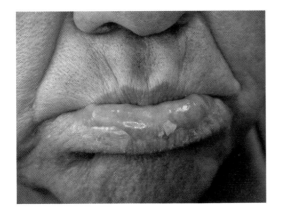

Figure 5.2. Actinic cheilitis: white scaly plaque.

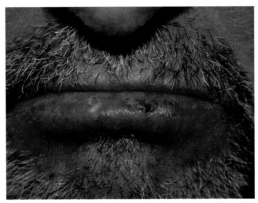

Figure 5.3. Actinic cheilitis: crusted erosions.

How is actinic cheilitis diagnosed?

Actinic cheilitis is usually diagnosed clinically. A skin biopsy may be taken if skin cancer or an inflammatory cause of cheilitis is suspected.

The pathological features of actinic cheilitis are variable thickening or atrophy of the lip, partial thickness epidermal dysplasia, solar elastosis and inflammation in the dermis.

What is the treatment for actinic cheilitis?

Smoking cessation and lifelong, year-round, daily sun protection are essential.

- Limit sun exposure.
- Wear a hat with a wide brim.
- Apply lip balm containing sunscreen frequently.

Men can consider growing a moustache.

Topical therapies for actinic cheilitis are unapproved. They include:

- topical retinoids.
- fluorouracil cream.
- imiquimod cream.
- photodynamic therapy.

Physical treatments for actinic cheilitis include:

- cryotherapy.
- electrocautery.
- vermilionectomy (surgical removal of the lip).
- laser ablation, e.g. with Er:YAG laser.

How can actinic cheilitis be prevented?

Actinic cheilitis can be prevented by protecting the lips from sun exposure.

What is the outlook for actinic cheilitis?

Actinic cheilitis can improve with effective sun protection and treatment. Continued sun exposure and lack of treatment increase the risk of squamous cell carcinoma, which is potentially life threatening.

5.2 Actinic keratosis

What is an actinic keratosis?

An actinic keratosis is a scaly spot found on sun-damaged skin (see *Figs 5.4–5.8*). It is also known as solar keratosis. It is considered precancerous or an early form of cutaneous squamous cell carcinoma.

Actinic keratoses should be distinguished from other scaly spots, such as seborrhoeic keratosis ("stuck on" appearance), porokeratosis (scaly rim) and keratosis pilaris (follicular prominence of upper arms and thighs).

Who gets actinic keratoses?

Actinic keratoses often affect people who have lived in the tropics or subtropics, and have predisposing factors such as:
- other signs of photoageing skin.
- fair skin with a history of sunburn.
- history of long hours spent outdoors for work or recreation.
- immune dysfunction.

What causes actinic keratoses?

Actinic keratoses are a reflection of abnormal skin cell development due to DNA damage by short wavelength UVB. They are more likely to appear if the immune function is poor, due to ageing, recent sun exposure, predisposing disease or certain drugs.

What are the clinical features of actinic keratosis?

Actinic keratosis may be solitary but there are often multiple keratoses. The appearance varies.

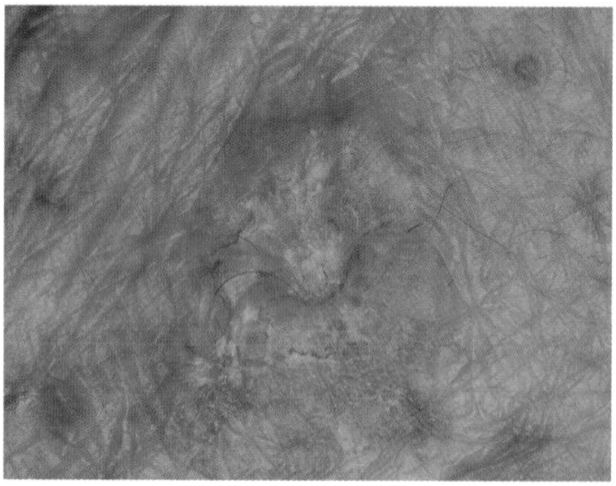

Figure 5.4. Actinic keratosis: indurated scaly papule on dorsum hand.

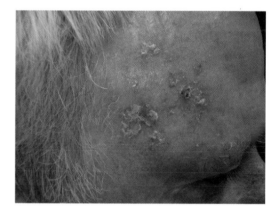

Figure 5.6. Actinic keratosis: diffuse scale crusted papules on temple.

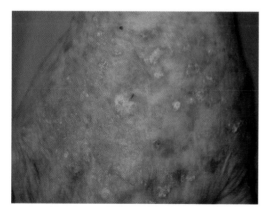

Figure 5.5. Actinic keratosis: diffuse scaly plaques on dorsum hand.

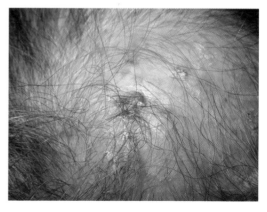

Figure 5.7. Actinic keratosis: scaly papules and plaques on bald scalp.

- A flat or thickened papule or plaque.
- White or yellow; scaly, warty or horny surface.
- Skin coloured, red or pigmented.
- Tender or asymptomatic.

Actinic keratoses are very common on sites repeatedly exposed to the sun, especially the backs of the hands and the face, most often affecting the ears, nose, cheeks, upper lip, vermilion of the lower lip, temples, forehead and balding scalp. In severely chronically sun-damaged individuals, they may also be found on the upper trunk, upper and lower limbs, and dorsum of feet.

Complications of actinic keratoses

The main concern is that actinic keratoses predispose to squamous cell carcinoma (SCC). It is rare for a solitary actinic keratosis to evolve to SCC, but the risk of SCC occurring at some stage in a patient with more than ten actinic keratoses is thought to be about 10–15%. A tender, thickened, ulcerated or enlarging actinic keratosis is suspicious of SCC.

Cutaneous horn may arise from an underlying actinic keratosis or SCC.

Because they are sun damaged, people with actinic keratoses are also at risk of developing actinic cheilitis, basal cell carcinoma (which is more common than SCC), melanoma and rare forms of skin cancer such as Merkel cell carcinoma.

How is actinic keratosis diagnosed?

Actinic keratosis is usually easy to diagnose clinically, by location on habitually sun-exposed sites, and adherent scale. Dermatoscopic features of actinic keratoses are described as "strawberry pattern" on facial skin (*Fig. 5.9*) and as white rosettes on the backs of the hands (*Fig. 5.10*).

Occasionally, biopsy is necessary, for example to exclude SCC, or if treatment fails.

What is the treatment for actinic keratoses?

Actinic keratoses are usually removed because they are unsightly or uncomfortable, or because of the risk that skin cancer may develop in them.

Treatment of an actinic keratosis requires removal of the defective skin cells. Epidermis regenerates from surrounding or follicular keratinocytes that have escaped sun damage.

Tender, thickened, ulcerated or enlarging actinic keratoses should be treated aggressively.

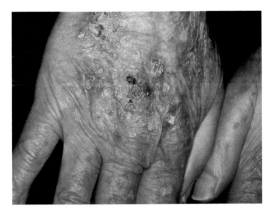

Figure 5.8. Actinic keratosis: tender dry patches on dorsum hand.

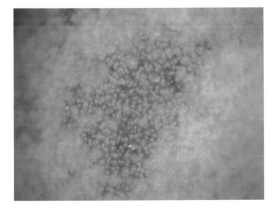

Figure 5.9. "Strawberry pattern" on dermatoscopy of facial actinic keratosis.

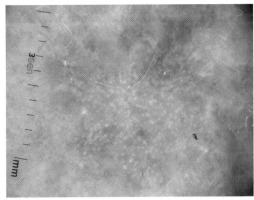

Figure 5.10. White rosettes on dermatoscopy of actinic keratosis on back of hand.

Asymptomatic flat keratoses may not require active treatment but should be kept under observation.

PHYSICAL TREATMENTS

Physical treatments are used to destroy individual keratoses that are symptomatic or have a thick hard surface scale. The lesions may recur in time, in which case they may be retreated by the same or a different method.

Cryotherapy using liquid nitrogen: Cryospray is required to ensure adequate depth and duration of freeze. This varies according to lesion location, width and thickness. Healing varies from 5–10 days on face, 3–4 weeks on the hands, and 6 weeks or longer on the legs. A light freeze for a superficial actinic keratosis usually leaves no mark, but longer freeze times result in hypopigmentation or scar.

Shave, curettage and electrocautery: Shave, curettage (scraping with a sharp instrument) and electrocautery (burning) may be necessary to remove a cutaneous horn or hypertrophic actinic keratosis. Healing of the wound takes several weeks or longer, depending on body site. A specimen is sent for pathological examination.

Excision: Excision ensures the actinic keratosis has been completely removed, which should be confirmed by pathology. The surgical wound is sutured. The sutures are removed after a few days, the time depending on the size and location of the lesion. The procedure leaves a permanent scar.

FIELD TREATMENTS

Creams are used to treat areas of sun damage and flat actinic keratoses, sometimes after physical treatments have been carried out. Field treatments are most effective on facial skin. Pretreatment with keratolytics (such as urea cream, salicylic acid ointment or topical retinoid) and thorough skin cleansing improve response rates. Results are variable and the course of treatment may need repeating from time to time. With the exception of diclofenac gel, field treatments result in local inflammatory reactions such as redness, blistering and discomfort for a varying length of time.

- Diclofenac is more often used as an anti-inflammatory drug. Applied as a gel twice daily for 3 months, it is well tolerated but less effective than the other options listed here.
- Fluorouracil cream is a cytotoxic agent. This is applied once or twice daily for 2–8 weeks (see *Fig. 5.11*).

- Imiquimod cream is an immune response modifier. 5% imiquimod cream is applied 2 or 3 times weekly for 4–16 weeks; 3.75% imiquimod cream is applied daily for 2 weeks. Treatment can be repeated after a break of 2–4 weeks (see *Fig. 5.12*).
- Photodynamic therapy (PDT) involves applying a photosensitiser (a porphyrin chemical) to the affected area prior to exposing it to daylight or an artificial source of visible light (*Fig. 5.13*).
- Ingenol mebutate gel is effective after only 2–3 applications (see *Fig. 5.14*).

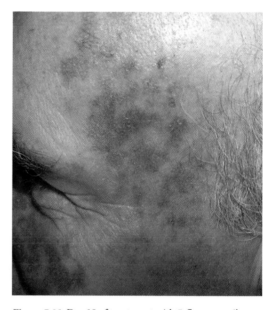

Figure 5.11. Day 12 of treatment with 5-fluorouracil cream.

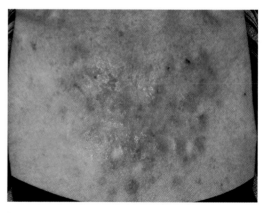

Figure 5.12. Treatment with imiquimod (after 10 applications).

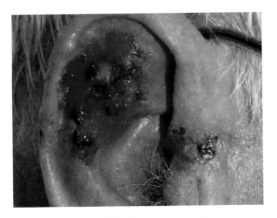

Figure 5.13. The day following treatment with photodynamic therapy.

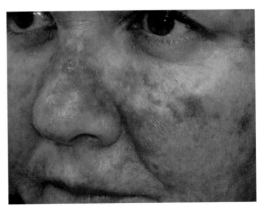

Figure 5.14. Day 3 of treatment with ingenol mebutate gel.

Prevention of actinic keratoses

Actinic keratoses are prevented by strict sun protection. If already present, keratoses may improve with very high sun protection factor (50+) broad-spectrum sunscreen applied at least daily to affected areas, year-round.

The number and severity of actinic keratoses can also be reduced by taking nicotinamide (vitamin B3) 500 mg twice daily.

What is the outlook for actinic keratoses?

Actinic keratoses may recur months or years after treatment. The same treatment can be repeated or another method used. Patients who have been treated for actinic keratoses are at risk of developing new keratoses. They are also at increased risk of other skin cancers, especially intraepidermal squamous cell carcinoma, invasive cutaneous squamous cell carcinoma, basal cell carcinoma and melanoma.

5.3 Ageing skin

What is ageing skin?

Ageing skin describes the changes in the appearance and characteristics of the skin that occur as people get older. Ageing changes are particularly pronounced on the skin of the face and hands (see *Figs 5.15–5.21*).

Who gets prematurely aged skin?

Skin appears prematurely aged in people who are chronically exposed to sunlight, a process known as sun damage or photoageing. Premature ageing of the skin also affects tobacco smokers and those chronically exposed to other environmental pollutants.

Photoageing is pronounced in people with the following characteristics.

- They live in the tropics or subtropics.
- They live at high altitude.
- They work outdoors or spend long periods outdoors for recreation.
- They are exposed to artificial sources of ultraviolet radiation (UV), such as indoor tanning.
- They have fair skin (skin phototype I and II), often with blond hair and blue eyes.
- They have genetic predisposition to premature ageing (most marked in progeria).

What causes the skin to age?

Intrinsic ageing

Intrinsic ageing of the skin is inevitable, and genetically predetermined. It occurs because of accumulation of reactive oxygen species, biological ageing of cells, and reduced cellular supply of nutrients and oxygen.

- The rate of epidermal cell proliferation reduces, affecting structure and function of the skin. The skin thins and flattens, with less resistance to shearing forces and injury.
- Water content in the stratum corneum reduces, with less transepidermal water loss.
- Hair thins and greys.
- The numbers of melanocytes reduce.
- Sebum production reduces.
- The dermis has reduced vascularity.
- There are fewer dermal mast cells and fibroblasts, and reduced glycosaminoglycans, hyaluronic acid and ground substance.
- There is reduced collagen and elastin turnover, and increased glycation.

- Volume of subcutaneous fat diminishes, especially on face, hands and feet—whereas it increases on thighs, waist and abdomen.
- Ageing is immune suppressing, leading to increased risk of skin cancer.

Menopause in females

In women, loss of oestrogen levels at menopause contribute to premature ageing, as compared with similarly aged men.

Photoageing

Photoageing is due to damage caused by solar radiation. Cell damage occurs because of the formation of reactive oxygen species.

- High energy, short wavelength UVB damages DNA and other components of the epidermis.
- Longer wavelength UVA is 100 times more prevalent than UVB at the earth's surface, but is of lower energy so is less damaging to DNA. UVA penetrates more deeply into the dermis, so also has effects on elastic tissue, collagen, blood vessels and immune cells.
- Infrared radiation penetrates to the deeper dermis and subcutaneous tissue, where it may also contribute to sun damage.

Smoking

Smoking exposes the skin to several damaging factors.

- Nicotine narrows blood vessels, reducing blood flow, and thus impairs oxygen and important nutrients reaching the cells.
- Many of the other numerous chemicals in tobacco smoke increase dermal matrix metalloproteinases, degrading collagen and elastin.
- The heat from burning cigarettes, and facial muscle movements associated with smoking, contribute to wrinkles.
- Nitrosamines and tar are carcinogens.

Immune dysfunction

Immune dysfunction also affects skin ageing. Examples include:

- immune deficiency diseases.
- immune suppressing treatments.
- chronic psychological stress.

What are the clinical features of ageing skin?

INTRINSIC AGEING

- Ageing skin is thin, and less elastic, tearing easily.
- It recovers more slowly from mechanical depression than younger skin.
- Women have thinner skin than men.
- Skin is dry, especially after frequent washing with soap and water.
- Dry skin increases the risk of asteatotic dermatitis.
- The barrier function of the skin is less effective.
- Pigmentation is uneven due to melanocyte activation and guttate hypopigmentation.

Genetically predisposed ageing skin may be also prone to:
- telangiectases and cherry angiomas.
- seborrhoeic keratosis.

PHOTOAGEING

Photoageing results in:
- fine lines and wrinkles.
- discoloration.
- textural changes.
- thin skin that easily blisters, tears and grazes (*Fig. 5.15*).
- solar elastosis/heliosis (*Fig. 5.16*).
- solar lentigos (*Fig. 5.17*).
- solar comedones (*Fig. 5.18*) and, rarely, colloid milia (*Fig. 5.19*).
- senile/solar purpura (*Fig. 5.20*).
- scarring.
- actinic keratosis (tender dry spots), see *Fig. 5.8*.
- skin cancer (destructive growths), see *Fig. 5.21*.

SMOKING

Compared to non-smokers of the same age, long-term smokers have:
- more facial lines.
- baggy eyelids and jawline.
- yellowish sallow complexion.
- open and closed comedones and cysts (Favre–Racouchot syndrome).
- greater risk of skin cancer.

Complications of ageing skin

Ageing skin is prone to keratinocytic skin cancer and melanoma. The most common form of skin cancer is basal cell carcinoma. However, excessively photoaged skin increases the risk

of intraepidermal carcinoma, squamous cell carcinoma, lentiginous forms of melanoma and rare skin cancers such as Merkel cell carcinoma.

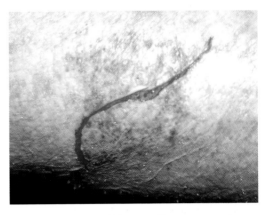

Figure 5.15. Photoaged skin is easily torn or grazed.

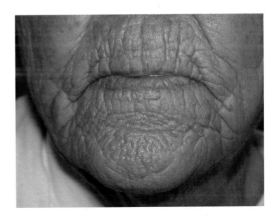

Figure 5.16. Solar elastosis.

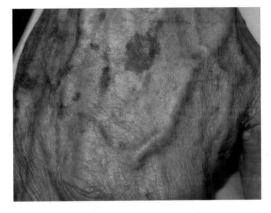

Figure 5.17. Solar lentigos.

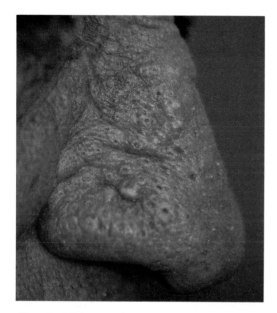

Figure 5.18. Solar comedones.

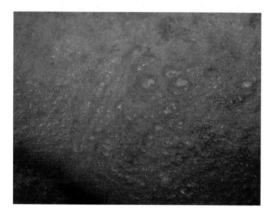

Figure 5.19. Colloid milia.

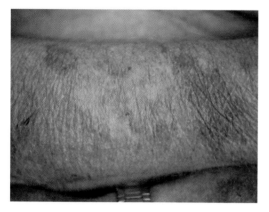

Figure 5.20. Senile/solar purpura.

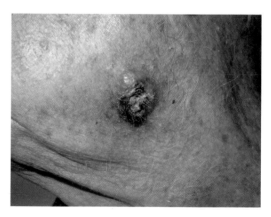

Figure 5.21. Skin cancer.

How are signs of ageing skin diagnosed?

The features of ageing skin are diagnosed clinically. Lesions suspicious of skin cancer may be growing lumps or sores that fail to heal. They often undergo diagnostic biopsy before or as part of treatment.

CLASSIFICATION OF PHOTOAGEING

Glogau classified the degree of sun damage by its clinical signs.

- Type I, mild, "no wrinkles".
  - Mild pigment changes
  - Minimal wrinkles
  - No keratoses
- Type II, moderate, "wrinkles in motion".
  - Appearance of lines only when face moves
  - Early lentigos
  - Skin pores more prominent
  - Early changes in skin texture
- Type III, advanced, "wrinkles at rest".
  - Prominent pigmentation
  - Noticeable solar lentigos
  - Prominent small blood vessels
  - Wrinkles present when face at rest
- Type IV, severe, "only wrinkles."
  - Wrinkles at rest or moving
  - Yellow–grey skin colour
  - Prior skin cancers
  - Actinic keratoses

How are the signs of ageing treated?

CANCER AND PRECANCEROUS LESIONS

- Actinic keratoses and intraepidermal carcinomas are most often removed by cryotherapy or treated topically.

- Basal cell carcinomas (BCC) are most often removed by minor surgery, but superficial BCC can be treated topically or by cryotherapy.
- Squamous cell carcinomas (SCC) and melanoma are nearly always removed surgically.

DRY AND DISCOLOURED SKIN

Moisturisers will help improve dry and flaky skin.

Alpha-hydroxy acids, vitamin C, lipoic acid, soy isoflavones or retinoid creams applied regularly long term reduce dryness. They may also reduce the number of fine wrinkles and even out pigmentation. Many other products are under investigation but their benefits are unclear.

FACIAL REJUVENATION

Procedures that aim to rejuvenate photoaged skin include:

- fillers (hyaluronic acid, polytetrafluoroethylene implants, fat grafts) to disguise facial expression lines.
- botulinum toxin injections to reduce frowning and lessen deep furrows.
- vascular laser and sclerotherapy to remove facial veins and angiomas.
- resurfacing procedures (dermabrasion, peels, and laser resurfacing).
- cosmetic surgery to remove redundant sagging skin, e.g. blepharoplasty for baggy eyelids, meloplasty (face lift) to tighten jowls.

How can the signs of ageing skin be prevented?

Intrinsic ageing is inevitable. In perimenopausal women, systemic hormone replacement may delay skin thinning; the skin is less dry, with fewer wrinkles, and wound healing is faster than prior to treatment. Replacement is less effective at improving skin ageing in the postmenopausal decades. The effects of topical oestrogens, phyto-oestrogens and progestins are under investigation.

Protection from solar UV is essential at all ages.

- Be aware of daily UV index levels.
- Avoid outdoor activities during the middle of the day.
- Wear sun protective clothing: broad-brimmed hat, long sleeves and trousers/skirts.
- Apply very high sun-protection factor, broad-spectrum sunscreens to exposed skin.

Do not smoke and where possible, avoid exposure to pollutants. Take plenty of exercise – active people appear younger. Eat fruit and vegetables daily to provide natural antioxidants.

Many oral supplements with antioxidant and anti-inflammatory properties have been advocated to retard skin ageing and to improve skin health. They include carotenoids, polyphenols, chlorophyll, aloe vera, vitamins B, C and E, red ginseng, squalene, and omega-3 fatty acids. Their role is unclear.

5.4 Basal cell carcinoma

What is basal cell carcinoma?

Basal cell carcinoma (BCC) is a common, locally invasive, keratinocytic, or non-melanoma, skin cancer. It is also known as rodent ulcer and basalioma. Multiple tumours are often diagnosed on a single occasion and over time.

Who gets basal cell carcinoma?

Risk factors for BCC include:
- age and gender – BCCs are particularly prevalent in elderly males; however, they also affect females and younger adults.
- previous BCC or other form of skin cancer (squamous cell carcinoma, melanoma).
- sun damage (photoageing, actinic keratoses).
- repeated prior episodes of sunburn.
- fair skin, blue eyes and blond or red hair; however, BCC can also affect darker skin types.
- previous cutaneous injury, thermal burn, disease (e.g. cutaneous lupus, sebaceous naevus).
- inherited syndromes – BCC is a particular problem for families with basal cell naevus syndrome (also called Gorlin syndrome, see *Fig. 5.22*), Bazex–Dupré–Christol syndrome, Rombo syndrome, Oley syndrome and xeroderma pigmentosum.
- other risk factors include ionising radiation, exposure to arsenic, and immune suppression.

What causes basal cell carcinoma?

The cause of BCC is multifactorial.
- Most often, there are DNA mutations in the patched (*PTCH*) tumour suppressor gene, part of hedgehog signalling pathway.
- These may be triggered by exposure to ultraviolet radiation.
- Various inherited gene defects predispose to BCC.

What are the clinical features of basal cell carcinoma?

BCC is a locally invasive skin tumour. The main characteristics are:
- slowly growing plaque or nodule.
- skin-coloured, pink or pigmented.
- varies in size from a few millimetres to several centimetres in diameter.
- spontaneous bleeding or ulceration (*Fig. 5.23*).

BCC is very rarely a threat to life. A small number of BCCs grow rapidly, invade deeply, and/or metastasise to local lymph nodes.

Types of basal cell carcinoma

There are several distinct clinical types of BCC, and over 20 histological growth patterns of BCC.

NODULAR BCC
- Most common type of facial BCC (see *Fig. 5.24*).
- Shiny or pearly nodule with a smooth surface.
- May have central depression or ulceration, so its edges appear rolled.
- Blood vessels cross its surface.
- Cystic variant is soft, with jelly-like contents.
- Micronodular, microcystic and infiltrative types are potentially aggressive subtypes.

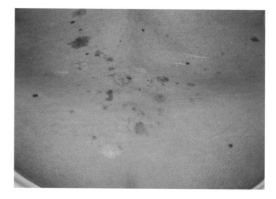

Figure 5.22. Multiple BCCs arising in patient with basal cell naevus syndrome (Gorlin syndrome).

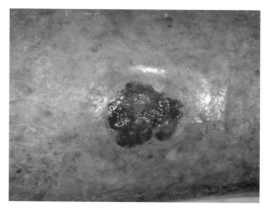

Figure 5.23. Ulcerated BCC.

Superficial BCC
- Most common type in younger adults (see *Fig. 5.25*).
- Most common type on upper trunk and shoulders.
- Slightly scaly, irregular plaque.
- Thin, translucent rolled border, best seen on stretching lesion.
- Multiple microerosions.

Morphoeic BCC
- Also known as morphoeiform or sclerosing BCC.
- Usually found in mid-facial sites (*Fig. 5.26*).
- Waxy, scar-like plaque with indistinct borders.
- Wide and deep subclinical extension.
- May infiltrate cutaneous nerves (perineural spread).

Basisquamous BCC
- Mixed or metatypical basal cell carcinoma (BCC) and squamous cell carcinoma (SCC).
- Infiltrative growth pattern.
- Potentially more aggressive than other forms of BCC.

Fibroepithelial tumour of Pinkus
- Warty plaque.
- Usually on trunk.

Pigmented BCC
- Any histological subtype.
- More common in darker skin (see *Fig. 5.27*).

Complications of basal cell carcinoma

Recurrent BCC
Recurrence of BCC after initial treatment is not uncommon. Characteristics of recurrent BCC often include:
- incomplete excision or narrow margins at primary excision.
- morphoeic, micronodular, and infiltrative subtypes.
- location on head and neck.

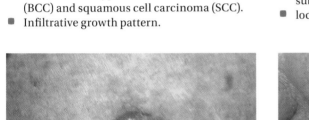

Figure 5.24. Nodular BCC.

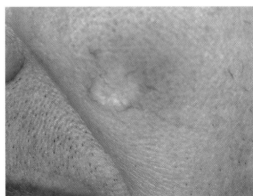

Figure 5.26. Morphoeic BCC.

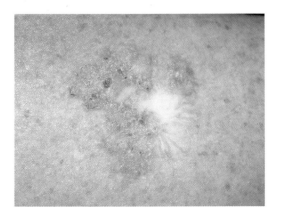

Figure 5.25. Superficial BCC.

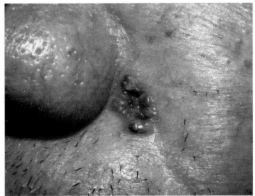

Figure 5.27. Pigmented BCC.

ADVANCED BCC

Advanced BCCs are large, often neglected tumours (see *Fig. 5.28*).

- They may be several centimetres in diameter.
- They may be deeply infiltrating into tissues below the skin.
- They are difficult or impossible to treat surgically.

METASTATIC BCC

- Very rare.
- Primary tumour is often large, neglected or recurrent, located on head and neck, with aggressive subtype.
- May have had multiple prior treatments.
- May arise in site exposed to ionising radiation.
- Can be fatal.

How is basal cell carcinoma diagnosed?

BCC is diagnosed clinically by the presence of a slowly enlarging skin lesion with typical appearance. The diagnosis and histological subtype is usually confirmed pathologically by a diagnostic biopsy or following excision.

Some typical superficial BCCs on trunk and limbs are clinically diagnosed and have non-surgical treatment without histology.

What is the treatment for primary basal cell carcinoma?

The treatment for a BCC depends on its type, size and location, the number to be treated, patient factors, and the preference or expertise of the doctor. Most BCCs are treated surgically. Long-term follow-up is recommended to check for new lesions and recurrence; the latter may be unnecessary if histology has reported wide clear margins.

EXCISION BIOPSY

Excision means the lesion is cut out and the skin stitched up (*Fig. 5.29*).

- Most appropriate treatment for nodular, infiltrative and morphoeic BCCs.
- Should include 3–5 mm margin of normal skin around the tumour.
- Very large lesions may require flap or skin graft to repair the defect.
- Pathologist will report deep and lateral margins.
- Further surgery is recommended for lesions that are incompletely excised.

MOHS MICROGRAPHICALLY CONTROLLED EXCISION

Mohs micrographically controlled surgery involves examining carefully marked excised tissue under the microscope, layer by layer, to ensure complete excision (see *Fig. 5.30*).

- Very high cure rates achieved by trained Mohs surgeons.
- Used in high-risk areas of the face around eyes, lips and nose.
- Suitable for ill-defined, morphoeic, infiltrative and recurrent subtypes.
- Large defects are repaired by flap or graft.

SUPERFICIAL SKIN SURGERY

Superficial skin surgery comprises shave, curettage, and electrocautery. It is a rapid technique using local anaesthesia and does not require sutures.

- Suitable for small, well-defined nodular or superficial BCCs.
- Lesions are usually located on trunk or limbs.

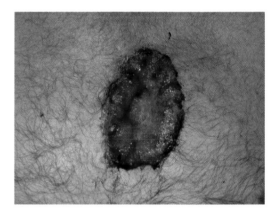

Figure 5.28. Advanced BCC.

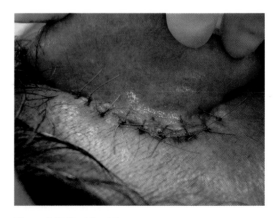

Figure 5.29. Excision biopsy.

- Wound is left open to heal by secondary intention.
- Moist wound dressings lead to healing within a few weeks.
- Eventual scar quality variable.

CRYOTHERAPY

Cryotherapy is the treatment of a superficial skin lesion by freezing it, usually with liquid nitrogen.

- Suitable for small superficial BCCs on covered areas of trunk and limbs.
- Best avoided for BCCs on head and neck, and distal to knees.
- Double freeze-thaw technique.
- Results in a blister that crusts over and heals within several weeks (see *Fig. 5.31*).
- Leaves permanent white mark (see *Fig. 5.22*).

PHOTODYNAMIC THERAPY

Photodynamic therapy (PDT) refers to a technique in which BCC is treated with a photosensitising chemical, and exposed to light several hours later (*Fig. 5.32*).

- Topical photosensitisers include aminolevulinic acid lotion and methyl aminolevulinate cream.
- Suitable for low-risk small, superficial BCCs.
- Best avoided if tumour in site of high recurrence.
- Results in inflammatory reaction, maximal 3–4 days after procedure.
- Treatment repeated 7 days after initial treatment.
- Excellent cosmetic results.

IMIQUIMOD CREAM

Imiquimod is an immune response modifier.

- 5% imiquimod cream is best used for superficial BCCs less than 2 cm diameter (see *Fig. 5.33*).
- Applied three to five times each week, for 6–16 weeks.
- Results in a variable inflammatory reaction, maximal at three weeks.
- Minimal scarring is usual.

FLUOROURACIL CREAM

Fluorouracil cream is a topical cytotoxic agent.

- Used to treat small superficial basal cell carcinomas.
- Requires prolonged course, e.g. twice daily for 6–12 weeks.
- Causes inflammatory reaction.
- Has high recurrence rates.

RADIOTHERAPY

Radiotherapy or X-ray treatment can be used to treat primary BCCs or as adjunctive treatment if margins are incomplete.

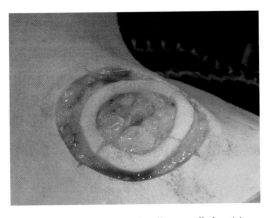

Figure 5.30. Mohs micrographically controlled excision.

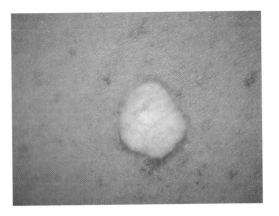

Figure 5.31. Ice-ball formation during cryotherapy.

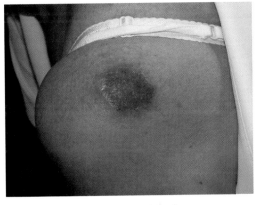

Figure 5.32. Reaction 24 hours after photodynamic therapy.

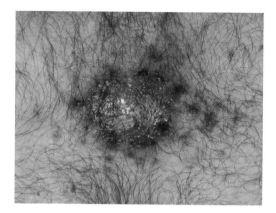

Figure 5.33. Effect of imiquimod cream on BCC after 3 weeks.

- Mainly used if surgery is not suitable.
- Best avoided in young patients and in genetic conditions predisposing to skin cancer.
- Best cosmetic results achieved using multiple fractions.
- Typically, patient attends once weekly for several weeks.
- Causes inflammatory reaction followed by scar.
- Risk of radiodermatitis, late recurrence, and new tumours.

What is the treatment for advanced or metastatic basal cell carcinoma?

Locally advanced primary, recurrent or metastatic BCC requires multidisciplinary consultation. Often a combination of treatments is used.
- Surgery.
- Radiotherapy.
- Targeted therapy.

Targeted therapy refers to the hedgehog signalling pathway inhibitors, vismodegib and sonedegib. These drugs have some important risks and side-effects.

How can basal cell carcinoma be prevented?

The most important way to prevent BCC is to avoid sunburn. This is especially important in childhood and early life. Fair-skinned individuals and those with a personal or family history of BCC should protect their skin from sun exposure daily, year-round and lifelong.
- Stay indoors or in the shade in the middle of the day.
- Wear covering clothing.
- Apply broad-spectrum sunscreens generously to exposed skin if outdoors.
- Avoid indoor tanning (sun beds and solaria).

Oral nicotinamide (vitamin B3) in a dose of 500 mg twice daily may reduce the number and severity of BCCs in people at high risk.

What is the outlook for basal cell carcinoma?

Most BCCs are cured by treatment. Cure is most likely if treatment is undertaken when the lesion is small.

About 50% of people with BCC develop a second one within 3 years of the first. They are also at increased risk of other skin cancers, especially melanoma. Regular self-skin examinations and long-term annual skin checks by an experienced health professional are recommended.

5.5 Cysts

What is a cyst?

A cyst is a benign, round, dome-shaped encapsulated lesion that contains fluid or semi-fluid material. It may be firm or fluctuant and often distends the overlying skin. There are several types of cyst.

What is a pseudocyst?

Cysts that are not surrounded by a capsule are better known as pseudocysts.

Who gets cysts?

Cysts are very common, affecting at least 20% of adults. They may be present at birth or appear later in life. They arise in all races. Most types of cyst are more common in males than in females.

What causes cysts?

The cause of many cysts is unknown.

- Epidermoid cysts are due to proliferation of epidermal cells within the dermis and originate from the follicular infundibulum. Multiple epidermoid cysts may indicate Gardner syndrome.
- The origin of a trichilemmal cyst is hair root sheath (see *Fig. 5.34*). Inheritance is autosomal dominant (the affected gene is within short arm of chromosome 3) or sporadic.
- The origin of steatocystoma is the sebaceous duct within the hair follicle. Steatocystoma multiplex is sometimes an autosomal dominantly inherited disorder due to mutations localised to the keratin 17 (*K17*) gene, when it may be associated

with pachyonychia congenita. More often, steatocysts are sporadic, when these mutations are not present.

- The origin of the eruptive vellus hair cyst is follicular infundibulum. It may be inherited as an autosomal dominant disorder due to mutations in the keratin gene.
- A dermoid cyst is a hamartoma.
- The origin of a ganglion cyst is degeneration of the mucoid connective tissue of a joint (see *Fig. 5.35*).
- A hidrocystoma is derived from an eccrine or apocrine duct.
- A milium is a pseudocyst due to failure to release keratin from an adnexal structure (see *Fig. 5.36*).
  - The origin of primary milium is infundibulum of a vellus hair follicle at the level of the sebaceous gland; a tiny version of an epidermoid cyst.

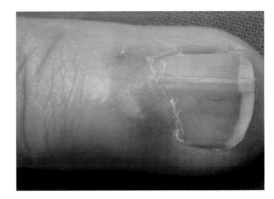

Figure 5.35. Ganglion cyst.

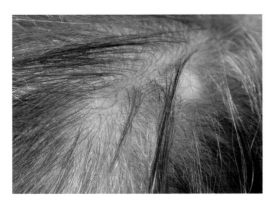

Figure 5.34. Trichilemmal cyst.

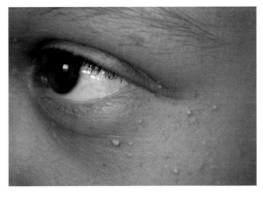

Figure 5.36. Milia.

◻ The origin of secondary milium is a retention cyst within a vellus hair follicle, sebaceous duct, sweat duct or epidermis.

◻ Occlusion of pilosebaceous units (hair follicles) or eccrine sweat ducts leads to a build-up of secretions. This can present as milia.

▪ An epidermal inclusion cyst is a response to an injury. Skin is tucked in to form a sac that is lined by normal epidermal cells that continue to multiply, mature and form keratin.

▪ Occlusion of the orifice of a mucous gland can lead to a fluid-filled cyst in a mucous membrane (lip, vulva, vagina).

▪ Pseudocysts in acne are formed by occlusion of the follicle by keratin and sebum.

What are the clinical features of cysts?

EPIDERMOID CYST

▪ Epidermoid cysts occur on face, neck, trunk or anywhere where there is little hair (see *Fig. 5.37*).

▪ Most epidermoid cysts arise in adult life.

▪ Cysts are more than twice as common in men than in women.

▪ They present as one or more flesh-coloured to yellowish, adherent, firm, round nodules of variable size.

▪ A central pore or punctum may be present.

▪ Keratinous contents are soft, cheese-like and malodorous.

▪ Scrotal and labial (see *Fig. 5.38*) cysts are frequently multiple and may calcify.

▪ Epidermoid cyst is also called follicular infundibular cyst, epidermal cyst and keratin cyst. Sebaceous cyst is a misnomer.

TRICHILEMMAL CYST (pilar cyst)

▪ 90% of trichilemmal cysts (see *Fig. 5.34*) occur on scalp; otherwise face, neck, trunk, and extremities.

▪ Most trichilemmal cysts arise in middle age.

▪ In 70% of cases, trichilemmal cysts are multiple.

▪ Adherent, round or oval, firm nodules.

▪ There is no punctum.

▪ The keratinous content is firm, white and easily enucleated.

▪ A trichilemmal cyst is also called pilar cyst.

STEATOCYSTOMA

▪ A solitary steatocystoma is known as steatocystoma simplex.

▪ More often, multiple cysts occur on chest, upper arms, axillae and neck (steatocystoma multiplex, see *Fig. 5.39*).

▪ The cysts arise in the late teens and twenties due to the effect of androgens, and persist lifelong.

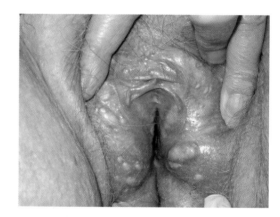

Figure 5.38. Labial cysts.

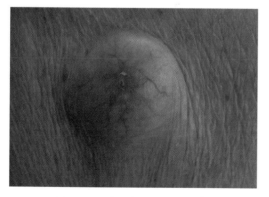

Figure 5.37. Epidermoid cyst.

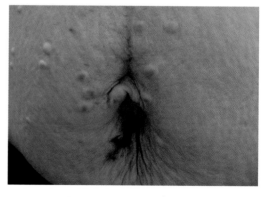

Figure 5.39. Steatocystoma multiplex.

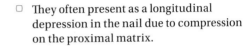

- They are freely moveable, smooth flesh to yellow colour papules 3–30 mm in diameter.
- There is no central punctum.
- Content of cyst is predominantly sebum.

ERUPTIVE VELLUS HAIR CYST
- Eruptive vellus hair cysts are present in childhood if familial, and later if sporadic.
- Multiple 2–3 mm papules develop over the sternum.
- The cysts contain vellus hairs.

DERMOID CYST
- A cutaneous dermoid cyst may include skin, skin structures and sometimes teeth, cartilage and bone.
- Most dermoid cysts are found on face, neck, scalp; often around eyelid, forehead and brow.
- It is a thin-walled tumour that ranges from soft to hard in consistency.
- The cyst is formed at birth but the patient may not present until an adult.

GANGLION CYST
- A ganglion cyst most often involves the scapholunate joint of the dorsal wrist.
- They arise in young to middle-aged adults.
- They are three times more common in women than in men.
- The cyst is a unilocular or multilocular firm swelling 2–4 cm in diameter that transilluminates.
- Cyst contents are mainly hyaluronic acid, a golden-coloured goo.
- Mucous/myxoid cysts are small lesions found in older adults on the distal phalanx.
  - They arise from the distal interphalangeal joint, associated with osteoarthritis.
  - They often present as a longitudinal depression in the nail due to compression on the proximal matrix.

LABIAL MUCOUS CYST/MUCOCOELE
- A cyst in the lip may be due to occlusion of the salivary duct.
- It is a soft to firm, 5–15 mm diameter, semi-translucent nodule (*Fig. 5.40*).

HIDROCYSTOMA
- A hidrocystoma is a translucent jelly-like cyst arising on an eyelid (*Fig. 5.41*).
- It is also known as cystadenoma, Moll gland cyst, and sudoriferous cyst.

MILIUM/MILIA
- They are 1–2 mm superficial (see *Fig. 3.36*) white dome-shaped papules that contain keratin.
- Primary milia arise in neonates (50%), adolescents and adults; they are rarely familial and sometimes eruptive.
- Primary milia occur on eyelids, cheeks, nose, mucosa (Epstein pearls) and palate (Bohn nodules) in babies; and eyelids, cheeks and nose of older children and adults.
- Transverse primary milia are sometimes noted across nasal groove or around areola.
- Secondary milia arise at the site of epidermal repair after blistering or injury, e.g. epidermolysis bullosa, bullous pemphigoid (see *Fig. 5.42*), porphyria cutanea tarda, thermal burn, dermabrasion.
- Secondary milia are reported as an adverse effect of topical steroids, fluorouracil cream, vemurafenib and dovitinib.

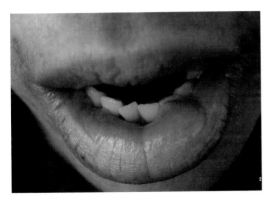

Figure 5.40. Labial mucous cyst/mucocoele.

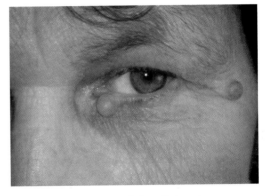

Figure 5.41. Hidrocystoma left medial canthus.

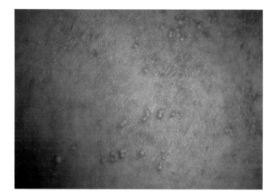

Figure 5.42. Milia arising after blisters have resolved in bullous pemphigoid.

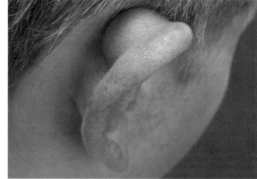

Figure 5.44. Pseudocyst of auricle.

PSEUDOCYST OF AURICLE
- Pseudocyst of auricle (external ear) follows trauma (see *Fig. 5.44*).

Complications of cysts

RUPTURE OF A CYST
- The contents of the cyst may penetrate the capsular wall and irritate surrounding skin.
- The area of tender, firm inflammation spreads beyond the encapsulated cyst (see *Fig. 5.45*).
- Sterile pus may be discharged.

SECONDARY INFECTION
- A ruptured cyst may infrequently become secondarily infected by *Staphylococcus aureus*, forming a furuncle (boil), see *Fig. 5.46*.

PRESSURE EFFECT
- A dermoid cyst can cause pressure on underlying bony tissue.
- A ganglion cyst can cause joint instability, weakness, limitation of motion and may compress a nerve.
- A digital mucous cyst may place pressure on the proximal matrix and cause malformation of the nail.

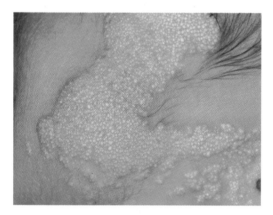

Figure 5.43. Milia en plaque.

- In milia en plaque, multiple milia arise on an erythematous plaque on face, chin or ears, see *Fig. 5.43*.

VULVAL MUCOUS CYST
- A vulval mucous cyst is due to occlusion of Bartholin or Skene duct.
- It presents as a soft swelling in the introitus of vagina: a posterior swelling is a Bartholin cyst and a periurethral swelling is a Skene cyst.

COMEDO AND ACNE PSEUDOCYST
- The open comedo (whitehead) and closed comedo (blackhead) are small, superficial uninflamed papules typical of acne vulgaris.
- Solar comedones arise in sun-damaged skin and are associated with smoking.
- Large uninflamed pseudocysts accompany inflammatory nodules in nodulocystic acne and hidradenitis suppurativa.

MALIGNANCY
- The vast majority of cysts are benign.
- Nodulocystic basal cell carcinoma is a common skin cancer that may initially be mistaken for a cyst, but steady enlargement, destruction of the epidermis with ulceration and bleeding occur eventually.
- Malignant proliferative trichilemmal cyst is extremely rare.

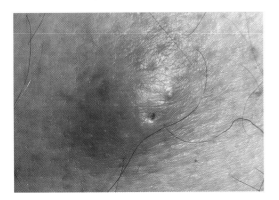

Figure 5.45. Rupture of a cyst.

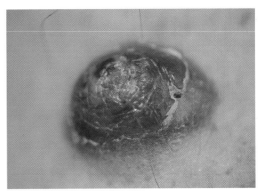

Figure 5.46. Secondary infection of a cyst.

How are cysts diagnosed?

Cysts are usually diagnosed clinically as they have typical characteristics. When a cyst is surgically removed, it should undergo histological examination. The type of lining of the wall of a cyst helps the pathologist classify it.

- Epidermoid cysts are lined with stratified squamous epithelium that contains a granular layer. Laminated keratin contents are noted inside the cyst. An inflammatory response may be present in cysts that have ruptured.
- Trichilemmal cysts have a palisaded peripheral layer without granular layer. Contents are eosinophilic hair keratin. Older cysts may exhibit calcification. The proliferating variety is considered a tumour.
- Steatocystoma has a folded cyst wall with prominent sebaceous gland lobules.
- Dermoid cyst contains fully mature elements of the skin including fat, hairs, sebaceous glands, eccrine glands, and in 20%, apocrine glands.

- The lining of the wall of a ganglion cyst or mucous cyst is collagen and fibrocytes.
- Hidrocystoma has a thin lining wall of eosinophilic bilaminar cells.

What is the treatment for cysts?

Asymptomatic epidermoid cysts do not need to be treated. In most cases, attempt to remove only the contents of a cyst is followed by recurrence. If desired, cysts may be fully excised. Recurrence even then is not uncommon, and re-excision may be surgically challenging.

Inflamed cysts are sometimes treated with:
- incision and drainage.
- intralesional injection with triamcinolone.
- oral antibiotics.
- delayed excision.

How can cysts be prevented?

Unknown.

What is the outlook for cysts?

Cysts generally persist unless surgically removed.

5.6 Dermatofibroma

What is a dermatofibroma?

A dermatofibroma is a common benign fibrous nodule that most often arises on the skin of the lower legs.

A dermatofibroma is also called a cutaneous fibrous histiocytoma.

Who gets dermatofibroma?

Dermatofibromas occur at all ages and in people of every ethnicity. They are more common in women than in men.

What causes dermatofibroma?

It is not clear if dermatofibroma is a reactive process or if it is a neoplasm. The lesions are made up of a proliferation of fibroblasts.

They are sometimes attributed to an insect bite or rose thorn injury, but not consistently. They may be more numerous in patients with altered immunity.

What are the clinical features of dermatofibroma?

Dermatofibromas most often occur on the legs and arms, but may also arise on trunk or any site of the body.

- People may have one or up to 15 lesions.
- Size varies from 0.5 to 1.5 cm diameter; most lesions are 7–10 mm diameter.
- They are firm nodules tethered to the skin surface but mobile over subcutaneous tissue (*Fig. 5.47*).
- The skin dimples on pinching the lesion (*Fig. 5.48*).

- Colour may be pink to light brown in white skin (*Fig. 5.49*), and dark brown to black in dark skin; some appear paler in the centre.
- They do not usually cause symptoms, but they are sometimes painful or itchy.

Complications of dermatofibroma

Because they are often raised lesions, they may be traumatised, for example by a razor.

Occasionally dozens of dermatofibromas may erupt within a few months, in the setting of immunosuppression (for example due to autoimmune disease, cancer or certain medications).

Dermatofibroma does not give rise to cancer. However, occasionally, it may be mistaken

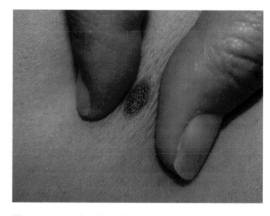

Figure 5.48. A dimple on lateral compression confirms a lesion to be a dermatofibroma.

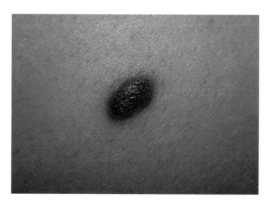

Figure 5.47. Pigmented dermatofibroma.

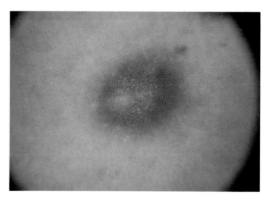

Figure 5.49. Dermatoscopy of dermatofibroma often reveals a central white zone.

for dermatofibrosarcoma or desmoplastic melanoma.

How is dermatofibroma diagnosed?

Dermatofibroma is usually easy to diagnose clinically, supported by dermatoscopy. The most common dermatoscopic pattern is a central white area surrounded by faint pigment network (*Fig. 5.49*).

Diagnostic excision or partial biopsy is undertaken if there is an atypical feature such as recent enlargement, ulceration, or asymmetrical structures and colours on dermatoscopy. The histology shows whirling fascicles of spindle cell proliferation with excessive collage deposition in the dermis.

There are several pathological variants of dermatofibroma. In case of doubt, immunohistochemical staining is used to confirm the diagnosis.

What is the treatment for dermatofibroma?

A dermatofibroma is harmless and seldom causes any symptoms. Usually only reassurance is needed.

If it is a nuisance or causing concern, the lesion can be removed surgically.

Cryotherapy, shave excision and laser treatments are rarely completely successful.

How can dermatofibroma be prevented?

Unknown.

What is the outlook for dermatofibroma?

Unless surgically excised, a dermatofibroma usually persists unchanged for years.

- Partial removal can lead to recurrence.
- An enlarging or changing lesion should be reassessed to consider another diagnosis.

5.7 Intraepidermal squamous cell carcinoma

What is intraepidermal squamous cell carcinoma?

Intraepidermal squamous cell carcinoma (SCC) is a common superficial form of skin cancer. It is also known as Bowen disease, intraepidermal carcinoma (IEC) and carcinoma *in situ* of the skin.

Intraepidermal SCC is derived from squamous cells, the flat epidermal cells that make keratin – the horny protein that makes up skin, hair and nails. "Intraepidermal" and "*in situ*" mean the malignant cells are confined to cell of origin, i.e. the epidermis.

Who gets intraepidermal carcinoma?

Risk factors for intraepidermal SCC include:
- age – intraepidermal SCC is increasingly prevalent with age.
- gender – it affects males and females, with lesions on the lower legs being more common in females.
- sun exposure – intraepidermal SCC is most often found in sun-damaged individuals.
- arsenic ingestion – intraepidermal SCC is common in populations exposed to arsenic.
- ionising radiation – intraepidermal SCC was common on unprotected hands of radiologists early in the 20th century.
- human papillomavirus (HPV) infection – this is implicated in intraepidermal SCC on the fingers and fingernails.
- immune suppression due to disease (e.g. chronic lymphocytic leukaemia) or medicines (e.g. azathioprine, ciclosporin).

Up to 50% of patients with intraepidermal SCC have other keratinocytic skin cancers, mainly basal cell carcinoma.

What causes intraepidermal SCC?

Ultraviolet radiation (UV) is the main cause of intraepidermal SCC. It damages the keratinocyte nucleic acids (DNA), resulting in a mutant clone of the gene *p53*. This sets off uncontrolled growth of the skin cells.

UV also suppresses the immune response, preventing recovery from damage.

What are the clinical features of intraepidermal SCC?

Intraepidermal SCC presents as one or more irregular scaly plaques of up to several centimetres in diameter (see *Figs 5.50–5.53*). They are most often red but may also be pigmented.

Although intraepidermal SCC may arise on any area of skin, it is most often diagnosed on sun-exposed sites of the ears, face, hands (*Fig 5.50*) and lower legs (*Fig. 5.52*). When there are multiple plaques, distribution is not symmetrical (unlike psoriasis).

Rarely, intraepidermal SCC may start to grow under a nail, when it results in a red streak (erythronychia) that later may destroy the nail plate (*Fig. 5.53*).

Complications of intraepidermal squamous cell carcinoma

Invasive cutaneous SCC arises in about 5% of intraepidermal SCC lesions. See *Section 5.12*.

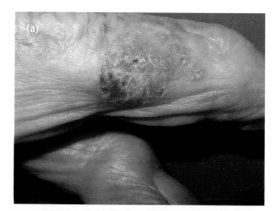

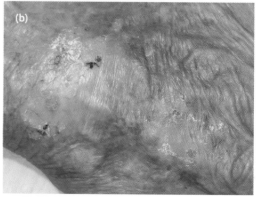

Figure 5.50. Intraepidermal SCC on (a) finger and (b) dorsum hand.

How is intraepidermal squamous cell carcinoma diagnosed?

Intraepidermal SCC is often recognised clinically because of an irregular scaly plaque (*Fig. 5.54a*). Dermatoscopy is supportive if it reveals crops of rounded or coiled blood vessels (*Fig. 5.54b*).

Diagnosis may be confirmed by biopsy; histology reveals full thickness dysplasia of the epidermis.

What is the treatment for intraepidermal squamous cell carcinoma?

As intraepidermal SCC is confined to the surface of the skin, there are various ways to remove it. Recurrence rates are high, whatever method is used, particularly in immunosuppressed patients.

OBSERVATION

As the risk of invasive SCC is low, it may not be necessary to remove all lesions, particularly

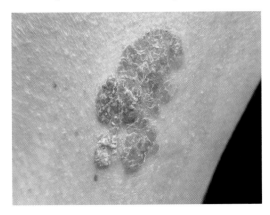

Figure 5.51. Intraepidermal SCC in axilla.

in elderly patients. Keratolytic emollients, e.g. containing urea or salicylic acid, may be sufficient to improve symptoms.

SUPERFICIAL SKIN SURGERY

Superficial skin surgery refers to shave, curettage and electrosurgery, and is a good choice for solitary or few hyperkeratotic lesions. The lesion is sliced off or scraped out, then the base is cauterised. Dressings are applied to the open wound to encourage moist wound healing over the next few weeks.

CRYOTHERAPY

Cryotherapy means removing a lesion by freezing it, usually with liquid nitrogen. Moderately aggressive cryotherapy is suitable for multiple, small, flat patches of intraepidermal SCC. It leaves a permanent white mark at the site of treatment.

FLUOROURACIL CREAM

Fluorouracil cream contains a cytotoxic agent and can be applied to multiple lesions. The cream is applied twice daily for 4 weeks, and repeated if necessary. It causes an inflammatory reaction that may ulcerate.

IMIQUIMOD CREAM

Imiquimod cream is an immune response modifier used off-licence to treat intraepidermal SCC. It is applied 3–5 times weekly for 4–16 weeks and causes an inflammatory reaction.

PHOTODYNAMIC THERAPY

Photodynamic therapy (PDT) refers to treatment with a photosensitiser (a porphyrin chemical)

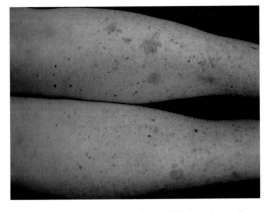

Figure 5.52. Multiple intraepidermal SCCs on lower legs.

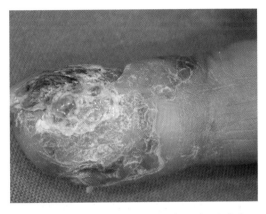

Figure 5.53. Intraepidermal SCC involving distal phalanx and nail unit.

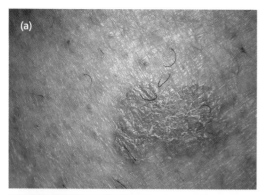

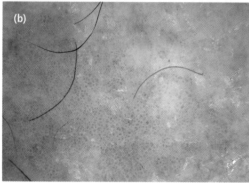

Figure 5.54. (a) Clinical and (b) dermatoscopic images of intraepidermal SCC.

that is applied to the affected area prior to exposing it to a strong source of visible light. The treated area develops an inflammatory reaction and then heals over a couple of weeks or so. The best studied, methyl levulinate cream PDT used off-licence, provides high cure rates for intraepidermal SCC on the face or lower legs, with excellent cosmetic results. The main disadvantage is the pain experienced by many patients during treatment.

OTHER

Other treatments occasionally used in the treatment of intraepidermal SCC include:
- combination treatments.
- diclofenac gel.
- topical retinoid (tazarotene, tretinoin).
- chemical peel.
- radiotherapy.
- electron beam therapy.
- carbon dioxide laser ablation.
- Erbium:YAG laser ablation.
- oral retinoid (acitretin, isotretinoin).

How can intraepidermal SCC be prevented?

Very careful sun protection at any time of life can reduce the number of intraepidermal SCCs. This is particularly important for ageing, sun-damaged, white skin; and in patients who are immunosuppressed.
- Stay indoors or in the shade in the middle of the day.
- Wear covering clothing.
- Apply high protection SPF 50+, broad-spectrum sunscreens generously to exposed skin, if outdoors.
- Avoid indoor tanning (sun beds and solaria).

What is the outlook for intraepidermal SCC?

Intraepidermal SCC may recur months or years after treatment. The same treatment can be repeated or another method used.

Patients who have been treated for intraepidermal SCC are at risk of developing new lesions of intraepidermal SCC. They are also at increased risk of other skin cancers, especially squamous cell carcinoma, basal cell carcinoma and melanoma.

5.8 Lentigo

What is a lentigo?

A lentigo is a pigmented flat or slightly raised lesion with a clearly defined edge. Unlike an ephilis (freckle), it does not fade in the winter months. There are several kinds of lentigo.

The name lentigo originally referred to its appearance resembling a small lentil. The plural of lentigo is lentigines, although lentigos is also in common use.

Who gets lentigines?

Lentigines can affect males and females of all ages and races. Solar lentigines are especially prevalent in fair-skinned adults. Lentigines associated with syndromes are present at birth or arise during childhood.

What causes lentigines?

Common forms of lentigo are due to exposure to ultraviolet radiation:
- sun damage including sunburn.
- indoor tanning.
- phototherapy, especially photochemotherapy (PUVA).

Ionising radiation, e.g. radiation therapy, can also cause lentigines.

Several familial syndromes associated with widespread lentigines originate from mutations in Ras-MAP kinase, mTOR signalling and *PTEN* pathways.

What are the clinical features of lentigines?

Lentigines have been classified into several different types depending on what they look like, where they appear on the body, causative factors, and whether they are associated to other diseases or conditions.

Lentigines may be solitary or, more often, multiple. Most lentigines are smaller than 5 mm in diameter.

LENTIGO SIMPLEX
- A precursor to junctional naevus.
- Arises during childhood and early adult life.
- Found on trunk and limbs.
- Small brown round or oval macule or thin plaque (*Fig. 5.55*).
- Jagged or smooth edge.
- May have a dry surface.
- May disappear in time.

SOLAR LENTIGO
- A precursor to seborrhoeic keratosis.
- Found on chronically sun-exposed sites such as hands, face (*Fig. 5.56*), lower legs.
- May also follow sunburn to shoulders.

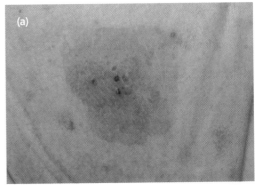

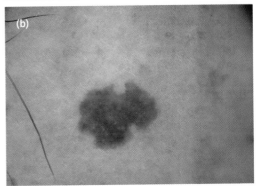

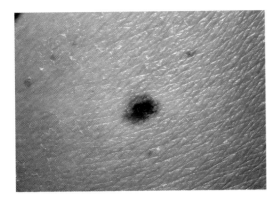

Figure 5.55. Lentigo simplex.

Figure 5.56. (a) Early seborrhoeic keratosis arising within facial solar lentigo. (b) Dermatoscopy of solar lentigo.

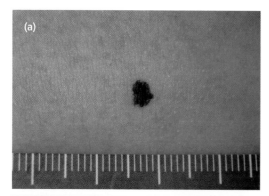

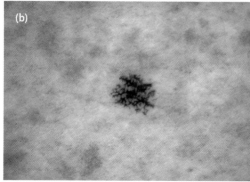

Figure 5.57. (a) Ink spot lentigo and (b) dermatoscopy of ink spot lentigo.

- Yellow, light or dark brown regular or irregular macule or thin plaque.
- May have a dry surface.
- Often has moth-eaten outline.
- Can slowly enlarge to several centimetres in diameter.
- May disappear, often through the process known as lichenoid keratosis.

INK SPOT LENTIGO
- Also known as reticulated lentigo.
- Few in number compared to solar lentigines.
- Follows sunburn in very fair-skinned individuals.
- Dark brown to black irregular ink spot-like macule (*Fig. 5.57*).

PUVA LENTIGO
- Similar to ink spot lentigo but follows photochemotherapy (PUVA).
- Location anywhere exposed to PUVA.

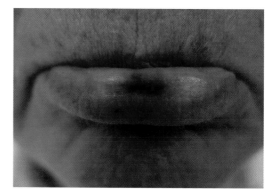

Figure 5.58. Melanotic macule on lower lip.

TANNING BED LENTIGO
- Similar to ink spot lentigo but follows indoor tanning.
- Location anywhere exposed to tanning bed.

RADIATION LENTIGO
- Occurs in site of irradiation (accidental or therapeutic).
- Associated with epidermal atrophy, subcutaneous fibrosis, keratosis, telangiectasia.

MELANOTIC MACULE
- Mucosal surfaces or adjacent glabrous skin, e.g. lip (*Fig. 5.58*), vulva, penis, anus.
- Also called mucosal melanosis.
- Light to dark brown.

GENERALISED LENTIGINES
- Found on any exposed or covered site from early childhood.
- Also called lentigines profusa, multiple lentigines.
- Not associated with syndromes.

AGMINATED LENTIGINES
- Naevoid eruption of lentigos confined to a single segmental area.
- Sharp demarcation in midline.
- May have associated neurological and developmental abnormalities.

PATTERNED LENTIGINES
- Inherited tendency to lentigines on face, lips, buttocks, palms, soles.
- Recognised mainly in dark-skinned individuals.

CENTROFACIAL NEURODYSRAPHIC LENTIGINOSIS

- Associated with mental retardation.

LENTIGINOSIS SYNDROMES

- Syndromes include LEOPARD/Noonan, Peutz–Jeghers, Laugier–Hunziker, Moynahan, xeroderma pigmentosa, myxoma syndromes (LAMB, NAME, Carney), Ruvalcaba–Myhre–Smith, Bannayan–Zonana syndrome, Cowden disease.
- Inheritance is autosomal dominant.
- Widespread lentigines present at birth or arising in early childhood.
- Associated with neural, endocrine and mesenchymal tumours.

Complications of lentigines

A lentigo is harmless. The main concern is cosmetic. However, it is important to identify lentiginosis syndromes, as tumours can include cancers.

How are lentigines diagnosed?

Lentigos are mainly diagnosed clinically by their typical appearance. Concern regarding possibility of melanoma may lead to:
- dermatoscopy.
- diagnostic excision biopsy.

Dermatoscopy may reveal pigment network or structureless pigmentation, depending on the type of lentigo and its body site. Histology of lentigo shows:
- thickened epidermis.
- an increased number of melanocytes along the basal layer of epidermis.
- unlike junctional melanocytic naevus, there are no nests of melanocytes.

- increased melanin pigment within the keratinocytes.
- additional features depending on type of lentigo.

In contrast, an ephilis (freckle) shows sun-induced increased melanin within the keratinocytes, without an increase in number of cells.

What is the treatment for lentigines?

Most lentigines are left alone. Attempts to lighten them may not be successful. The following approaches are used:
- SPF 50+ broad-spectrum sunscreen.
- hydroquinone bleaching cream.
- alpha hydroxy acids.
- vitamin C.
- retinoids.
- azelaic acid.
- chemical peels.

Individual lesions can be permanently removed using:
- cryotherapy.
- intense pulsed light.
- pigment laser.

How can lentigines be prevented?

Lentigines associated with exposure to ultraviolet radiation can be prevented by very careful sun protection. Clothing is more successful at preventing new lentigines than are sunscreens.

What is the outlook for lentigines?

Lentigines usually persist. They may increase in number with age and sun exposure. Some in sun-protected sites may fade and disappear.

5.9 Melanoma

What is melanoma?

Melanoma is a potentially serious type of skin cancer, in which there is uncontrolled growth of melanocytes (pigment cells). Melanoma is sometimes called malignant melanoma.

MELANOCYTES

Normal melanocytes are found in the basal layer of the epidermis (the outer layer of skin). Melanocytes produce a protein called melanin, which protects skin cells by absorbing ultraviolet (UV) radiation. Melanocytes are found in equal numbers in black and in white skin, but melanocytes in black skin produce much more melanin. People with dark brown or black skin are very much less likely to be damaged by UV radiation than those with white skin.

Non-cancerous growth of melanocytes results in moles (properly called benign melanocytic naevi) and freckles (ephelides and lentigines). Cancerous growth of melanocytes results in melanoma. Melanoma is described as:

- *in situ*, if the tumour is confined to the epidermis.
- invasive, if the tumour has spread into the dermis.
- metastatic, if the tumour has spread to other tissues.

Who gets melanoma?

The highest reported rates of melanoma in the world are in Australia and New Zealand; about 1 in 15 white-skinned New Zealanders are expected to develop melanoma in their lifetime, compared with:

- 1 in 40 white-skinned Americans.
- 1 in 54 white-skinned people in the UK.

In 2012, invasive melanoma was the 3rd most common cancer in males (after prostate and colorectal cancers) and in females (after breast and colorectal cancers). In the UK, melanoma is the 7th most common cancer in males and the 5th most common cancer in females. Melanoma is the 6th most common cancer in the USA. Although less common in the UK and USA, melanoma is increasing in incidence.

Melanoma can occur in adults of any age but is very rare in children. Median age at diagnosis:

- 61 years in New Zealand.
- 63 years in the USA.
- 65 years in the UK.

Invasive melanomas are diagnosed slightly more frequently in males and more males than females die from melanoma.

The main risk factors for developing the most common type of melanoma (superficial spreading melanoma) include:

- increasing age (see above).
- previous invasive melanoma or melanoma *in situ*.
- previous basal or squamous cell carcinoma.
- many melanocytic naevi (moles; see *Fig. 5.59*).
- multiple (>5) atypical naevi (large or histologically dysplastic moles).
- strong family history of melanoma with two or more first-degree relatives affected.
- white skin that burns easily.

These risk factors are not important for rare types of melanoma.

What causes melanoma?

Melanoma is thought to begin as uncontrolled proliferation of melanocytic stem cells that have undergone genetic transformation.

Superficial forms of melanoma spread out within the epidermis (*in situ*). A pathologist may report this as the radial or horizontal growth phase.

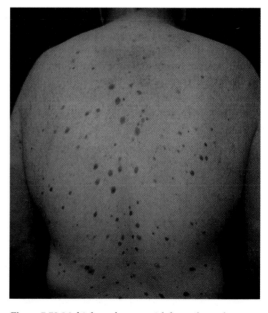

Figure 5.59. Multiple moles are a risk factor for melanoma.

Further genetic changes promote the tumour to invade through the basement membrane into surrounding dermis, when it becomes an invasive melanoma.

Nodular melanoma has a vertical growth phase, which is potentially more dangerous than the horizontal growth phase. It may arise within a previously healthy dermis, or within the invasive portion of a pre-existing more superficial kind of melanoma.

Once the melanoma cells have reached the dermis, they may spread to other tissues via the lymphatic system to the local lymph nodes or via the blood stream to other organs such as the lungs or brain. This is known as metastatic disease or secondary spread. The chance of this happening mainly depends on how deep the cells have penetrated into the skin.

What are the clinical features of melanoma?

Melanoma can arise from otherwise normal-looking skin (in about 75% of melanomas) or from within a mole or freckle, which starts to grow larger and change in appearance. Precursor lesions include:
- benign melanocytic naevus (normal mole).
- atypical or dysplastic naevus (funny-looking mole).
- atypical lentiginous junctional naevus (unstable lentigo in heavily sun-damaged skin).
- large or giant-sized congenital melanocytic naevus (brown birthmark).

Melanomas can occur anywhere on the body, not only in areas that get a lot of sun. The most common site in men is the back (around 40% of melanomas in men), and the most common site in women is the leg (around 35% of melanomas in women).

Although melanoma usually starts as a skin lesion, it can also rarely grow on mucous membranes such as the lips or genitals. Occasionally it occurs in other parts of the body such as the eye, brain, mouth or vagina.

The first sign of a melanoma is usually an unusual-looking freckle or mole. A melanoma may be detected at an early stage when it is only a few millimetres in diameter, but it may grow to several centimetres in diameter before it is diagnosed.
- A melanoma may have a variety of colours including tan, dark brown, black, blue, red and, occasionally, light grey.

- Melanomas that are lacking pigment are called amelanotic melanoma.
- There may be areas of regression that are the colour of normal skin, or white and scarred.

During its horizontal phase of growth, a melanoma has a flat surface. As the vertical phase develops, the melanoma becomes thickened and raised.

Some melanomas are itchy or tender. More advanced lesions may bleed easily or crust over.

Most melanomas have characteristics described by the Glasgow 7-point checklist or by the ABCDEs of melanoma. Not all lesions with these characteristics are malignant. Not all melanomas show these characteristics.

GLASGOW 7-POINT CHECKLIST

Major features	Minor features
Change in size	Inflammation
Irregular shape	Oozing
Irregular colour	Change in sensation
Diameter >7 mm	

THE ABCDEs OF MELANOMA

A   Asymmetry
B   Border irregularity
C   Colour variation
D   Diameter >6 mm
E   Evolving (enlarging, changing)

Subtypes of melanoma

CONVENTIONAL CLASSIFICATION

Melanomas are described according to their appearance and behaviour. Those that start off as a flat patch (i.e. they have a horizontal growth phase) include:
- superficial spreading melanoma (*Fig. 5.60*).
- lentigo maligna, lentigo maligna melanoma and lentiginous melanoma (in sun-damaged skin, see *Fig. 5.61*).
- acral lentiginous melanoma (on soles of feet, palms of hands or nails, see *Fig. 5.62*).

These superficial forms of melanoma tend to grow slowly, but at any time, they may develop a nodule (i.e. they progress to a vertical growth phase).

Melanomas that quickly involve deeper tissues include:
- nodular melanoma (*Fig. 5.63*).
- spitzoid melanoma (*Fig. 5.64*).
- mucosal melanoma (*Fig. 5.65*).

- neurotropic and desmoplastic melanoma (*Fig. 5.66*).
- ocular melanoma (*Fig. 5.67*).

Combinations may arise, e.g. nodular melanoma arising within a superficial spreading melanoma or desmoplastic melanoma arising below lentigo maligna.

CLASSIFICATION BY AGE, SUN EXPOSURE AND NUMBER OF NAEVI

Melanoma can be classified according to its relationship with age, sun exposure, and number of melanocytic naevi.

Childhood melanomas (below 10 years of age):
- extremely rare.

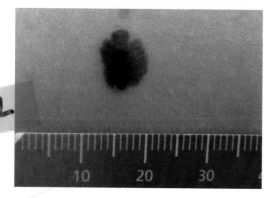

Figure 5.60. Superficial spreading melanoma.

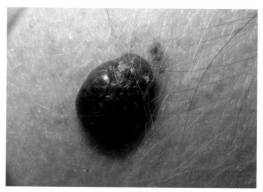

Figure 5.63. Nodular melanoma.

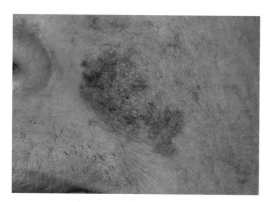

Figure 5.61. Lentigo maligna.

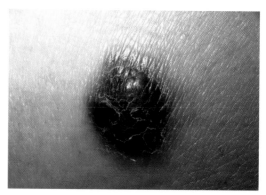

Figure 5.64. Spitzoid melanoma.

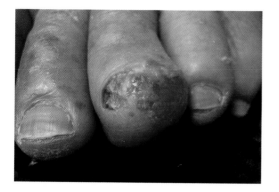

Figure 5.62. Acral lentiginous melanoma.

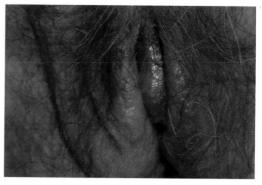

Figure 5.65. Mucosal melanoma.

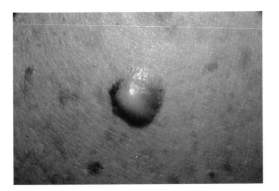

Figure 5.66. Neurotropic melanoma.

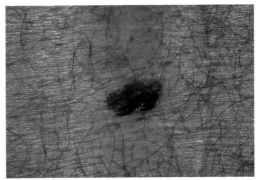

Figure 5.68. Superficial spreading melanoma.

- infrequently associated with excessive sun exposure.
- compared to melanoma in adults, they are more often amelanotic (flesh coloured, pink or red), nodular, bleeding and ulcerated.
- may arise within giant congenital melanocytic naevi >40 cm diameter.

Early-onset melanomas:
- more common in women than in men.
- most common clinical subtype is superficial spreading.
- associated with many melanocytic naevi.
- tend to be seen on lower extremity.
- tend to have BRAF V600E genetic mutation.
- associated with intermittent sun exposure.

Late-onset melanomas:
- more common in men than in women.
- most common clinical subtype is lentigo maligna.
- often occur on head and neck.
- associated with accumulated, lifelong sun exposure.

Melanoma is usually epithelial in origin, i.e. starting in the skin, or, less often, mucous membranes. But very rarely, melanoma can start in an internal tissue such as the brain (primary CNS melanoma) or the back of the eye (one type of ocular melanoma).

How is melanoma diagnosed?

Some melanomas are extremely difficult to recognise clinically. Melanoma may be suspected because of a lesion's clinical features (see *Fig. 5.68*) or because of a history of change. The dermatoscopic appearance is helpful in the diagnosis of featureless early melanoma (*Fig. 5.69*).

The suspicious lesion is surgically removed with a 2–3 mm clinical margin for pathological examination (diagnostic excision). Partial biopsy is best avoided, but may be considered in large lesions.

The pathological diagnosis of melanoma can be very difficult. Histological features of superficial spreading melanoma *in situ* include the presence of buckshot (pagetoid) scatter of atypical melanocytes within the epidermis.

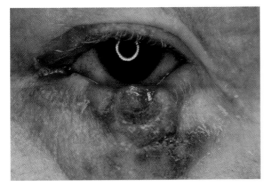

Figure 5.67. Ocular melanoma.

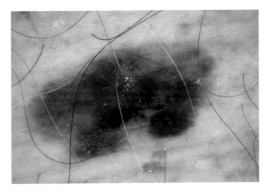

Figure 5.69. Dermatoscopy of melanoma from *Fig. 5.98*.

These cells may be enlarged with unusual nuclei. Dermal invasion results in melanoma cells within the dermis or deeper into subcutaneous fat.

Immunohistochemical stains may be necessary to confirm melanoma.

Pathology report
The pathologist's report should include a macroscopic description of the specimen and melanoma (the naked eye view), and a microscopic description. The following features should be reported if there is invasive melanoma:
- diagnosis of primary melanoma.
- Breslow thickness to the nearest 0.1 mm.
- Clark level of invasion.
- margins of excision, i.e. the normal tissue around the tumour.
- mitotic rate – a measure of how fast the cells are proliferating.
- whether or not there is ulceration.

The report may also include comments about the cell type and its growth pattern, invasion of blood vessels or nerves, inflammatory response, regression and whether there is associated *in situ* disease and/or associated naevus (original mole).

What is breslow thickness?
Breslow thickness is reported for invasive melanomas. It is measured vertically in millimetres from the top of the granular layer (or base of superficial ulceration) to the deepest point of tumour involvement. It is a strong predictor of outcome; the thicker the melanoma, the more likely it is to metastasise (spread).

What is the clark level of invasion?
The Clark level indicates the anatomic plane of invasion.

Level 1	*In situ* melanoma
Level 2	Melanoma has invaded papillary dermis
Level 3	Melanoma has filled papillary dermis
Level 4	Melanoma has invaded reticular dermis
Level 5	Melanoma has invaded subcutaneous tissue

Deeper Clark levels have a greater risk of metastasis. It is useful in predicting outcome in thin tumours. It is less useful than Breslow thickness for thick tumours.

What is the treatment for melanoma?
Following confirmation of the diagnosis, wide local excision is carried out at the site of the primary melanoma. The extent of surgery depends on the thickness of the melanoma and its site. Margins recommended are shown below:

Melanoma *in situ*:	5–10 mm
Melanoma <1 mm:	10 mm
Melanoma 1–2 mm:	10–20 mm
Melanoma >2 mm:	20 mm

Staging
Melanoma staging means finding out if the melanoma has spread from its original site in the skin. Most melanoma specialists refer to the American Joint Committee on Cancer (AJCC) cutaneous melanoma staging guidelines (2016). In essence, the stages are:

Stage	Characteristics
Stage 0	*In situ* melanoma
Stage 1	Thin melanoma <2 mm in thickness
Stage 2	Thick melanoma >2 mm in thickness
Stage 3	Melanoma spread to involve local lymph nodes
Stage 4	Distant metastases have been detected

Should the lymph nodes be removed?
If the local lymph nodes are enlarged due to metastatic melanoma, they should be completely removed. This requires a surgical procedure, usually under general anaesthetic. If they are not enlarged, they may be tested to see if there is any microscopic spread of melanoma. The test is known as a sentinel node biopsy.

Many surgeons recommend (based on AJCC Guidelines) sentinel node biopsy for melanomas thicker than 1 mm, especially in younger people. Although the biopsy may help in staging the cancer, it does not offer any survival advantage.

Lymph nodes containing metastatic melanoma often increase in size quickly. An involved node is usually non-tender and firm to hard in consistency.

Treatment of advanced melanoma
If the melanoma is widespread, treatment is not always successful in eradicating the cancer. Some patients may be offered new or experimental treatments, such as:
- immunotherapy – interleukin-2, interferon alpha 2b.
- BRAF inhibitors – dabrafenib and vemurafenib.

- MEK inhibitors – trametinib, cobimetinib.
- C-KIT inhibitors – imatinib, nilotinib.
- CTLA-4 antagonist – ipilimumab.
- PD-1 blocking antibodies – nivolumab, pembrolizumab.

What happens at follow-up?

The main purpose of follow-up is to detect recurrences early but it also offers an opportunity to diagnose a new primary melanoma at the first possible opportunity. A second invasive melanoma occurs in 5–10% of melanoma patients, and melanoma *in situ* in more than 20% of melanoma patients.

The Australian and New Zealand Guidelines for the Management of Melanoma (2008) make the following recommendations for follow-up for patients with invasive melanoma.
- Self skin examination.
- Regular routine skin checks by patient's preferred health professional.
- Follow-up intervals are preferably six-monthly for five years for patients with stage 1 disease, three- or four-monthly for five years for patients with stage 2 or 3 disease, and yearly thereafter for all patients.
- Individual patients' needs should be considered before appropriate follow-up is offered.
- Provide education and support to help patient adjust to their illness.

In the UK, refer to NICE Guidelines (NG14, 2015). In the USA, refer to the American Academy of Dermatology Clinical Guidelines (2011).

The follow-up appointments may be undertaken by the patient's general practitioner and/or specialist.

Follow-up appointments may include:

- a check of the scar where the primary melanoma was removed (see *Fig. 5.70*, metastatic melanoma within the scar).
- a feel for the regional lymph nodes.
- general skin examination.
- full physical examination.
- in those with many moles or atypical moles, baseline whole body imaging and sequential macro and dermatoscopic images of melanocytic lesions of concern (mole mapping; see *Fig. 5.71*).

In those with more advanced primary disease, follow-up may include:
- blood tests, including LDH.
- imaging – ultrasound, X-ray, CT, MRI and/or PET scan.

Tests are not worthwhile for patients with stage 1 or 2 melanoma unless there are signs or symptoms of disease recurrence or metastasis. No tests are necessary for healthy patients who have remained well for 5 years or longer after removal of their melanoma.

What is the outlook for patients with melanoma?

Melanoma *in situ* is cured by excision because it has no potential to spread round the body.

The risk of spread and ultimate death from invasive melanoma depends on several factors, but the main one is the Breslow thickness of the melanoma at the time it was surgically removed.

Metastases are rare for melanomas <0.75 mm and the risk for tumours 0.75–1 mm thick is about 5%. The risk steadily increases with thickness so that melanomas >4 mm have a risk of metastasis of about 40%.

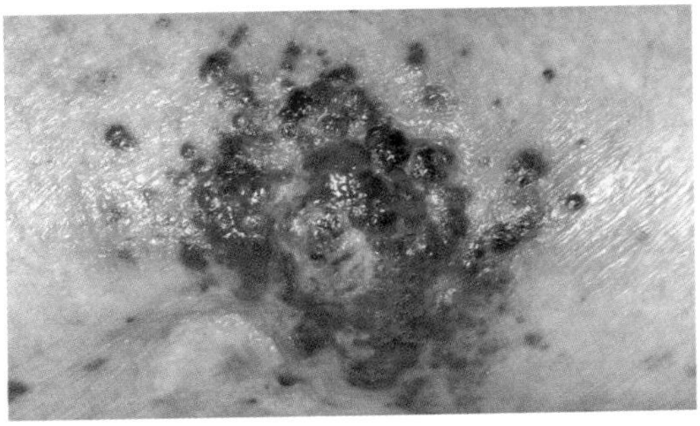

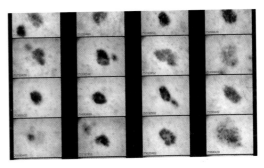

Figure 5.70. Primary melanoma removal scar (recurrent melanoma). Metastatic melanoma arising at site of primary excision.

Figure 5.71. Dermatoscopic images of atypical naevi displayed during mole mapping.

5.10 Moles

What is a mole?

A mole is a common benign skin lesion due to a local proliferation of pigment cells (melanocytes). It is more correctly called a melanocytic naevus (US spelling 'nevus'), and is sometimes also called a naevocytic naevus. A brown or black mole contains the pigment melanin, so may also be called a pigmented naevus.

A mole can be present at birth (congenital naevus) or appear later (acquired naevus). There are various kinds of congenital and acquired naevi.

Who gets moles?

Almost everyone has at least one mole.
- About 1% of individuals are born with one or more congenital melanocytic naevi. This is usually sporadic, with rare instances of familial congenital naevi.
- Fair-skinned people tend to have more moles than darker-skinned people.
- Moles that appear during childhood (aged 2–10 years) tend to be the most prominent and persistent moles throughout life.
- Moles that are acquired later in childhood or adult life often follow sun exposure.

Most white-skinned New Zealanders have 20–50 moles, but individuals in Northern Europe and the USA tend to have fewer.

What causes moles?

Although the exact reason for local proliferation of naevus cells is unknown, it is clear that the number of moles a person has depends on genetic factors, on sun exposure, and on immune status.
- People with many moles tend to have family members who also have many moles, and their moles may have a similar appearance.
- Somatic mutations in *RAS* genes are associated with congenital melanocytic naevi.
- New melanocytic naevi may erupt following the use of *BRAF* inhibitor drugs.
- People living in Australia and New Zealand have many more naevi than their relatives residing in Northern Europe.
- Immunosuppressive treatment leads to an increase in numbers of naevi.

What are the clinical features of moles?

Moles vary widely in clinical, dermatoscopic and histological appearance.
- They may arise on any part of the body.
- Moles differ in appearance depending on the body site of origin.
- They may be flat or protruding.
- They vary in colour from pink or flesh tones to dark brown, steel blue, or black.
- Light-skinned individuals tend to have light-coloured moles and dark-skinned individuals tend to have dark brown or black moles.
- Although mostly round or oval in shape, moles are sometimes unusual shapes.
- They range in size from a couple of millimetres to several centimetres in diameter.

Classification of melanocytic naevi

Congenital melanocytic naevi are classified according to their actual or predicted adult size in maximum dimension.
- A small congenital melanocytic naevus is <1.5 cm.
- A medium congenital melanocytic naevus is 1.5–19.9 cm.
- A large or giant congenital melanocytic naevus is ≥20 cm.

Special types of congenital naevi include:
- hairy melanocytic naevus (*Fig. 5.72*).
- bathing trunk naevus (*Fig. 5.73*).
- café au lait macule (*Fig. 5.74*).
- speckled lentiginous naevus (*Fig. 5.75*).
- dermal melanocytosis – Mongolian spot (*Fig. 5.76*), naevus of Ota (*Fig. 5.77*) naevus of Ito, Hori naevus.

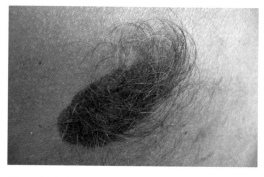

Figure 5.72. Hairy melanocytic naevus.

The pathological classification of melanocytic naevi relates to where naevus cells are found in the skin.

- A junctional naevus has groups or nests of naevus cells at the junction of the epidermis and the dermis; a flat mole (*Fig. 5.78*).
- A dermal or intradermal naevus has naevus cell nests in the dermis. A papule, plaque or nodule with a pedunculated, papillomatous (Unna naevus; *Fig. 5.79*) or smooth surface (Miescher naevus; *Fig. 5.80*).

- A compound naevus has nests of naevus cells at the epidermal–dermal junction as well as within the dermis; a central raised area surrounded by a flat patch (*Fig. 5.81*).
- A blue naevus has elongated, fusiform naevus cells in the deep dermis. Flat or papular, the name describes its usual colour (*Fig. 5.82*).
- A combined naevus has two distinct types of mole within the same lesion – usually blue naevus and compound naevus (see *Fig. 5.83*).

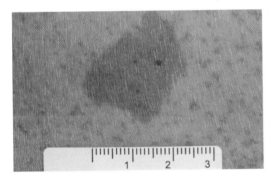

Figure 5.73. Bathing trunk naevus.

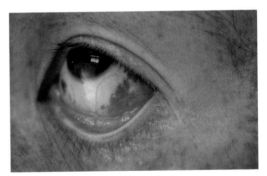

Figure 5.76. Mongolian spot.

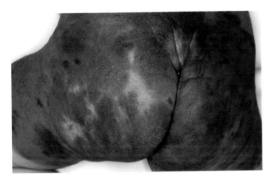

Figure 5.74. Café au lait macule.

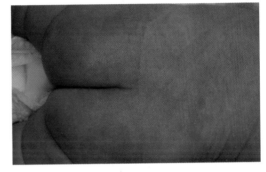

Figure 5.77. Naevus of Ota.

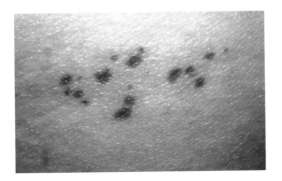

Figure 5.75. Speckled lentiginous naevus.

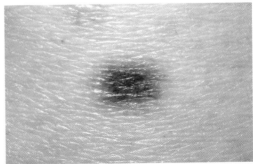

Figure 5.78. Junctional naevus.

Dermatoscopy has given rise to a new classification based on the pigment patterns of melanocytic naevi. Examples include:

- a junctional naevus described with reticular pattern of intersecting brown lines (*Fig. 5.86*).
- a dermal naevus described with aggregated cobblestones (*Fig. 5.90*) or globules (*Fig. 5.87*).
- a blue naevus is hazy steel blue and uniform structureless lesion (*Fig. 5.89*).

Signature naevi are the predominant type of naevus in an individual with multiple moles.

Descriptive terms for signature naevi include solid brown (*Fig. 5.84*), solid pink (*Fig. 5.85*), eclipse/annular (*Fig. 5.88*), cockade/bull's eye (*Fig. 5.91*), naevus with perifollicular hypopigmentation (*Fig. 5.93*), more easily seen by dermoscopy (*Fig. 5.96*), naevus with eccentric pigmentation, fried-egg naevus, and lentiginous naevus (see *Fig. 5.55*).

Uncommon types of melanocytic naevi include:

- Spitz naevus or epithelioid cell naevus – a pink (classic Spitz; *Fig. 5.94*) or brown

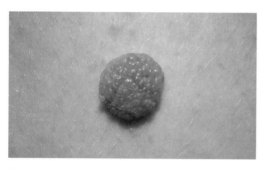

Figure 5.79. Unna or papillomatous naevus.

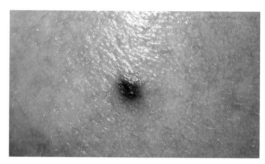

Figure 5.82. Blue naevus.

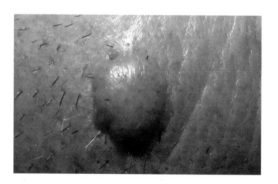

Figure 5.80. Miescher naevus.

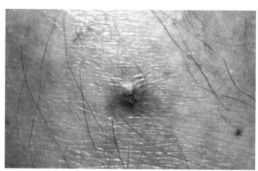

Figure 5.83. Combined naevus.

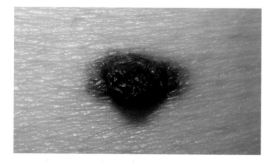

Figure 5.81. Compound naevus.

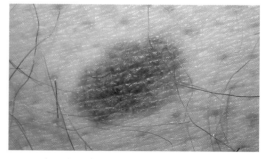

Figure 5.84. Solid brown compound naevus.

(pigmented Spitz; *Fig. 5.92*) dome-shaped mole that arises in children and young adults.

- Reed naevus – darkly pigmented type of Spitz naevus with starburst dermatoscopic pattern (*Fig. 5.95*).
- Agminated naevi – a cluster of similar moles (*Fig. 5.97*).

The term atypical naevus may be used in several ways.

- A benign mole that has some clinical or histopathological characteristics of melanoma.

- A mole with specific characteristics: large (>5 mm); ill-defined or irregular borders; varying shades of colour; with flat and bumpy components (*Fig. 5.98*).
- Or, any funny-looking mole; large, or different from the patient's other moles.

Atypical naevi usually occur in fair-skinned individuals when they are due to sun exposure. They may be solitary or numerous. Pathology is reported as dysplastic junctional or compound

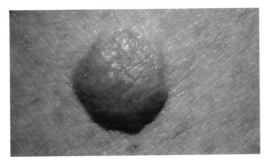

Figure 5.85. Solid pink naevus.

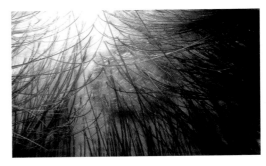

Figure 5.88. Annular naevus on scalp.

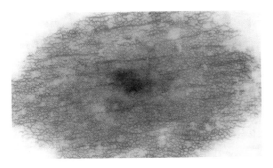

Figure 5.86. Dermatoscopic appearance of junctional naevus (reticular pattern).

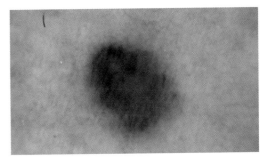

Figure 5.89. Dermatoscopic appearance of blue naevus with structureless, steel-grey colour.

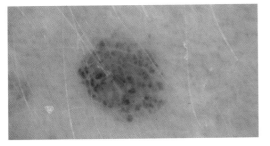

Figure 5.87. Dermatoscopic appearance of dermal naevus with globules.

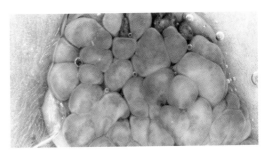

Figure 5.90. Dermatoscopic appearance of dermal naevus with aggregated cobblestones.

naevus and has specific histological features (the Clark naevus).

What are the complications of moles?

People worry about moles because they have heard about melanoma, a malignant proliferation of melanocytes that is the most common reason for death from skin cancer.

- At first, melanoma may look similar to a harmless mole, but in time it becomes more disordered in structure and tends to enlarge.

- People with a greater number of moles have a higher risk of developing melanoma than those with few moles, especially if they have over 100 of them.

Moles sometimes change for other reasons than melanoma, for example, due to normal ageing, or following sun exposure or during pregnancy. They can enlarge, regress or involute (disappear).

- A Meyerson naevus is itchy and dry because it is surrounded by eczema (*Fig. 5.99*).

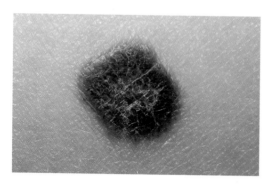

Figure 5.91. Cockade naevus.

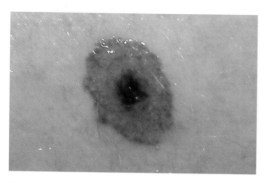

Figure 5.92. Pigmented Spitz naevus.

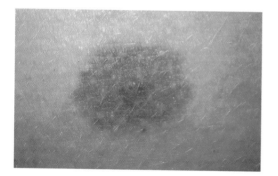

Figure 5.93. Naevus with perifollicular hypopigmentation.

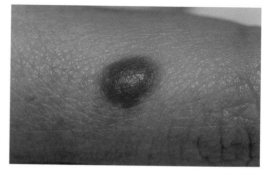

Figure 5.94. Classic Spitz naevus.

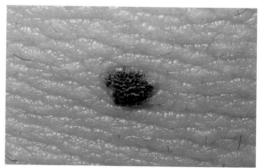

Figure 5.95. Reed naevus.

Figure 5.96. Naevus with perifollicular hypopigmentation seen by dermatoscopy.

- Sutton or halo naevus is surrounded by a white patch, and fades away over several years (*Fig. 5.100*).
- A recurrent naevus is one that appears in a scar following surgical removal of a mole – this may have odd clinical and dermatoscopic features (*Fig. 5.101*).

How is a mole diagnosed?

Moles are usually diagnosed clinically by their typical appearance. If there is any doubt about the diagnosis, an expert may be consulted in person or with the help of clinical and dermatoscopic images. This is especially important if:

- a mole changes size, shape, structure or colour.
- a new mole develops in adult life (>40 years).
- it appears different from the person's other moles (a so-called ugly duckling).
- it has ABCD characteristics (Asymmetry, Border irregularity, Colour variation, Diameter >6 mm).
- it is bleeding, crusted or itchy.

Most skin lesions with these characteristics are actually harmless when evaluated by an expert using dermatoscopy. Short-term digital dermatoscopic imaging may be used in equivocal flat lesions to check for change over time.

Naevi that remain suspicious for melanoma are excised for histopathology (diagnostic biopsy). Partial biopsy is not recommended, as it may miss an area of cancerous change.

What is the treatment for moles?

Most moles are harmless and can be safely left alone. Moles may be removed in the following circumstances:

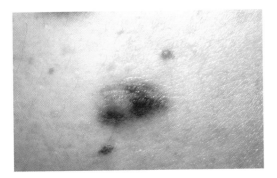

Figure 5.97. Agminated naevi.

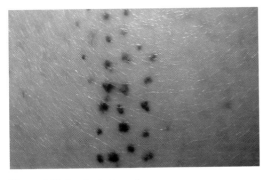

Figure 5.98. Atypical naevus; large, irregular shape and colour.

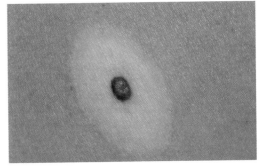

Figure 5.100. Sutton or halo naevus.

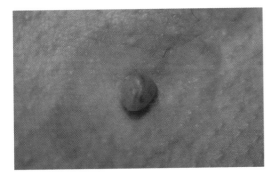

Figure 5.99. Meyerson naevus.

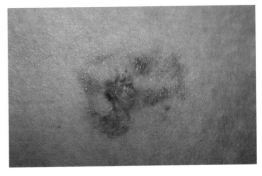

Figure 5.101. Recurrent naevus following shave excision of benign dermal naevus.

- to exclude cancer.
- the mole is a nuisance – perhaps irritated by clothing, comb or razor.
- cosmetic reasons – the mole is unsightly.

Surgical techniques include:
- excision biopsy of flat or suspicious mole.
- shave biopsy of protruding mole.
- electrosurgical destruction.
- laser to lessen pigment or remove coarse hair.

Can moles be prevented?

The number of moles can be minimised by strict protection from the sun, starting from birth. Sunscreen alone is not sufficient to prevent new moles from appearing.

At any age, sun protection is important to reduce skin ageing and the risk of skin cancer.
- In New Zealand, the SunSmart's Sun Protection Alert advises when protection is required. Smartphone apps provide UV protection advice specific for any geographical location.
- Cover up. Wear a hat, long sleeves and long skirt or trousers. Choose fabrics designed for the sun (UPF 40+) when outdoors.
- Apply sunscreen to areas you can't cover. Choose broad-spectrum high protection (SPF 50+) sunscreens, applied frequently to exposed areas.

What is the outlook for moles?

Most moles that appear in childhood remain forever. Teenagers and young adults tend to have the greatest number of moles. There are fewer in later life because some of them slowly fade away.

To increase the chance of spotting melanoma early, recommend:
- self-skin examination monthly.
- significant changes in moles or new lesions are reported to doctor or dermatologist.
- regular skin examinations in patients with many moles, atypical naevi or previous skin cancer.
- total body photography and digital dermatoscopic imaging (mole mapping) for patients at high risk of melanoma, especially if they have many moles.

5.11 Seborrhoeic keratoses

What is a seborrhoeic keratosis?

A seborrhoeic keratosis is a harmless warty spot that appears during adult life as a common sign of ageing. Some people have hundreds of them.

Seborrhoeic keratosis (or seborrheic keratosis, using US spelling) is also called SK, basal cell papilloma, senile wart, brown wart or barnacle.

Who gets seborrhoeic keratoses?

Seborrhoeic keratoses are extremely common. It has been estimated that over 90% of adults over the age of 60 years have one or more of them. They occur in males and females of all races, typically beginning to erupt in the 30s or 40s. They are uncommon under the age of 20 years.

What causes seborrhoeic keratoses?

The precise cause of seborrhoeic keratoses is not known.

The name is misleading, because they are not limited to a seborrhoeic distribution (scalp, mid-face, chest, upper back) as in seborrhoeic dermatitis, nor are they formed from sebaceous glands, as is the case with sebaceous hyperplasia.

Seborrhoeic keratoses are considered degenerative in nature, appearing as part of the skin ageing process. As time goes by, seborrhoeic keratoses become more numerous. Some people inherit a tendency to develop a very large number of them. Researchers have noted the following:

- Eruptive seborrhoeic keratoses can follow sunburn or dermatitis.
- Skin friction may be the reason they appear in body folds.

- Viral cause (e.g. human papillomavirus) seems unlikely.
- Stable and clonal mutations or activation of *FRFR3*, *PIK3CA*, *RAS*, *AKT1* and *EGFR* genes are found in seborrhoeic keratoses.
- *FRFR3* mutations are associated with increased age and location on the head and neck, suggesting a role of ultraviolet radiation.
- Seborrhoeic keratoses do not harbour tumour suppressor gene mutations.
- Epidermal growth factor receptor inhibitors (used to treat cancer) often result in an increase in verrucal (warty) keratoses.

What are the clinical features of seborrhoeic keratoses?

Seborrhoeic keratoses can arise on any area of skin, covered or uncovered, with the exception of palms and soles (*Figs 5.102–5.107*). They do not arise from mucous membranes.

Seborrhoeic keratoses have highly variable appearance.

- Flat or raised papule or plaque.
- 1 mm to several cm in diameter.
- Skin-coloured (*Fig. 5.103*), yellow (*Fig. 5.104*), grey, light brown (*Fig. 5.105*), dark brown, black or mixed colours.
- Smooth, waxy or warty surface (see *Figs 5.106* and *5.107*).
- Solitary or grouped (see *Fig. 5.102*) in certain areas, such as within the scalp, under the breasts, over the spine or in the groin.

They appear to stick on to the skin surface like barnacles.

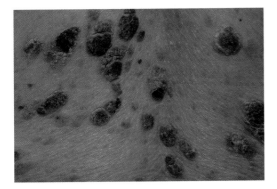

Figure 5.102. Multiple seborrhoeic keratosis.

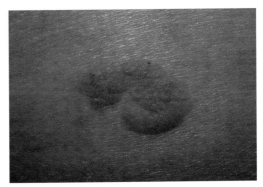

Figure 5.103. Skin-coloured seborrhoeic keratosis.

Variants of seborrhoeic keratoses include:

- solar lentigines – flat circumscribed pigmented patches in sun exposed sites (see *Fig. 5.17*). Thicker seborrhoeic keratoses may arise within solar lentigos.
- dermatosis papulosa nigra – small, pedunculated and heavily pigmented seborrhoeic keratoses on head and neck of darker-skinned individuals (*Fig. 5.108*).

- stucco keratosis – grey, white or yellow papules on the lower extremities (*Fig. 5.109*).
- inverted follicular keratosis.
- large cell acanthoma.
- lichenoid keratosis: an inflammatory phase preceding involution of some seborrhoeic keratoses and solar lentigines (*Fig. 5.110*), with characteristic grey dots on dermatoscopy (*Fig. 5.111*).

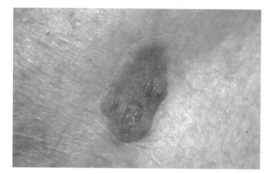

Figure 5.104. Yellowish seborrhoeic keratosis.

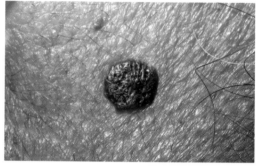

Figure 5.107. Melanoacanthoma: a brown seborrhoeic keratosis with a waxy surface.

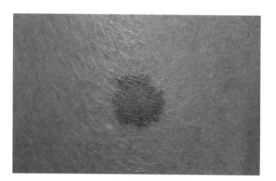

Figure 5.105. Flat brown seborrhoeic keratosis.

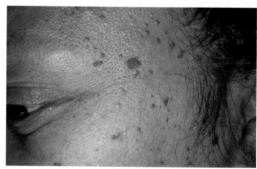

Figure 5.108. Dermatosis papulosa nigra.

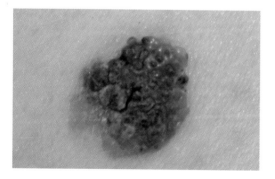

Figure 5.106. Seborrhoeic keratosis with warty surface.

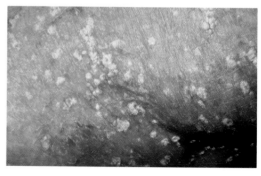

Figure 5.109. Stucco keratosis.

Complications of seborrhoeic keratoses

Seborrhoeic keratoses are not premalignant tumours. However:

- skin cancers are sometimes difficult to tell apart from seborrhoeic keratoses.
- a skin cancer may by chance arise within or collide with a seborrhoeic keratosis.

Very rarely, eruptive seborrhoeic keratoses may denote an underlying internal malignancy, most often gastric adenocarcinoma. The paraneoplastic syndrome is known as the sign of Leser–Trélat. Eruptive seborrhoeic keratoses that are not associated with cancer are sometimes called pseudo-sign of Leser–Trélat.

An irritated seborrhoeic keratosis is an inflamed, red and crusted lesion (*Fig. 5.112*). It may give rise to dermatitis around the seborrhoeic keratosis. Dermatitis may also trigger new seborrhoeic keratoses to appear.

How is a seborrhoeic keratosis diagnosed?

The diagnosis of seborrhoeic keratosis is often easy.

- A stuck-on, well-demarcated warty plaque.
- Other similar lesions.

Sometimes, seborrhoeic keratosis may resemble a skin cancer, such as basal cell carcinoma, squamous cell carcinoma or melanoma.

Dermatoscopy often shows a disordered structure in a seborrhoeic keratosis, as is the case in skin cancers. There are diagnostic dermatoscopic clues to seborrhoeic keratosis, such as multiple orange or brown clods (due to keratin in skin surface crevices), white "milia-like" clods (*Fig. 5.113*), curved thick ridges and furrows forming a brain-like or cerebriform pattern (*Fig. 5.114*).

If doubt remains, a seborrhoeic keratosis may undergo partial shave or punch biopsy or diagnostic excision.

The dominant histopathological features of seborrhoeic keratosis may be described as:

- melanoacanthoma (deeply pigmented, see *Fig. 5.107*).
- acanthotic.
- hyperkeratotic or papillomatous.
- adenoid or reticulated.

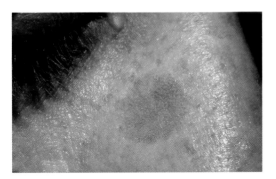

Figure 5.110. Solar lentigo evolving into lichenoid keratosis (*Fig. 5.111*).

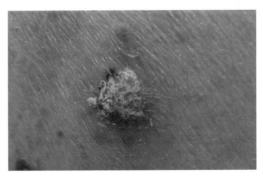

Figure 5.112. Irritated seborrhoeic keratosis.

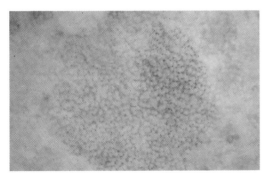

Figure 5.111. Lichenoid keratosis (*Fig. 5.110*) confirmed by grey dots on dermatoscopy.

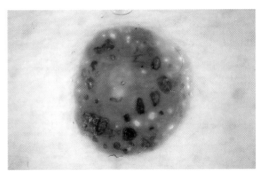

Figure 5.113. Orange and white clods seen on dermatoscopy of seborrhoeic keratosis.

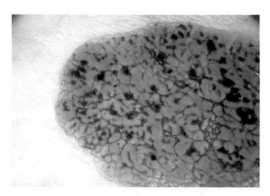

Figure 5.114. Cerebriform dermatoscopic pattern in seborrhoeic keratosis.

- clonal or nested.
- adamantinoid or mucinous.
- desmoplastic.
- irritated.

What is the treatment for seborrhoeic keratoses?

An individual seborrhoeic keratosis can easily be removed if desired. Reasons for removal may be that it is unsightly, itchy, or catches on clothing.

Methods used to remove seborrhoeic keratoses include:

- cryotherapy (liquid nitrogen) for thinner lesions (repeated if necessary).
- curettage and/or electrocautery.
- ablative laser surgery.
- shave biopsy (shaving off with a scalpel).
- focal chemical peel with trichloracetic acid.

All methods have disadvantages. Treatment-induced loss of pigmentation is a particular issue for dark-skinned patients. There is no easy way to remove multiple lesions on a single occasion.

How can seborrhoeic keratoses be prevented?

Unknown.

What is the outlook for seborrhoeic keratoses?

Seborrhoeic keratoses tend to persist. From time to time, individual or multiple lesions may remit spontaneously or via the lichenoid keratosis mechanism.

Those associated with dermatitis may regress after it has been controlled.

5.12 Squamous cell carcinoma – cutaneous

What is cutaneous squamous cell carcinoma?

Cutaneous squamous cell carcinoma (SCC) is a common type of keratinocytic or non-melanoma skin cancer. It is derived from keratinising cells within the epidermis. Keratin is the horny protein that makes up skin, hair and nails.

Cutaneous SCC is an invasive disease, referring to cancer cells that have grown beyond the epidermis. SCC can sometimes metastasise and may prove fatal.

Intraepidermal carcinoma (SCC *in situ*) and mucosal SCC are considered elsewhere.

Who gets cutaneous squamous cell carcinoma?

Risk factors for cutaneous SCC include the following.

- Age and gender: SCCs are particularly prevalent in elderly males. However, they also affect females and younger adults.
- Previous SCC or other form of skin cancer (basal cell carcinoma, melanoma).
- Actinic keratosis.
- Smoking.
- Fair skin, blue eyes and blond or red hair.
- Previous cutaneous injury, thermal burn, disease (e.g. cutaneous lupus, epidermolysis bullosa, leg ulcer).
- Inherited syndromes: SCC is a particular problem for families with xeroderma pigmentosum and albinism.
- Other risk factors include ionising radiation, exposure to arsenic, and immune suppression due to disease (e.g. chronic lymphocytic leukaemia) or treatment. Organ transplant recipients have a massively increased risk of developing SCC.

What causes cutaneous squamous cell carcinoma?

More than 90% of cases of SCC are associated with DNA mutations in the *p53* tumour suppressor gene, caused by exposure to ultraviolet radiation (UV), especially UVB. Mutations in signalling pathways including epidermal growth factor receptor, RAS, Fyn, or p16INK4a signalling are also implicated.

Beta-genus human papillomaviruses (wart virus) are thought to play a role in SCC arising in immunosuppressed populations. β-HPV and HPV subtypes 5, 8, 17, 20, 24, and 38 have also been associated with an increased risk of cutaneous SCC in immunocompetent individuals.

What are the clinical features of cutaneous squamous cell carcinoma?

Cutaneous SCCs present as enlarging scaly or crusted lumps (*Figs 5.115–5.116*). They usually arise within pre-existing actinic keratosis or intraepidermal carcinoma.

- Grow over weeks to months.
- May ulcerate (*Fig. 5.115*).
- Often tender or painful.
- Often located on sun-exposed sites, particularly the face, lips, ears, hands, forearms and lower legs.
- Size varies from a few millimetres to several centimetres in diameter.

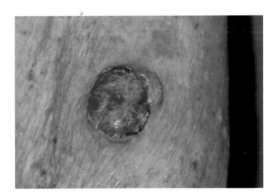

Figure 5.115. Ulcerated cutaneous SCC.

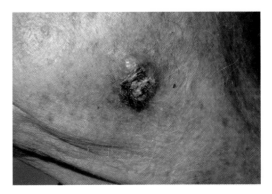

Figure 5.116. Crusted cutaneous SCC.

Types of cutaneous squamous cell carcinoma

Distinct clinical types of invasive SCC include:
- cutaneous horn – the horn is due to excessive production of keratin (see *Fig. 5.118*).
- keratoacanthoma – a rapidly growing keratinising nodule that may resolve without treatment (see *Figs 5.117* and *5.119*).
- carcinoma cuniculatum ('verrucous carcinoma'), a slow-growing, warty tumour on the sole of the foot (*Fig. 5.120*).

The pathologist may classify the SCC as well differentiated, moderately well differentiated, poorly differentiated or anaplastic. There are other variants.

HIGH-RISK CUTANEOUS SQUAMOUS CELL CARCINOMA

Cutaneous SCC is classified as low-risk or high-risk, depending on the chance of tumour recurrence and metastasis. Characteristics of high-risk SCC include:
- diameter ≥2 cm.

- location on the ear, vermilion of lip (see *Fig. 5.1*), central face, hands, feet, genitalia.
- arising in elderly or immune suppressed patient.
- histological thickness >2 mm, poorly differentiated histology, or with invasion of the subcutaneous tissue, nerves and blood vessels.

Metastatic SCC is found in regional lymph nodes (80%), lungs, liver, brain, bones and skin.

Staging SCC

In 2011, the American Joint Committee on Cancer (AJCC) published a new staging system for cutaneous SCC for the 7th edition of the AJCC Manual. This evaluates the dimensions of the original primary tumour (T) and its metastases to lymph nodes (N).

TUMOUR STAGING FOR CUTANEOUS SCC

TX   Primary tumour cannot be assessed
T0   No evidence of primary tumour

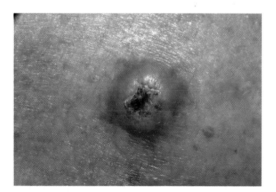

Figure 5.117. Keratoacanthoma.

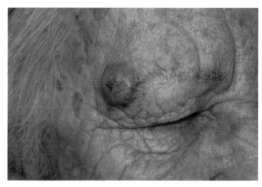

Figure 5.119. Keratoacanthoma.

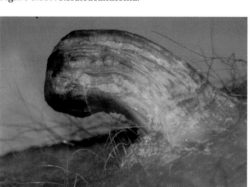

Figure 5.118. Cutaneous horn.

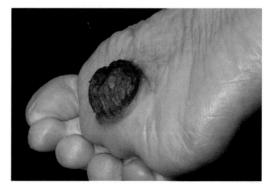

Figure 5.120. Carcinoma cuniculatum.

Tis Carcinoma *in situ*
T1   Tumour ≤2 cm without high-risk features
T2   Tumour ≥2 cm
     Tumour ≤2 cm with high-risk features
T3   Tumour with invasion of maxilla, mandible, orbit or temporal bone
T4   Tumour with invasion of axial or appendicular skeleton or perineural invasion of skull base

NODAL STAGING FOR CUTANEOUS SCC
NX Regional lymph nodes cannot be assessed
N0 No regional lymph node metastasis
N1 Metastasis in one local lymph node ≤3 cm
N2 Metastasis in one local lymph node ≥3 cm
    Metastasis in >1 local lymph node ≤6 cm
N3 Metastasis in lymph node ≥6 cm

How is squamous cell carcinoma diagnosed?

Diagnosis of cutaneous SCC is based on clinical features. The diagnosis and histological subtype is confirmed pathologically by diagnostic biopsy or following excision.

Patients with high-risk SCC may also undergo staging investigations to determine whether it has spread to lymph nodes or elsewhere. These may include:
- ultrasound scan, X-rays, CT scans, MRI scans.
- lymph node or other tissue biopsy.

What is the treatment for cutaneous squamous cell carcinoma?

Cutaneous SCC is nearly always treated surgically. Most cases are excised with a 3–10 mm margin of normal tissue around the visible tumour. A flap or skin graft may be needed to repair the defect.

Other methods of removal include:
- shave, curettage and electrocautery for low-risk tumours on trunk and limbs.
- aggressive cryotherapy for very small, thin, low-risk tumours.
- Mohs micrographic surgery for large facial lesions with indistinct margins or recurrent tumours.
- radiation therapy for inoperable tumour, patients unsuitable for surgery, or as adjuvant.

What is the treatment for advanced or metastatic squamous cell carcinoma?

Locally advanced primary, recurrent or metastatic SCC requires multidisciplinary consultation. Often a combination of treatments is used.
- Surgery.
- Radiotherapy.
- Experimental targeted therapy using epidermal growth factor receptor inhibitors.

Many thousands of New Zealanders are treated for SCC each year, and more than 100 die from their disease. In the UK, more than 750 non-melanoma skin cancer deaths were recorded in 2014, mostly due to cutaneaous SCC.

How can cutaneous squamous cell carcinoma be prevented?

There is a great deal of evidence to show that very careful sun protection at any time of life reduces the number of SCCs. This is particularly important in ageing, sun-damaged, fair skin; in patients who are immunosuppressed; and in those who already have actinic keratoses or previous SCC.
- Stay indoors or in the shade in the middle of the day.
- Wear covering clothing.
- Apply broad-spectrum sunscreens generously to exposed skin if outdoors.
- Avoid indoor tanning (sun beds and solaria).

Oral nicotinamide (vitamin B3) in a dose of 500 mg twice daily may reduce the number and severity of SCCs in people at high risk.

Patients with multiple squamous cell carcinomas may be prescribed an oral retinoid (acitretin or isotretinoin). These reduce the number of tumours but have some nuisance side effects.

What is the outlook for cutaneous squamous cell carcinoma?

Most SCCs are cured by treatment. Cure is most likely if treatment is undertaken when the lesion is small.

About 50% of people at high risk of SCC develop a second one within 5 years of the first. They are also at increased risk of other skin cancers, especially melanoma. Regular self-skin examinations and long-term annual skin checks by an experienced health professional are recommended.

5.13 Vascular lesions

Introduction

Terminology of vascular conditions can be confusing, with several lesions being incorrectly named or classified. Vascular skin lesions include:

1. Vascular naevi.
2. Angiomas.
3. Telangiectasias.
4. Vascular sarcomas.

A paediatric dermatologist, paediatrician, vascular specialist or surgeon should assess significant infantile capillary malformations or proliferative haemangiomas, especially when large, symptomatic (e.g. ulcerated), located on the head and neck or close to eye, nose or mouth.

Vascular naevi

Vascular naevi or anomalies are present at birth or appear in early childhood. They are classified according to the size and type of vessel. They may remain stable or become more prominent with maturity. There are various associated syndromes (see *DermNet NZ*).

- Capillary malformation – salmon patch (*Fig. 5.121*) and port wine stain (*Fig. 5.122*).
- Venous malformations – glomovenous malformation, arteriovenous malformations, blue rubber bleb syndrome (*Fig. 5.123*) (associated gastrointestinal lesions).
- Arteriovenous malformations: of mixed blood vessel origin.
- Lymphatic malformation: Lymphangioma circumscriptum, cavernous lymphangioma (*Fig. 5.124*).
- Angioma serpiginosa: a crop of swirling vascular papules (*Fig. 5.125*).
- Naevus anaemicus – in this naevus, blood flow is interrupted resulting in pale areas (*Fig. 5.126*).

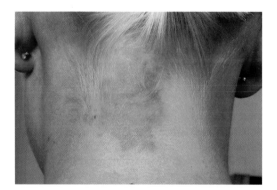

Figure 5.121. Capillary malformation.

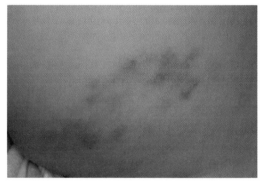

Figure 5.123. Blue rubber bleb syndrome.

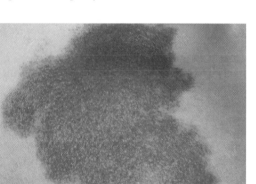

Figure 5.122. Port wine stain.

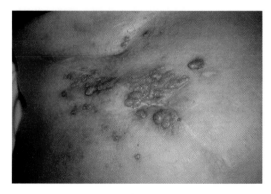

Figure 5.124. Cavernous lymphangioma.

Angiomas

Angiomas are benign tumours formed by dilation of blood vessels or formation of new ones by proliferation of endothelial cells.

- Infantile proliferative haemangioma (capillary, cavernous or mixed): proliferates in the first few weeks of life, followed by involution later in childhood (*Fig. 5.127*).
- Congenital haemangioma is at full size at birth and may rapidly involute (RICH) or persist (NICH).
- Kaposiform haemangioendothelioma is a rare aggressive haemangioma that results in platelet trapping – the Kasabach–Merritt phenomenon.
- Tufted angioma: rare childhood tumour with characteristic histology.
- Cherry angioma (*Fig. 5.128*) adult onset, common degenerative lesions, usually multiple. Dermatoscopy shows red, purple or blue clods (*Fig. 5.131*).

- Angiokeratoma: acquired scaly angiomas, usually on vulva or scrotum, or in association with Fabry disease (see *Fig. 5.129*).
- Glomus tumour: tender papule on nail bed or palm arising in young to middle-aged adult (*Fig. 5.130*).

Pyogenic granuloma (see *Fig. 5.132*) occurs in children and young adults on skin and mucosa, most often lower lips, fingers and toes in response to a minor, often unnoticed, injury. It grows rapidly and may become pedunculated or polypoid and surrounded by a collarette of normal skin. It bleeds and crusts.

Bacillary angiomatosis is a rare opportunistic bacterial infection due to *Rochalimaea henselae*.

Telangiectasias

Prominent cutaneous blood vessels can be physiological or pathological (e.g. feeding a tumour such as basal cell carcinoma, and they are a common sign of rosacea). There are some named conditions in which telangiectasia is characteristic.

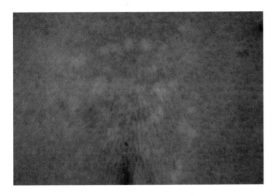

Figure 5.125. Angioma serpiginosa.

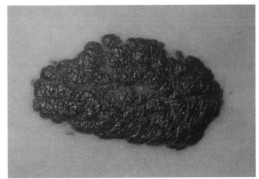

Figure 5.127. Infantile proliferative haemangioma.

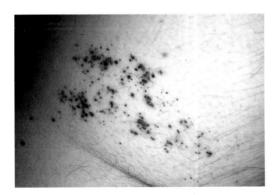

Figure 5.126. Naevus anaemicus.

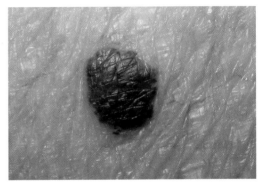

Figure 5.128. Cherry angioma.

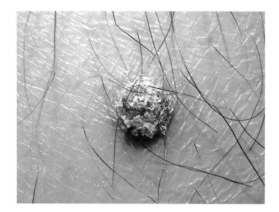

Figure 5.129. Angiokeratoma seen on dermatoscopy.

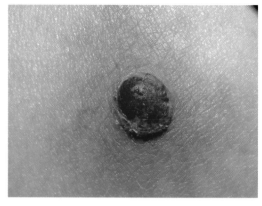

Figure 5.132. Pyogenic granuloma.

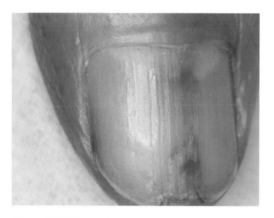

Figure 5.130. Glomus tumour.

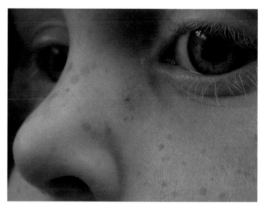

Figure 5.133. Spider angioma.

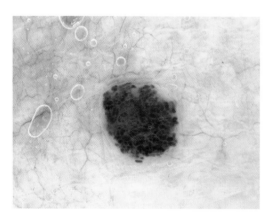

Figure 5.131. Purple clods of angioma seen on dermatoscopy.

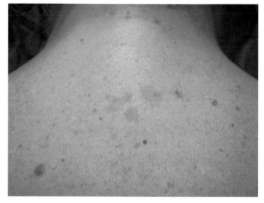

Figure 5.134. Benign hereditary telangiectasia.

- Spider angioma (*Fig. 5.133*) or spider telangiectasis consists of central arteriole and radiating capillaries. Very common in healthy individuals, but more arise in response to oestrogen, e.g. pregnancy, liver disease.

- Venous lake (*Fig. 5.136*): blue or purple compressible papule due to venous dilation, often on lower lip or ear.
- Unilateral acquired telangiectasia: telangiectasia with naevoid distribution.

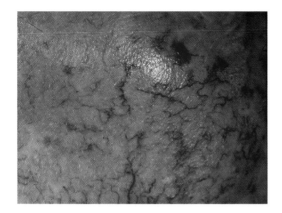

Figure 5.135. Essential telangiectasia.

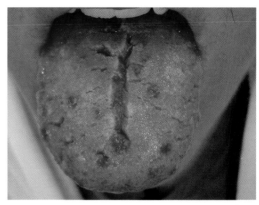

Figure 5.137. Hereditary haemorrhagic telangiectasia.

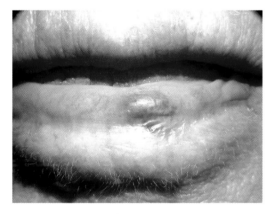

Figure 5.136. Venous lake.

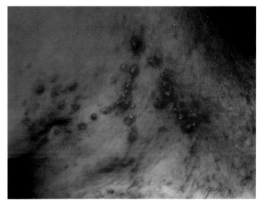

Figure 5.138. Acquired lymphangiectasia.

- Essential telangiectasia: idiopathic telangiectasia and venulectasia (see *Fig. 5.135*).
- Benign hereditary telangiectasia: familial condition in which matt telangiectases appear (*Fig. 5.134*).
- Hereditary haemorrhagic telangiectasia: telangiectasia on skin and mucous membranes associated with bleeding from nose and gut causing anaemia (see *Fig. 5.137*).
- Acquired lymphangiectasia: "frog-spawn" appearance that follows lymphatic obstruction, e.g. tumour or surgery (see *Fig. 5.138*).

Malignant vascular tumours

- Kaposi sarcoma: due to human herpesvirus 8 (HHV8) and immunosuppression, e.g. infection with human immunodeficiency virus (HIV). There are four types. Kaposi sarcoma presents with multiple purple macules, papules and plaques on skin and mucous membranes (see *Fig. 5.139*).
- Angiosarcoma: idiopathic or secondary to chronic lymphoedema or radiation. Often an aggressive cancer, it mostly presents in elderly people with spreading purple patches and plaques that may bleed and ulcerate (*Fig. 5.140*).

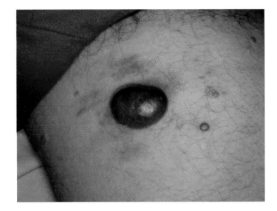

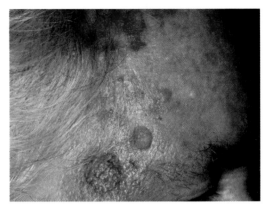

Figure 5.139. Kaposi sarcoma.

Figure 5.140. Angiosarcoma.

Chapter 6

Investigations and treatments

6.1 Dermatological investigations: general

An experienced clinician can often diagnose a skin condition without the need for investigations. However, at times, skin swabs, scrapings and nail clippings, biopsies and blood samples are sent to the laboratory, and allergy testing or imaging is arranged. Investigations may also be used to monitor the effects of systemic treatments.

Microbiology

- Standard skin or wound swabs have a cotton tip on a plastic shaft and are typically placed in Amies (charcoal) gel transport medium for routine bacterial culture, and if appropriate, antibiotic sensitivities.
- Low vaginal, male meatal or urine swabs may be sent in buffer for polymerase chain reaction (PCR), a molecular biology technique used to detect chlamydia, gonorrhoea, trichomonas and other organisms.
- Skin scrapings, nail clippings and extracted hair are treated with potassium hydroxide (KOH) and examined by direct microscopy before being plated out for fungal culture. An interim report may describe hyphae, arthrospores and mycelia typical of dermatophyte or yeast. Culture results and the specific organisms identified are reported about four weeks later.
- Viral transport medium is used to detect herpes simplex and herpes zoster by culture, immunofluorescence or PCR.
- Skin specimens in a small amount of sterile saline may also be processed for Gram stain, microscopy and culture, including low-temperature culture for atypical mycobacteria and identification of organisms such as leishmaniasis and deep fungi.

Histology

- Most skin biopsy samples are sent to the laboratory in 10% buffered formalin, with 24-hour fixation and processing time prior to examination by a histopathologist. Reports are issued in about a week. Interpretation of skin biopsies requires considerable training and experience.
- Samples for immunofluorescence should be placed in culture medium, saline or liquid nitrogen and should be sent to the laboratory urgently.
- Frozen sections do not have fixative and can be quickly viewed by a pathologist in a hospital setting. In dermatology, they are mainly used to determine if a basal cell carcinoma has been fully surgically removed by Mohs surgery (microscopically controlled excision). Considerable skill and training is required to interpret frozen sections.
- Cell cytology of the base of a blister can be assessed on a smear of tissue applied to a glass slide and fixed by air-drying, i.e. Tzanck smear. It is quick, but is not very reliable for diagnosis.

Blood tests

Haematology

- Neutrophilia is typical of infection but may also accompany severe inflammatory disorders including pustular psoriasis, and neutrophilic dermatoses such as Sweet syndrome or pyoderma gangrenosum.
- Eosinophilia is associated with atopic eczema, scabies, bullous disease and lymphoma. It can be quite non-specific in patients with erythroderma.
- Lymphocytosis is associated with viral infections and certain bacterial infections such as tuberculosis and syphilis.

Other

- Renal, hepatic and thyroid function, and iron status may be evaluated in patients with generalised pruritus, vasculitis or systemic symptoms.
- Blood glucose and glycosylated haemoglobin detect and monitor diabetes, which may be of relevance in infection, or skin diseases associated with metabolic syndrome.
- Antinuclear and extractable nuclear antigen antibodies and tissue autoantibodies are assessed in patients with suspected connective tissue or autoimmune disease.
- Proteins, including immunoglobulins, cryoproteins/cryoglobulins and complement, are assessed in patients with vasculitis or connective tissue disease.
- Specific serology is requested for infections, e.g. hepatitis B, hepatitis C, human immunodeficiency virus (HIV), syphilis.

- Additional tests in vasculitis include anti-neutrophil cytoplasmic antibodies (ANCA), antiphospholipids, thrombophilia screen.
- Hormonal tests are occasionally arranged in females with acne, hirsutism and androgenetic alopecia if symptoms indicate these tests are warranted, or if virilism is present.
- Urinary and faecal or serum porphyrins are requested in patients who may have a cutaneous porphyria.

Allergy tests

Determination of allergy requires a careful history and examination, and testing should have a specific question in mind.

PRICK TESTS

Prick tests for immediate hypersensitivities are sometimes undertaken in patients with suspected contact urticaria or latex allergy. They are not useful in atopic dermatitis or acute/chronic spontaneous urticaria.

PATCH TESTS

Patch tests are undertaken by specialist clinics for patients with suspected contact allergic dermatitis; they detect delayed hypersensitivity reactions. Patients should have a chronic or relapsing dermatitis.

- A baseline series of common allergens and additional batteries of test substances are selected, depending on the site of rash or occupational exposures.
- Standardised concentrations of allergens are sourced from specialised companies.
- Test patches are applied to the upper back on Day 0, removed on Day 2, and reviewed on Day 4, and sometimes Day 7.
- Photopatch tests require a duplicate set of photoallergens to be applied, with exposure to ultraviolet radiation to one of the sets of allergens on the day of removal.
- Interpretation of equivocal results can be challenging.

Imaging

RADIOLOGICAL EXAMINATIONS

X-rays, CT scans, MRI scans and ultrasound tests are not routinely requested in dermatology, but may be arranged for systemic symptoms or monitoring treatment.

BLACK LIGHT EXAMINATION

Exposure to long wavelength UVA emitted by a Wood lamp is mainly used to investigate pigmentary disorders and chronic superficial skin infections, where fluorescence supports a specific cause.

DIGITAL DERMATOSCOPY

Digital dermatoscopy is digital imaging of skin lesions under dermatoscopy. Ideally, these are accompanied by macroscopic and location images. Dermatoscopic images can be taken using a variety of dermatoscopes, adapters and video and still cameras using contact and non-contact, polarised and unpolarised systems.

Mole mapping is a system in which the location of melanocytic naevi is mapped to a mannequin, total body photographs are taken, and macroscopic and digital images are recorded for lesions of clinical concern. The procedure is repeated at intervals to monitor patients with high risk of melanoma, particularly if they have many naevi or naevi with an unusual appearance.

OTHER

Optical coherence tomography and reflectance confocal microscopy are *in vivo* techniques for cutaneous diagnoses. They are mainly used in research centres.

6.2 Skin biopsy

What is a skin biopsy?

A skin biopsy is the removal and histopathological examination of a sample of skin to identify the presence, cause or extent of a disease or condition.

Why have a skin biopsy?

One or more skin biopsies are performed to make or confirm a diagnosis, which often helps determine the correct treatment.

- There may be several distinct skin conditions with similar clinical appearance but different time course and management.
- Complex treatment may be under consideration.
- It may be unclear if a skin lesion is benign, and can be left alone, or if it is malignant, when it should be completely removed.
- The clinician may be attempting to find the edge of a tumour.

Choosing the site for a biopsy

It is crucial that the site of a biopsy is chosen carefully, or the pathological diagnosis could be incorrect or misleading.

- Excoriated lesions will show nonspecific inflammation and wound healing.
- Ulcerated areas are often very inflamed and secondarily infected, whatever the original cause of the ulcer.
- A fresh lesion is often the most suitable for evaluation of an inflammatory skin condition, particularly if vasculitis is a consideration.
- The edge of an enlarging lesion is often the best site to detect basal cell or squamous cell skin cancer.
- A small intact blister may show more useful information than the corner of a large one.
- Diagnostic clues are found in the skin adjacent to a scarred or ulcerated area.

Completing the request form

The clinician should ensure the pathology request form includes patient information (including age and identification details), the site and type of biopsy, time and date, clinical information and a range of possible diagnoses.

The sample pot should be labelled with patient identification details, the body site of the biopsy, time and date.

What happens to the biopsy sample?

Most skin biopsies are placed in formalin in a small pot and are sent to the lab for paraffin fixation, processing and histopathology.

- If considering deep fungal infection or mycobacteria, the sample may be divided so that one part of the sample is sent in formalin for histopathology and the other is placed on a saline-soaked gauze swab for microbiology.
- Samples for direct immune fluorescence are placed in transport media, snap frozen in liquid nitrogen, or sent "fresh" (e.g. placed on a moistened gauze swab).

Types of skin biopsy

Skin biopsy is usually undertaken using a local anaesthetic injection into the surrounding skin to numb the area. The injection stings transiently. After the procedure, a dressing will usually be applied to the site of the biopsy. This should be left in place for the first 24 hours and replaced if necessary. There will be a small scar left after the skin biopsy site has healed.

PUNCH BIOPSY

A punch biopsy is quick to perform, convenient, and only produces a small wound. The pathologist can evaluate the full thickness of skin.

The disposable skin biopsy punch has a round stainless steel blade ranging from 2–6 mm in diameter; 3 and 4 mm are the most common sizes used for inflammatory skin disease. The clinician holds the instrument perpendicular to the skin and rotates it to pierce the skin and removes a cylindrical core of epidermis, dermis and sometimes, subcutaneous tissue.

A suture is often used to close the wound, or, if the wound is small, it may heal adequately without it.

SHAVE BIOPSY

A shave biopsy may be used if the skin lesion is superficial, for example to confirm a suspected diagnosis of intraepidermal squamous cell carcinoma or basal cell carcinoma.

A tangential shave of skin is taken using a scalpel, special shave-biopsy instrument or razor blade. No stitches are required. The wound forms a scab that should heal in 1–3 weeks.

A scoop biopsy is a deep form of shave biopsy, used to remove a skin lesion such as a benign mole by "scooping" it out. It is also called "saucerisation" or "tangential excision."

CURETTAGE
A skin curette may be used to scrape off a superficial skin lesion, such as basal cell carcinoma or seborrhoeic keratosis. Some of the curettings are sent for histopathology. These samples are not suitable for determining if a lesion has been completely removed.

INCISIONAL BIOPSY
Incisional biopsies refer to removal of a larger ellipse of skin for diagnosis, using a scalpel blade. Stitches are usually required after an incisional biopsy.

EXCISION BIOPSY
Excision biopsy refers to complete removal of a skin lesion, such as a skin cancer. A margin of surrounding skin is taken, as a precaution. Smaller lesions are most often removed using a scalpel blade as an ellipse, with primary closure using sutures. Larger excisions may be repaired using a skin flap (moving adjacent skin to cover the wound) or graft (skin taken from another site to patch the wound).

Complications of skin biopsy

Skin biopsy is usually straightforward and complications are uncommon.

BLEEDING
Intraoperative or postoperative bleeding can occur in anyone, but can be particularly troublesome in those with a bleeding tendency, or taking blood-thinning medications such as warfarin or aspirin.

INFECTION
Bacterial wound infection affects about 1 to 5% of surgeries. It is more likely in ulcerated or crusted skin lesions. The risk of infection is greater than usual in diabetics, elderly patients, and in people taking immunosuppressive medicines.

DELAYED HEALING
Delayed healing is most likely in biopsies taken from the lower legs, especially if the leg is swollen, the arterial or venous circulation is impaired, or there is a skin condition that predisposes to ulceration after skin injury (e.g. pyoderma gangrenosum).

NERVE INJURY
The blade may cut a superficial nerve, causing pain or numbness. This is most likely to occur where the skin is thin, for example on the face or back of hand.

SCARRING
It is usual for a biopsy site to form a permanent scar. Some people form excessive or hypertrophic scars, particularly in certain body sites such as the centre of the chest.

PERSISTENCE OR RECURRENCE OF THE SKIN LESION
Many biopsies are deliberately partial, so that the underlying skin condition remains. In other cases, complete removal is intended but not achieved; in time, the lesion may recur at the same site.

Obtaining the results of the biopsy

It usually takes about one week to obtain the result from the pathology laboratory, but can sometimes take longer if special stains are required. The pathologist describes what is observed under light microscopy in several sections of the biopsy sample, and provides the likely diagnosis. Sometimes it is not possible to make an exact diagnosis on the biopsy sample provided.

CLINICOPATHOLOGICAL CORRELATION
Skin diseases and conditions can at times be very difficult to diagnose accurately. The various specialists involved may need to consult with each other. This is called clinicopathological correlation (CPC). Larger organisations hold regular multidisciplinary meetings (MDMs) at which clinical information, clinical and dermatoscopic photographs, and pathology slides are reviewed by a team of experts to determine the best diagnosis and treatment for the patient.

6.3 Interpreting dermatopathology reports

*See www.DermNetNZ.org for
dermatopathological glossary.*

What is dermatopathology?

Dermatopathology involves the microscopic
examination, description and interpretation of
biopsy specimens obtained from the skin.

The interpretation of skin specimens can
be complicated and difficult, as many diverse
inflammatory skin diseases share the same
basic inflammatory process or pattern. The
final diagnosis requires clinical input and
clinicopathological correlation.

How are skin biopsy specimens examined?

Skin biopsy specimens are processed and then
stained with haematoxylin and eosin (H&E).
With this stain, eosinophilic or acidophilic
structures stain red, e.g. cytoplasm, while
basophilic or acidic structures stain purplish-
blue in colour, e.g. nuclei. Depending on the
observed dermatopathological pattern present
and/or the clinical features, special stains
may be requested to identify agents causing
the condition (e.g. bacteria or fungi), specific
substances deposited in the skin (e.g. amyloid,
iron or melanin) or specific markers to identify
the origin, nature and distribution of cells in the
specimen being examined.

The specimen is systematically examined by
looking at the structure of the epidermis, dermis,
subcutis, fascia and underlying structures.
Based on the findings, the pathologist may come
up with a definitive diagnosis, or list several
possible explanations, creating a differential
diagnosis. The integration of clinical information
in conjunction with the pathological findings
generates the final diagnosis.

Potential errors in diagnosis

Pathologists depend on the clinician supplying a
good history and differential diagnosis, and their
job is easier with a large biopsy sample than with
a small one. Even then, the sample may not be
representative of the disease as a whole.

- The biopsy may have been taken from the
  wrong lesion.
- The biopsy may not contain diagnostic
  material.
- The biopsy may be fragmented or crushed.
- There may be processing errors.

- Incorrect diagnosis may arise because of lack
  of information on the request form.
- The microscopy may appear normal despite
  quite obvious clinical disease.
- Changes may be too subtle to diagnose if the
  lesion is very early in its development.
- Secondary changes obscure primary pathology.
  These include excoriation, ulceration, healing,
  infection, necrosis and fibrosis.
- The thin section examined by the pathologist
  may not contain any part of the lesion
  present in another portion of the original
  specimen.
- Dense cellular infiltration may obscure the
  presence of another pathological feature,
  preventing its identification.
- Two quite different skin diseases might
  appear similar under the microscope.

Common inflammatory skin diseases

Histological patterns of eczema, psoriasis, lichen
planus, bullous pemphigoid, vasculitis and
granuloma annulare are described below.

ECZEMA/DERMATITIS

The histological features of eczema are:

- spongiosis in acute eczema with associated
  lymphocyte exocytosis (see *Fig. 6.1*).
- acanthosis in chronic eczema.
- parakeratosis and perivascular
  lymphohistiocytic infiltrate.
- excoriation and signs of rubbing (irregular
  acanthosis and perpendicular orientation of
  collagen in dermal papillae) in chronic cases
  (lichen simplex), see *Fig. 6.2*.

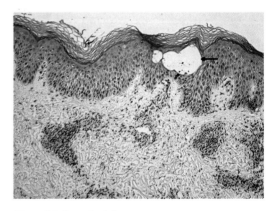

Figure 6.1. Spongiosis in acute eczema
(×100 magnification).

PSORIASIS

Typical histological features of chronic plaque psoriasis (see *Figs 6.3* and *6.4*) are:

- hyperkeratosis – mainly parakeratosis, some orthokeratosis.
- neutrophils in stratum corneum and squamous cell layer.
- hypogranulosis.
- epidermis is thin over dermal papillae.
- regular acanthosis, often with clubbed rete ridges.
- relatively little spongiosis.
- dilated capillaries in dermal papillae.
- perivascular lymphohistiocytic infiltrate.

LICHEN PLANUS

The histological features of lichen planus (see *Figs 6.5* and *6.6*) are:

- orthokeratosis.
- hypergranulosis.
- irregular acanthosis with saw-toothed rete ridges (older lesions).

- colloid or Civatte bodies in lower epidermis and upper dermis.
- liquefaction degeneration of the basal layer.
- lichenoid lymphohistiocytic infiltrate in upper dermis (interface dermatitis) and sometimes within the epidermis.
- melanin incontinence.

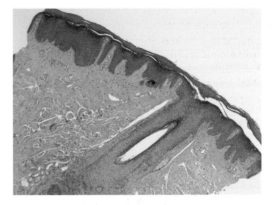

Figure 6.4. Psoriasis (×40 magnification).

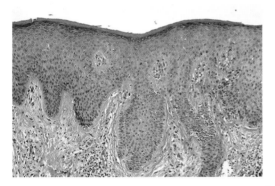

Figure 6.2. Acanathosis in chronic eczema (×100 magnification).

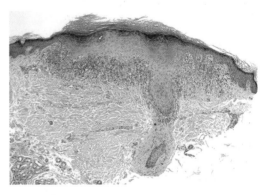

Figure 6.5. Lichen planus (×40 magnification).

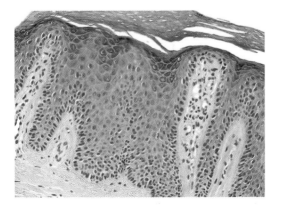

Figure 6.3. Psoriasis (×200 magnification).

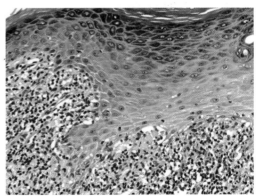

Figure 6.6. Lichen planus (×200 magnification).

Bullous pemphigoid

The histological features of bullous pemphigoid (*Figs 6.7* and *6.8*) are:
- subepidermal blister.
- viable roof over new blister, necrotic over an old blister.
- variable perivascular infiltrate (lymphocytes, histiocytes, eosinophils).
- pre-bullous lesions may show spongiosis with eosinophil exocytosis (eosinophilic spongiosis).

Vasculitis

Note: vascular damage can be a secondary feature of conditions that are not primarily a vasculitis.

The histological features of leucocytoclastic vasculitis (*Figs 6.9* and *6.10*) are:
- vessel wall damage – necrosis, hyalinisation, fibrin.
- invasion of inflammatory cells into vessel walls.
- red cell extravasation.
- nuclear dust from leucocytoclasia of neutrophils.
- severe cases may show ischaemic necrosis of the epidermis.

Granuloma annulare

The histological features of granuloma annulare (*Figs 6.11* and *6.12*) are:
- normal epidermis.
- central foci of dermal collagen degeneration (necrobiosis) and mucin accumulation.
- palisading of histiocytes.
- multinucleate giant cells.
- single-filing of inflammatory cells between collagen bundles ('busy' dermis).

Common cutaneous tumours

Histology of the common cutaneous tumours seborrhoeic keratosis, basal cell carcinoma, squamous cell carcinoma *in situ*

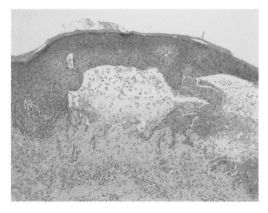

Figure 6.7. Bullous pemphigoid (×40 magnification).

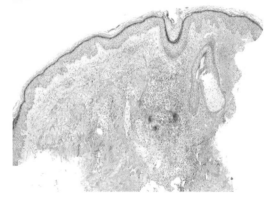

Figure 6.9. Leucocytoclastic vasculitis (×4 magnification).

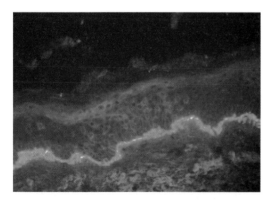

Figure 6.8. Bullous pemphigoid (direct immune fluorescence).

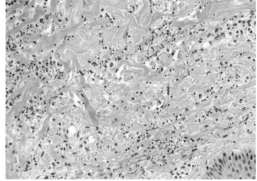

Figure 6.10. Leucocytoclastic vasculitis (×20 magnification).

(intraepidermal carcinoma), squamous cell carcinoma, cysts, lentigo, melanocytic naevus, melanoma and dermatofibroma are described below.

SEBORRHOEIC KERATOSIS

The histological features of seborrhoeic keratoses (*Figs 6.13* and *6.14*) may be quite varied and can overlap with solar lentigo, but typically show:

- hyperkeratosis, papillomatosis, acanthosis.
- basaloid keratinocytes.
- horn cysts.
- abundant melanin in basal layer or throughout epidermis.
- sharp demarcation of base of epidermal hyperplasia.
- largely located above the surrounding epidermis.

Irritated seborrhoeic keratoses may show many features suggestive of malignancy, and can be difficult at times to differentiate from squamous carcinoma.

BASAL CELL CARCINOMA

The histological features of basal cell carcinoma (*Figs 6.15* and *6.16*) are typically:

- cohesive nests of basaloid tumour cells (sometimes with a small amount of squamous differentiation).
- peripheral palisading of nuclei at the margins of cell nests.
- retraction artefact (clefts) around cell nests.
- variable inflammatory infiltrate and ulceration.

ACTINIC KERATOSIS

The histological features of actinic keratosis (*Figs 6.17* and *6.18*) are:

- hyperkeratosis and/or ulceration.
- columns of parakeratosis, overlying atypical keratinocytes, separated by areas of orthokeratosis.

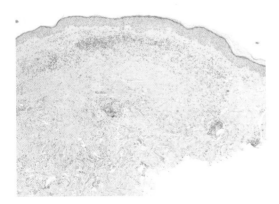

Figure 6.11. Granuloma annulare (×4 magnification).

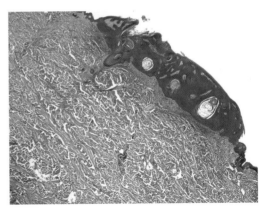

Figure 6.13. Seborrhoeic keratosis (×20 magnification).

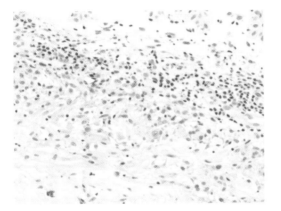

Figure 6.12. Granuloma annulare (×40 magnification).

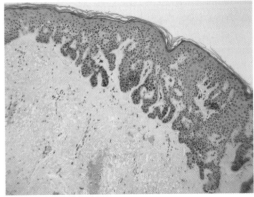

Figure 6.14. Seborrhoeic keratosis (×10 magnification).

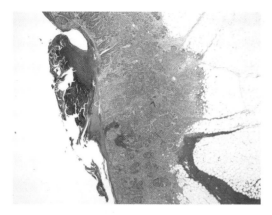

Figure 6.15. Basal cell carcinoma (×20 magnification).

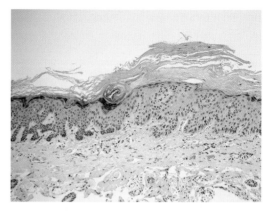

Figure 6.17. Actinic keratosis (×20 magnification).

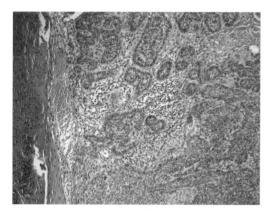

Figure 6.16. Basal cell carcinoma (×100 magnification).

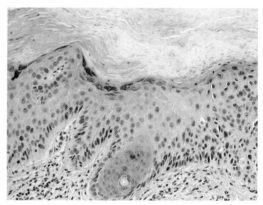

Figure 6.18. Actinic keratosis (×40 magnification).

- basal atypical keratinocytes with varying degrees of overlying loss of maturation, hyperchromatism, pleomorphism, increased and abnormal mitoses, dyskeratosis – full thickness change may be called 'Bowenoid actinic keratosis'.
- variable superficial perivascular or lichenoid chronic inflammatory infiltrate.
- solar elastosis.

IN SITU SQUAMOUS CELL CARCINOMA
The histological features of *in situ* squamous cell carcinoma (*Figs 6.19* and *6.20*) show extensive overlap with actinic keratosis and are:
- hyperkeratosis, parakeratosis.
- acanthosis.
- full thickness epidermal involvement by atypical keratinocytes, with pale vacuolated or multinucleated cells.
- in some lesions, pagetoid spread at the margins.

INVASIVE SQUAMOUS CELL CARCINOMA
Histological features of invasive squamous cell carcinomas (*Figs 6.21* and *6.22*) can vary, but in general are:
- proliferation of atypical keratinocytes.
- invasion of dermis.
- variable degrees of keratinisation, sometimes squamous eddies or keratin pearls.

EPIDERMOID AND PILAR CYSTS
The histological features of epidermal inclusion cysts (epidermoid cysts, see *Fig. 6.23*) are:
- cyst lined by squamous epithelium, sometimes flattened, with a granular layer.
- lamellated keratin within cyst.
- milia are very small epidermoid cysts.

Dermoid cysts differ by showing hair follicles and sebaceous glands in the wall and hair shafts in the contents.

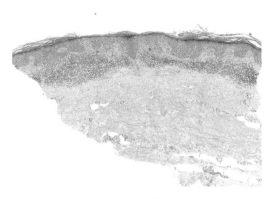

Figure 6.19. In situ squamous cell carcinoma (×4 magnification).

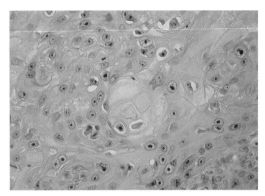

Figure 6.22. Invasive squamous cell carcinoma (×40 magnification).

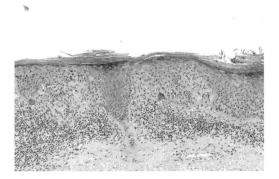

Figure 6.20. In situ squamous cell carcinoma (×20 magnification).

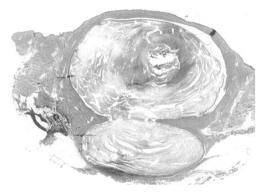

Figure 6.23. Epidermal inclusion cyst (×2 magnification).

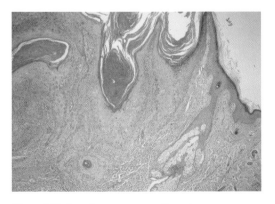

Figure 6.21. Invasive squamous cell carcinoma (×10 magnification).

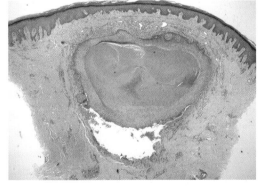

Figure 6.24. Trichilemmal cyst (×4 magnification).

Trichilemmal (pilar) cysts (see *Fig. 6.24*) show:
- a squamous lining but no granular layer.
- dense keratin content.
- frequent calcification.

LENTIGO

The histological features of lentigines (*Fig. 6.25*) are:
- hyperpigmented elongated rete ridges.
- increased melanocytes.

MELANOCYTIC NAEVUS

The histological features of melanocytic naevi (see *Figs 6.26–6.28*) are:

- variable epidermal changes – atrophy, hyperplasia, papillomatosis, horn cysts.
- nests of melanocytes/naevus cells at the dermo-epidermal junction (junctional naevus, see *Fig. 6.26*) and/or in the dermis (compound naevus, see *Fig. 6.27*, and dermal naevus, see *Fig. 6.28*).
- naevus cells in the epidermis confined to the basal layer, usually at the tips of the rete ridges.
- generally round naevus cells that show decreasing size of both the cells and the cell nests with increasing depth in the dermis (so-called maturation).
- little inflammation unless traumatised (except halo and dysplastic naevi).

MELANOMA

The histological features of melanoma differ, depending on the type of tumour, but in general terms show (*Fig. 6.29*):

- asymmetrical proliferation of melanocytes.
- atypical melanocytes invading upwards through epidermis and downwards into dermis.
- variable cytological atypia: loss of maturation, pleomorphism, hyperchromatism, increased mitoses, prominent nucleoli.

DERMATOFIBROMA

The histological features of dermatofibroma (*Fig. 6.30*) are:

- epidermal hyperplasia (sometimes mimicking basal cell carcinoma).
- hyperpigmented basal layer.
- circumscribed but poorly demarcated proliferation of spindled fibroblasts.
- histiocytes and few giant cells.
- variable amounts of collagen.

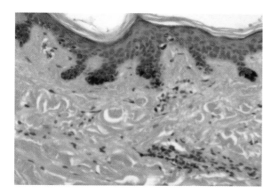

Figure 6.25. Solar lentigo (×20 magnification).

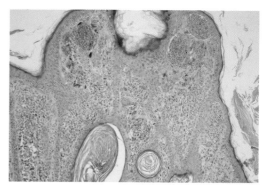

Figure 6.27. Compound naevus (×10 magnification).

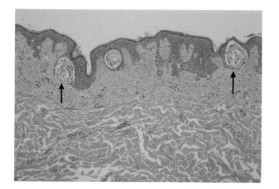

Figure 6.26. Melanocytic naevus: arrows show junctional nests of melanocytes (×10 magnification).

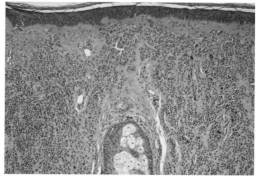

Figure 6.28. Dermal naevus (×10 magnification).

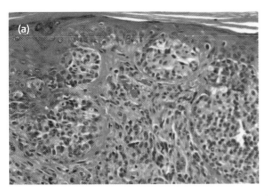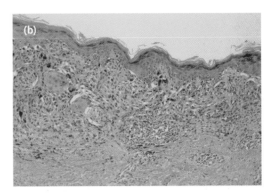

Figure 6.29. (a) Invasive melanoma (×100 magnification). (b) Melanoma *in situ.*

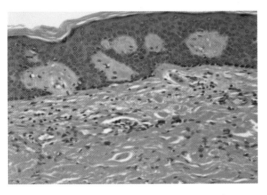

Figure 6.30. Dermatofibroma (×40 magnification).

6.4 Treatments: introduction

In dermatology, we have innumerable diseases, but not very many treatments. Our topical treatments may be expensive, messy, irritating and tedious to apply. Systemic treatments may have troublesome side-effects and require monitoring. It is not surprising that many patients fail to adhere to treatment recommendations.

- Plan for prolonged and repeated consultations for patients with chronic skin diseases.
- Find out how the condition and its treatment affect the patient at home and at work or school.
- Stress and anxiety are common causes and common effects of skin diseases and should be acknowledged.
- Keep detailed and meticulous notes.
- Clinical photography is useful for the clinical record and follow-up.
- Do no harm; many skin conditions are self-limiting.
- Keep treatment regimens as simple as possible.
- Patient education (verbal and written) is essential – www.DermNetNZ.org topic pages are free for anyone to download and print.
- Expect to be asked about diet, clothing and bathing.
- Tell the patient or caregiver who to contact for advice, and how to contact them.

There is no need to try every drug in the pharmacopoeia. Refer to a dermatologist for help when you are stuck – there are now many opportunities for online advice from your colleagues, even though face-to-face consultations for the patient may be scarce. I have aimed to cover most common drugs used in the UK, USA and Australasia; however, you should be aware that although the drugs detailed will all be appropriate for treatment, not all will be available on prescription in all territories. Please refer to your local prescribing guidelines and datasheets for detailed pharmacology and therapeutics about the drugs described. In dermatology, be aware that many treatments are used off-licence.

Cosmetic treatments are not discussed among the treatment options which follow in *Sections 6.5–6.15*. These and other options are described on www.DermNetNZ.org.

6.5 Topical formulations

General principles

Topical formulations are applied directly to the skin. Advantages of this include:

- increased dose of medication where it is needed.
- reduced side-effects and toxicity to other organs.

Disadvantages include:

- time-consuming.
- complicated.
- may be messy or uncomfortable.

Topical formulations are made up in a vehicle, or base, which may be optimised for a particular site of the body or type of skin condition. The product may be designed to be moisturising or to maximise the penetration of an active ingredient, a medicine, into or through the skin.

The amount of the active ingredient that is absorbed through the skin varies.

- Thin skin absorbs more than thick skin – skin thickness varies with body site, age and skin disorder.
- Skin barrier function disrupted by dermatitis, ichthyosis and keratolytic agents (such as salicylic acid) absorbs more than intact, normal skin.
- Occlusion increases absorption in skin folds, under dressings and greasy ointments.
- Small molecules are more easily absorbed through the skin than large molecules.
- Lipophilic compounds are better absorbed than hydrophilic compounds.
- Higher concentrations may penetrate more than lower concentrations.
- Other ingredients in the formulation may interact to increase or reduce potency or absorption rates.

Minor differences in formulation may make surprising differences to the effectiveness of a topical medication.

Quantities

How much topical medication to prescribe can challenge the most experienced dermatologist. It depends on:

- vehicle.
- thickness of application.
- total area to be treated.
- frequency of application.
- duration of treatment.

Expect 1 gram of cream to spread out over a 10 cm^2 area of skin; an ointment spreads a little further. The fingertip unit (0.5 g) is a guide to the amount of a cream or ointment needed to treat an area for a certain time. One fingertip unit (see *Fig. 6.37*) covers one side of two flat hands and 1 gram covers both sides of the patient's two hands.

It takes 20–30 g of cream or ointment to cover an adult once.

Vehicles

Topical formulations contain an active ingredient, often a medication or botanical, and a vehicle. The vehicle contains water, oil, alcohol or propylene glycol mixed with preservatives, emulsifiers, absorption promoters and fragrances.

Manufacturers interpret the definitions in various ways so a similar preparation might be called lotion, gel or cream.

CLASSIFICATION OF TOPICAL FORMULATIONS

- Solution: water or alcoholic lotion containing a dissolved powder.
- Lotion: usually considered thicker than a solution and more likely to contain oil as well as water or alcohol. A shake lotion separates into parts with time so needs to be shaken into suspension before use.
- Cream: thicker than a lotion, maintaining its shape, e.g. 50/50 emulsion of oil and water. Requires preservative to extend shelf life. Often moisturising.
- Ointment: semi-solid, water-free or nearly water-free (80% oil). Greasy, sticky, emollient, protective, occlusive. No need for preservative so contact allergy is rare. May include hydrocarbon (paraffin), wool fat, beeswax, macrogols, emulsifying wax, cetrimide or vegetable oil (olive oil, arachis oil, coconut oil).
- Gel: aqueous or alcoholic monophasic semisolid emulsion, often based on cellulose. Liquefies upon contact with skin. Often includes preservatives and fragrances.
- Paste: concentrated suspension of oil, water and powder.
- Aerosol foam or spray: solution with pressurised propellant.
- Powder: solid, e.g. talc (a mineral) or corn starch (vegetable).

- Solid: may melt on reaching body temperature, e.g. suppository.
- Transdermal patch: drug delivery system that allows precise dosing; includes an adhesive.

Other terms used by cosmetic and pharmaceutical manufacturers include emulsion, paint, suspension, milk, syrup, collodion, balm and mist. Formulae may have mixed ingredients with more than one type of vehicle.

When a pharmacist makes up a mixture, it is extemporaneously compounded. The crude ingredients (often natural in origin) are called galenicals. They may be added to a vehicle or to a brand-name product.

NATURE OF THE DERMATOSIS

- Wet or oozy skin conditions: creams, lotions, drying pastes.
- Dry scaly skin conditions: ointments, oils.
- Inflamed skin: wet compresses, soaks followed by creams or ointments.
- Cracks and sores: bland applications – avoid alcohol and acidic preparations.

SITE

- Palms and soles: ointment or cream.
- Skin folds: cream or lotion.
- Hairy areas: lotion, solution, gel, foam.
- Mucosal surfaces: non-irritating formulations.

Special circumstances

NEWBORN BABIES

Topically applied medications can be more likely to result in side-effects and toxicity in newborn babies.

- Although the skin barrier function of full-term newborn babies is nearly the same as in older children and adults, the barrier function in premature babies is markedly impaired.
- The surface area of a baby is proportionally much greater than that of an adult.

- Liver, kidneys, blood and central nervous system are not fully developed.

PREGNANCY AND LACTATION

Like oral medicines, some topical medications may be unsafe during pregnancy. These include:

- podophyllin.
- dithranol.
- fluorouracil.
- salicylic acid.

Medications are classified according to their risk. The US FDA classification system is often used. Refer to local formulary and manufacturer datasheets.

Tips for using topical agents

- Topical steroids and emollients are more effective if the skin is slightly wet, e.g. within 3 minutes after a bath or shower.
- Apply the steroid to active areas only. If you are also prescribed emollient, wait a few minutes for the topical steroid to penetrate, then apply emollient widely.
- Complaints that products sting on facial skin are common, especially if the skin is damp at the time of application. Wait 20 minutes and the stinging is often much less troublesome.
- Stinging is common with lotions and creams and sometimes also occurs with ointments. A change of formulation rather than medicament may solve the problem. Sometimes it is best to put up with stinging, which often only lasts a few minutes, because after a few applications of an effective treatment the skin heals and stinging lessens.
- If it is difficult to squeeze out a cream or ointment, cut off the end of the tube. Note that this may invalidate the expiry date and increase the chance of contamination of the product.

6.6 Emollients and moisturisers

What are emollients and moisturisers?

Emollients are products used to soften skin. Moisturisers are products used to add moisture to the skin. There are numerous emollients and moisturisers on sale at supermarkets and pharmacies. Options include:

- oils.
- lotions.
- creams.
- ointments.

Emollients and moisturisers are most effective when applied immediately after bathing but can also be applied at other times.

Why use emollients and moisturisers?

Uses of emollients and moisturisers include:

- to relieve dryness and scaling of the skin.
- to disguise fine lines and wrinkles.
- to treat mild irritant contact dermatitis.
- as a base for make-up.

What do emollients and moisturisers contain?

Active ingredients of emollients and moisturisers are occlusives and humectants.

They often include other ingredients such as surfactants (non-soap cleansers), fragrances and preservatives.

OCCLUSIVE MOISTURISERS

Occlusives are oils of non-human origin, often mixed with water and an emulsifier to form a lotion or cream. They provide a layer of oil on the surface of the skin to reduce water loss from the stratum corneum.

- Bath oil deposits a thin layer of oil on the skin upon rising from the water.
- Directly applied creamy lotions are more occlusive than soaking in an oily bath.
- Creams are more occlusive again. Thicker barrier creams containing dimeticone are particularly useful for hand dermatitis.
- Ointments are the most occlusive, and include pure oil preparations such as equal parts of white soft and liquid paraffin or petroleum jelly.

The choice of occlusive emollient depends upon the area of the body and the degree of dryness and scaling of the skin.

- Aqueous lotions are used for the scalp and other hairy areas and for mild dryness elsewhere.

- Creams are used when more emollience is required.
- Ointments are prescribed for dry, thick, scaly areas, but many patients find them too greasy.

Typical general-purpose moisturisers that are cheap and available in bulk without prescription include cetomacrogol (non-ionic) cream and emulsifying ointment.

The minimum quantity for an occlusive emollient is 250 g (or ml) and often 500 g or 1 kg is needed: liberal and regular usage is to be encouraged. How frequently it is applied depends on how dry the skin is: very dry skin may benefit from a greasy emollient (such as 50% white soft paraffin, 50% liquid paraffin) every couple of hours, but slightly dry skin may only need a light moisturiser at night.

HUMECTANTS

Humectants increase the water-holding capacity of the stratum corneum. They include:

- glycerine.
- urea.
- lactic acid.
- glycolic acid.
- salicylic acid.

Urea and the acidic preparations often sting if applied to scratched or fissured skin. They are also keratolytic, i.e. they have a descaling or peeling effect, important in management of ichthyosis.

Adverse reactions to emollients

IRRITANT REACTIONS

People with sensitive skin associated with atopic dermatitis or rosacea often describe irritant reactions to emollients and moisturisers, such as burning and stinging. If irritation is transient, the product can continue to be used. It should be discontinued if contact dermatitis appears.

CONTACT ALLERGY

Contact allergy to moisturisers and emollients is rare. Suspected contact allergy to preservative, fragrance or vehicle can be investigated by patch testing.

FOLLICULITIS

Occlusive emollients can cause or aggravate acne, perioral dermatitis, folliculitis and boils.

6.7 Topical steroids

What are topical steroids?

Topical steroids are safe and effective anti-inflammatory preparations used to control eczema/dermatitis and many other skin conditions. They are available in creams, ointments and other vehicles.

Topical steroids are sometimes combined with other active ingredients, including antibacterial agents, antifungal agents and calcipotriol.

Topical steroids are also called topical corticosteroids, glucocorticosteroids, and cortisones.

Background information

The effects of topical steroids on various cells in the skin are:
- anti-inflammatory.
- immunosuppressive.
- anti-proliferative.
- vasoconstrictive.

POTENCY OF TOPICAL STEROIDS

The potency of topical steroids depends on:
- the specific molecule.
- amount that reaches the target cell.
- absorption through the skin (0.25–3%).
- formulation.

There is little point in diluting a topical steroid, as their potency does not depend much on concentration. After the first two or three applications, there is no additional benefit from applying a topical steroid more than once daily.

Steroids are absorbed at different rates depending on skin thickness.
- The greatest absorption occurs through thin skin of eyelids, genitals, skin creases, when potent topical steroids are best avoided.
- The least absorption occurs through the thick skin of palms and soles, where mild topical steroids are ineffective.

Absorption also depends on the vehicle in which the topical steroid is delivered and is greatly enhanced by occlusion.

FORMULATIONS

Several formulations are available to suit the type of skin lesion and its location. Creams and lotions are general purpose and are the most popular formulations.

OINTMENT
- Most suitable formulation for dry, non-hairy skin.
- No requirement for preservative, reducing risk of irritancy and contact allergy.
- Occlusive, increasing risk of folliculitis and miliaria.

GEL OR SOLUTION
- Useful in hair-bearing skin.
- Has an astringent (drying) effect.
- Stings inflamed skin.

As a general rule, use the weakest possible steroid that will do the job. On the other hand, it is often appropriate to use a potent preparation for a short time to ensure the skin condition clears completely.

Which topical steroids are widely available?

Topical steroids are medicines regulated by Health Authorities. They are classified according to their strength. The products listed here are those widely available in New Zealand, the UK and the USA in January 2017.

MILD
Hydrocortisone
Hydrocortisone acetate

MODERATE POTENCY
Clobetasone butyrate
Triamcinolone acetonide
Fludoxycortide

POTENT
Betamethasone valerate
Betamethasone dipropionate
Diflucortolone valerate
Fluocinolone
Hydrocortisone 17-butyrate
Mometasone furoate
Methylprednisolone aceponate

VERY POTENT
Clobetasol propionate
Betamethasone dipropionate in optimised vehicle

What are the side-effects of topical steroids?

Side-effects are uncommon or rare when topical steroids are used appropriately under medical supervision. Topical steroids may be falsely blamed for a sign when underlying disease or another condition is responsible (e.g. hypopigmentation, which is in fact post-inflammatory).

CUSHING SYNDROME

Internal side-effects similar to those due to systemic steroids are rarely reported after long-term use of large quantities of topical steroid (e.g. >50 g of clobetasol propionate or >500 g of hydrocortisone per week).

CUTANEOUS SIDE-EFFECTS

Local side-effects of topical steroids may arise when potent topical steroids are applied daily for long periods of time (months). Most reports of side-effects describe prolonged use of unnecessarily potent topical steroids for inappropriate indications.

- Skin thinning (atrophy).
- Stretch marks (striae) in armpits or groin (*Fig. 6.31*).
- Easy bruising (senile/solar purpura) and tearing of the skin (*Fig. 6.32*).
- Enlarged blood vessels (telangiectasia, see *Fig. 6.33*).
- Localised increased hair thickness and length (hypertrichosis, see *Fig. 6.34*).

Topical steroids can cause, aggravate or mask skin infections, e.g. impetigo, tinea (known as tinea incognito, see *Fig. 6.35*), herpes simplex, malassezia folliculitis and molluscum contagiosum. Note: topical steroids remain the first-line treatment for infected eczema.

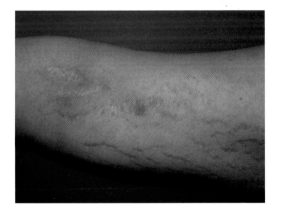

Figure 6.31. Striae.

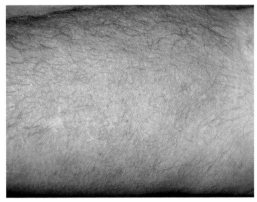

Figure 6.33. Telangiectasia.

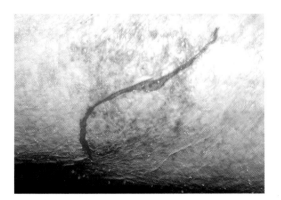

Figure 6.32. Purpura and laceration due to thin, fragile skin.

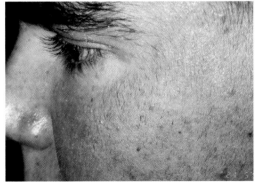

Figure 6.34. Hypertrichosis.

Potent topical steroids applied for weeks to months or longer can lead to:

- periorificial dermatitis (common, see *Fig. 6.36*).
- steroid rosacea.
- rebound redness.
- pustular psoriasis.

Stinging is not infrequent when a topical steroid is first applied, due to underlying inflammation and broken skin. Contact allergy to steroid molecule, preservative or vehicle is uncommon, but may occur after the first application of the product, or after many years of its use.

OCULAR SIDE-EFFECTS

Topical steroids should be used cautiously on eyelid skin. Potentially, their excessive use over weeks to months might lead to glaucoma or cataracts.

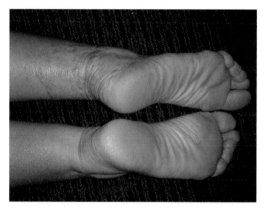

Figure 6.35. Tinea incognito.

How to use topical steroids

Topical steroid is applied once daily (usually at night) to inflamed skin for a course of 5 days to several weeks. After that, it is usually stopped, or the strength or frequency of application is reduced.

Emollients can be applied before or after the application of topical steroid, to relieve irritation and dryness or as a barrier preparation. Infection may need additional treatment.

FINGERTIP UNITS

Fingertip units guide the amount of topical steroid to be applied to a body site. One unit describes the amount of cream squeezed out of its tube onto the volar aspect of the terminal phalanx of the index finger (*Fig. 6.37*).

The quantity of cream in a fingertip unit varies with age:

- adult male – one fingertip unit provides 0.5 g.
- adult female – one fingertip unit provides 0.4 g.
- child aged 4 years – approximately 1/3 of adult amount.
- infant 6 months to 1 year – approximately 1/4 of adult amount.

The amount of cream that should be used varies with the body part:

- one hand – apply 1 fingertip unit.
- one arm – apply 3 fingertip units.
- one foot – apply 2 fingertip units.
- one leg – apply 6 fingertip units.
- face and neck – apply 2.5 fingertip units.
- trunk, front and back – 14 fingertip units.
- entire body – about 40 units.

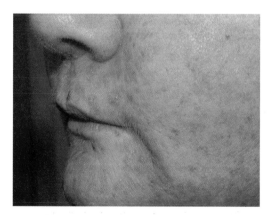

Figure 6.36. Periorificial dermatitis.

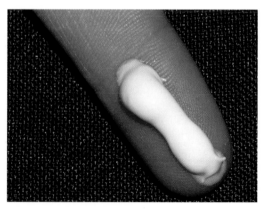

Figure 6.37. Fingertip unit.

6.8 Other topical drugs

Acne treatments

Topical acne treatments for mild to moderate acne include salicylic acid, benzoyl peroxide, retinoids (tretinoin, adapalene) and antibiotics. They are not curative.

- They should be applied to all areas affected by acne (not just to individual spots).
- They take several weeks to start working, and are most effective after several months of use.
- Conventional acne treatments are irritating to sensitive skin (see *Fig. 6.38*).
- Patients should be advised to test tolerance, and to wash off after increasing periods of time.
- Topical antibiotics risk bacterial resistance, which is reduced by co-prescribing benzoyl peroxide or a retinoid.
- Some non-prescription acne treatments appear better tolerated than benzoyl peroxide and topical retinoids; their efficacy is unproven.

Topical antiseptics and antibiotics

Topical antiseptics are used pre-surgery, for wound care and in patients with recurrent skin infections, often in the form of a skin cleanser.

- Concern has been expressed about the effect of antiseptics on normal skin microbiome and they should not be recommended as a routine or long term without careful consideration of the pros and cons.
- Antiseptics are sometimes used as a 7-day course to treat mild skin infections.
- Antiseptics and preservatives cause irritant and allergic contact dermatitis in some people.

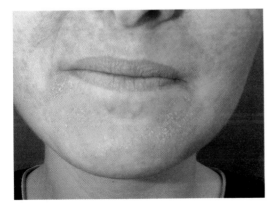

Figure 6.38. Irritant contact dermatitis from topical tretinoin.

- Twice-weekly bath with antiseptic oils, or bleach baths, using 2 ml of 2.2% household bleach per litre of water (or swims in a chlorinated pool) reduce the incidence of secondary staphylococcal infection in atopic dermatitis and recurrent impetigo/boils.
- The use of topical antibiotics is generally discouraged except short-term as a treatment of impetigo or a definite wound infection. This is mainly to minimise bacterial antibiotic resistance, but topical antibiotics are also prone to induce contact allergic dermatitis.

Topical antifungal agents

There are many topical antifungal agents available as gels, sprays, creams, solutions and lacquers. They are suitable for mild or localised dermatophyte and yeast infections. Although frequently prescribed for dermatophyte fungal nail infection (onychomycosis), they are much less effective than oral antifungal agents and must be used for prolonged periods of up to 2 years even for mild distal nail infection. They are not effective for dermatophyte scalp infections (tinea capitis).

- When in doubt about the diagnosis of a scaly skin condition, take scrapings for mycology (confirm infection in nail dystrophy prior to commencing treatment).
- Patients should be advised of the need to apply topical therapy widely and to continue treatment for several days after apparent clearance of a skin infection.

Calcipotriol

Calcipotriol is a vitamin D derivative, mainly used to treat psoriasis. It can be useful in some other scaly conditions.

- Solution, cream or ointment is applied twice daily to psoriasis plaques.
- Calcipotriol can be irritating, particularly to facial skin. It causes peeling.
- It is available in combination with the ultrapotent topical steroid betamethasone diproprionate as gel and ointment, which are more effective and better tolerated than calcipotriol alone for short-term and once-daily use on scalp, trunk and limbs.
- Cycles of the combination treatment for 4 weeks followed by calcipotriol alone for 4 weeks are often recommended.

Coal tar

Coal tar is still occasionally used for scalp psoriasis and less often for chronic plaque psoriasis and atopic dermatitis (see *Fig. 6.39*).

- Its anti-inflammatory effects are established but poorly understood.
- It is messy, malodorous, and generally unpopular with patients.
- It can provoke folliculitis.

Fluorouracil

Fluorouracil is a cytotoxic agent available as a cream to treat actinic keratosis (see *Fig. 6.40*), intraepidermal squamous cell carcinoma (squamous cell carcinoma *in situ*) and, with less efficacy, small, superficial basal cell carcinomas.

- Patients need considerable counselling and follow-up for optimal results.
- Hyperkeratotic lesions should be pre-treated with cryotherapy, and pre-treatment of larger areas using tretinoin and topical keratolytic agents such as urea or salicylic acid improves results.
- Direct exposure of treated areas to the sun should be avoided.
- The cream is applied once or twice daily for 2–6 weeks until a brisk inflammatory reaction is experienced, and then discontinued.
- Tolerance varies.
- Severe local or systemic adverse reactions should be considered a contraindication to further use.
- The course can be repeated if necessary.

Imiquimod

Imiquimod is an immune response modulator used to treat actinic keratosis (see *Fig. 6.41*),

small superficial basal cell carcinomas and genital warts. Side-effects and results are highly variable.

- Patients need considerable counselling and follow-up for optimal results.
- Hyperkeratotic lesions should be pre-treated with cryotherapy, and pretreatment of larger areas using tretinoin and topical keratolytic agents such as urea or salicylic acid improves results.

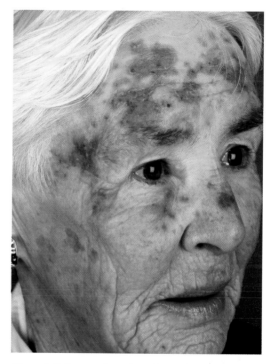

Figure 6.40. Expected reaction after applying fluorouracil cream to facial actinic keratoses for 2 weeks.

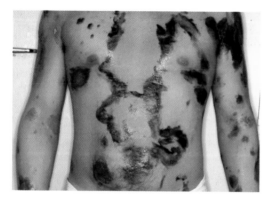

Figure 6.39. Coal tar treatment.

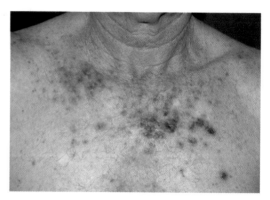

Figure 6.41. Expected reaction after applying imiquimod cream to actinic keratoses for 3 weeks.

- Direct exposure of treated areas to the sun should be avoided.
- The cream is applied at night 2–5 times per week to maintain a moderate inflammatory reaction.
- Research-based manufacturer recommendations are 4-week courses of 5% imiquimod cream for actinic keratosis and 6-week courses for superficial basal cell carcinoma, but experienced practitioners continue until adequate results have been achieved (i.e. cure) – which is highly variable. A 3.75% strength is also available to treat larger areas affected by actinic keratoses. Follow local prescribing guidelines.
- Tolerance varies.
- Severe local or systemic adverse reactions should lead to temporary cessation. Once the reaction has settled, imiquimod cream is recommended until the end-point has been reached or it has clearly been ineffective.
- The course can be repeated if necessary.

Ingenol mebutate

Ingenol mebutate gel is used to treat actinic keratosis (*Fig. 6.42*).

- Pre-treatment with cryotherapy, tretinoin and topical keratolytic agents improves results.
- Facial keratoses are treated on three consecutive evenings with 0.015% gel.
- Actinic keratoses elsewhere are treated on two consecutive evenings with 0.05% gel.
- Tolerance varies.
- Erythema, dryness, blistering, oedema are expected on treated areas but resolve within 14 days.
- The course can be repeated if necessary.

Sunscreens

Sunscreens are a vital part of the management of patients with phototype 1–3 skin and with photosensitivity disorders to protect them from the damaging effects of exposure to ultraviolet radiation. They should be applied when outdoors when the ultraviolet index is greater than 3; the ultraviolet index varies according to latitude and altitude and patients should be reminded to check with local metereological services or to use a smartphone app to check UV levels.

- Numerous different formulations of sunscreens are available for different skin types, body sites and personal preference.
- There are differing standards for manufacture and sale of sunscreens in Europe, USA, Australasia and elsewhere.
- Patient education is essential.
- Sunscreens do not protect skin as well as closely-woven fabrics.
- In general, broad-spectrum, water-resistant, sun protection factor (SPF) 50+ products should be selected, which provide UVA and UVB protection.
- Sunscreens should be applied liberally to all exposed skin before going outdoors and every 2 hours if remaining outdoors and after bathing.
- Contact allergy and photoallergy to sunscreens are rare and may be due to the sunscreen chemicals themselves, to preservatives, fragrances or other ingredients (see *Fig. 6.43*).

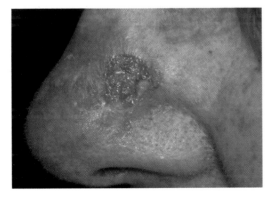

Figure 6.42. Expected reaction after applying ingenol gel to facial actinic keratoses for 2 days.

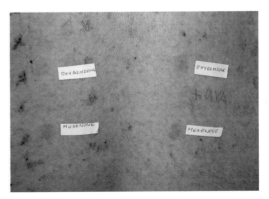

Figure 6.43. Positive patch and photopatch tests to multiple sunscreen ingredients.

6.9 Tetracyclines

What are tetracyclines?

Tetracyclines are oral antibiotics often used to treat skin diseases. There has been over 50 years' experience with these medications, which were originally derived from soil bacteria *Streptomyces aureofaciens*.

The original base medicines, chlortetracycline, tetracycline and oxytetracycline, have been replaced by products that are better absorbed and more lipophilic, with excellent tissue distribution. These include:

- doxycycline.
- lymecycline.
- minocycline.

Doxycycline is the most commonly prescribed tetracycline in New Zealand, with lymecycline more common in the UK.

Chemically modified tetracyclines are under development to reduce antibiotic activity and to increase their non-antibiotic, anti-inflammatory effect.

What are tetracyclines used for?

Tetracyclines are broad-spectrum antibiotics often used to treat skin, chest, urethral, and pelvic infections. Doxycycline is indicated in a wide range of infections including syphilis, Lyme disease, Q fever, Rocky Mountain spotted fever and plague. It is also widely used for malaria prophylaxis.

Tetracyclines are also effective at controlling non-infectious, inflammatory skin and mucosal diseases, including:

- acne.
- rosacea.
- perioral dermatitis.
- hidradenitis suppurativa.
- recurrent aphthous stomatitis.
- bullous pemphigoid.
- pyoderma gangrenosum.
- Sweet syndrome.
- granulomatous disorders.

How do tetracyclines work?

As antibiotics, tetracyclines interfere with protein synthesis of susceptible bacteria. They are also anti-inflammatory agents.

- They inhibit matrix metalloproteinases (MMPs) – these enzymes are active in dermal inflammatory skin disorders.
- They reduce production of pro-inflammatory cytokines.
- They are antioxidants, reducing free radical production and nitric oxide.
- They inhibit angiogenesis and granuloma formation.

What is the usual dose?

The antibiotic dose of doxycycline is 100 mg once or twice daily. It should be taken while upright, with plenty of water. The usual dose of lymecycline is 408 mg once daily (300 mg base tetracycline dose). Minocycline 50–100 mg is less often prescribed due to its greater potential for serious adverse effects, and has a "black triangle" warning in the UK.

Lower doses of doxycycline have been shown to be effective in rosacea (20 mg twice daily or 40 mg once daily). The lowest dose of doxycycline available in New Zealand is 50 mg. The side effect of low-dose doxycycline in other skin disorders is unknown.

For how long are tetracyclines taken?

Infections are treated for 7 to 28 days, depending on the condition being treated.

Inflammatory disorders take several weeks or months to respond to tetracyclines such as doxycycline. They are often prescribed for months or years for inflammatory skin disorders. They are not curative for these conditions.

What are the side-effects and risks of tetracyclines?

Tetracyclines must not be taken by pregnant or breast-feeding women, or by children under 12 years, because they discolour growing teeth and may cause enamel hypoplasia (malformed permanent teeth). Staining of permanent teeth is usually temporary but can persist for long periods.

Doxycycline is usually tolerated very well, particularly in subantibiotic dose. Allergy can occur, but is rare. There are some important precautions.

- It must be taken when upright and with copious water, to reduce oesophagitis.
- Patients should protect skin and nails from sun exposure, as it is photosensitising (see *Figs 6.44* and *6.45*).

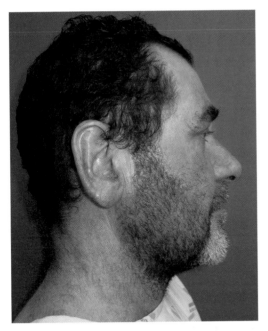

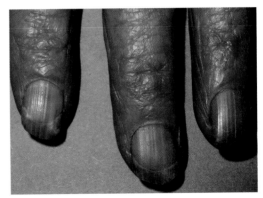

Figure 6.47. Minocycline pigmentation of nails.

- It can cause nausea, vomiting and diarrhoea; it is better tolerated when taken after food rather than on an empty stomach.
- Women prone to vulvovaginal thrush with broad-spectrum antibiotics should consider prophylactic treatment with intermittent topical or systemic azole antifungal agent.

Side-effects of minocycline include:
- drug hypersensitivity syndrome.
- autoimmune reactions.
- dizziness and headache.
- after prolonged use, blue pigmentation of skin and nails (see *Figs 6.46* and *6.47*).

Minocycline is less likely than doxycycline to cause photosensitivity.

DRUG INTERACTIONS
Important drug interactions with tetracyclines include:
- risk of raised intracranial hypertension with systemic retinoids (acitretin, isotretinoin, altretinoin).
- reduced bioavailability of tetracyclines with iron, aluminium, magnesium, calcium, rifampicin, celestipol and anticonvulsants.
- increased renal toxicity with diuretics.

Figure 6.44. Phototoxic reaction after sun exposure in patient taking doxycycline.

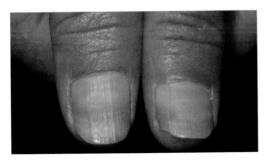

Figure 6.45. Photo-onycholysis due to doxycycline.

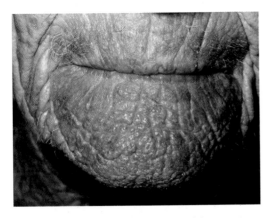

Figure 6.46. Minocycline pigmentation of skin.

6.10 Systemic steroids

What are systemic steroids?

Corticosteroids taken by mouth or given by intramuscular injection are often called systemic steroids. They are synthetic derivatives of the natural steroid, cortisol, produced by the adrenal glands, and have profound anti-inflammatory effects.

Systemic (cortico) steroids are also called glucocorticoids or cortisones. They include prednisone, prednisolone, methylprednisolone, beclometasone, betamethasone, dexamethasone, hydrocortisone and triamcinolone. Fludrocortisone is predominantly a mineralocorticoid and its anti-inflammatory effects are minimal.

Prednisone and prednisolone are equivalent, and are the most commonly prescribed oral corticosteroids for inflammatory skin diseases.

What are systemic steroids used for in dermatology?

They are used for a few days (short-term) to indefinitely (long-term) in a wide variety of skin conditions including:
- eczema/dermatitis.
- bullous diseases.
- lupus erythematosus.
- sarcoidosis.
- vasculitis.

Systemic steroids are best avoided in patients with psoriasis.

How do systemic steroids work?

Systemic steroids work in the same way as natural cortisol. Natural cortisol has important effects in the body, including regulation of:
- protein, carbohydrate, lipid and nucleic acid metabolism.

- inflammation and immune response.
- distribution and excretion of water and solutes.
- secretion of adrenocorticotrophic hormone (ACTH) from the pituitary gland.

How do systemic steroids differ?

Systemic steroids differ in dose, mineralocorticoid potency, half-life (duration of action) and how effectively they suppress the hypothalamic–pituitary–adrenal (HPA) axis (suppression leads to reduced production of natural cortisol); see Table 6.1.

What is the usual dose of systemic steroid?

Generally, a higher dose of prednisone or prednisolone, such as 40–60 mg daily, is prescribed at first, to gain control of the skin condition. In 2–4 weeks, the dose is reduced.

Prednisone is best taken as a single dose in the morning, which is thought to reduce steroid-induced suppression of the hypothalamic-pituitary–adrenal axis compared to evening dosing.

The maintenance dose should be kept as low as possible to minimise adverse effects.

Steroid dose is commonly characterised into:
- low dose, e.g. <10 mg/day of prednisone.
- medium dose, e.g. 10–20 mg/day of prednisone.
- high dose, e.g. >20 mg/day of prednisone, sometimes more than 100 mg/day.

Treatment for less than one month is considered short-term treatment. Corticosteroids for a few days or weeks are relatively safe when prescribed for acute dermatitis. Treatment continuing for more than 3 months is regarded as long term, and results in the majority of undesirable side-effects.

Table 6.1. Comparison of systemic steroids.*					
Drug	**Cortisone**	**Hydro-cortisone**	**Prednis-o(lo)ne**	**Methylpred-nisolone**	**Dexametha-sone**
Equivalent dose	25	20	5	4	0.75
Mineralocorticoid potency	2+	2+	1+	0–0.5+	0
Biological half-life (hours)	8–12	8–12	24–36	24–36	36–54
Daily dose causing HPA axis suppression (mg)	25–30	20–30	7.5	7.5	1–1.5

*Information from Vancouver Coastal Health Formulary tool [Accessed 12 July 2014].

What are the side-effects and risks of short-term systemic steroids?

Side-effects are rarely serious if systemic steroids have been prescribed for one month or less. The following problems may arise, particularly when higher doses are taken:

- sleep disturbance.
- increased appetite.
- weight gain.
- psychological effects, including increased or decreased energy.

Rare but more worrisome side-effects of a short course of corticosteroids include: serious infection, mania, psychosis, delirium, depression with suicidal intent, heart failure, peptic ulceration, diabetes and avascular necrosis of the hip. The risk increases with increasing dose.

What are the side-effects and risks of long-term systemic steroids?

Nearly everyone on systemic steroids for more than a month suffers from some adverse effects, depending on daily dose and how long they have been on systemic steroids. The main concerns are infections, hypertension, diabetes, osteoporosis, avascular necrosis, myopathy, cataracts and glaucoma. The list that follows is incomplete.

CUTANEOUS ADVERSE EFFECTS

Cutaneous adverse effects from long-term systemic steroids may include:

- bacterial infections – cellulitis, wound infections.
- fungal infections – tinea, candida, pityriasis versicolor.
- viral infections – herpes zoster.
- skin thinning, purpura, fragility, telangiectasia and slow wound healing, especially in sun-damaged areas (*Fig. 6.48*).
- stretch marks (striae) under the arms and in the groin or anywhere (*Fig. 6.49*).
- steroid acne (malassezia folliculitis; see *Fig. 6.50*).
- hypertrichosis and hair loss.

EFFECTS ON BODY FAT

- Redistribution of body fat: moon face, buffalo hump, truncal obesity.
- Weight gain: increased appetite and food intake.

EFFECTS ON THE EYE

- Glaucoma.
- Posterior subcapsular cataracts; children are more susceptible than adults.

- Eyelid oedema and exophthalmos.
- Central serous chorioretinopathy.

VASCULAR DISEASE

- Hypertension.
- Ischaemic heart disease.
- Stroke and transient ischaemic attack (TIA).

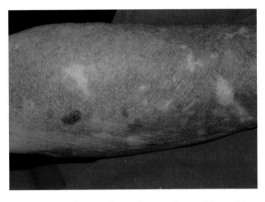

Figure 6.48. Adverse effects of systemic steroids on skin of an arm.

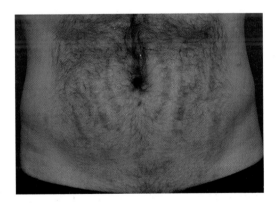

Figure 6.49. Stretch marks following systemic steroid use.

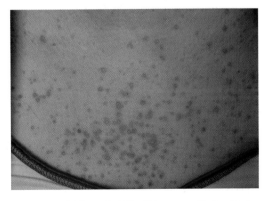

Figure 6.50. Malassezia folliculitis as a result of systemic steroid use.

The effects of systemic steroids on atherosclerotic vascular disease may be due to complex metabolic changes, including:
- hyperlipidaemia.
- peripheral insulin resistance and hyperinsulinaemia.

GASTROINTESTINAL TRACT
- Dyspepsia, gastritis, peptic ulceration and perforation of the gut, especially in patients also taking NSAIDs.
- Acute pancreatitis.
- Fatty liver.

FLUID BALANCE
- Sodium and fluid retention cause leg swelling and weight increase.
- Potassium loss causes general weakness.

REPRODUCTIVE SYSTEM
- Irregular menstruation.
- Hirsutism.
- Lowered fertility in men and women.
- Possible fetal growth retardation in women taking prolonged courses of steroids during pregnancy.
- Breast-feeding can usually continue but infant should be monitored for adrenal suppression if mother on >40 mg prednisone daily.

MUSCULOSKELETAL SYSTEM
- Bone fractures.
- Osteoporosis.
- Osteonecrosis, especially hip.
- Myopathy affecting shoulders and thighs.
- Tendon ruptures.
- Growth restriction in children.

Osteoporosis is particularly common in smokers, postmenopausal women, the elderly, underweight or immobile, and patients with diabetes or lung problems. Osteoporosis may result in fractures of the spine, ribs or hip joint with minimal trauma. These occur after the first year in 10–20% of patients treated with more than 7.5 mg prednisone daily. It is estimated that up to 50% of patients on long-term prednisone will develop bone fractures. Vertebral fractures are more common in patients on steroids, even in those with normal bone density.

NERVOUS SYSTEM
- Psychological effects: mood changes, increased energy, excitement, euphoria.
- Less often: hypomania, psychosis, delirium, memory loss, depression.
- Insomnia and sleep disturbance.
- Shakiness and tremor.
- Headaches.

METABOLIC EFFECTS
- Transient or persistent diabetes in previously non-diabetic patients.
- Higher blood sugar levels in patients with diabetes mellitus.
- Cushing syndrome.

IMMUNE RESPONSE
- Raised neutrophil and total white cell count are usual on prednisone.
- Impaired innate and acquired immunity.
- Increased susceptibility to tuberculosis.
- Increased severity of measles, varicella.
- Reduced efficacy and increased risk of vaccines.

Live vaccines such as polio or MMR (measles, mumps, rubella) should not be given to patients taking ≥20 mg prednisone daily. It is safe and advisable to have other routine immunisations, such as annual influenza vaccination.

RISKS DURING INTERCURRENT ILLNESS OR SURGERY

Significant intercurrent illness, trauma or surgical procedure requires a temporary increase in corticosteroid dose, or if already stopped, a temporary re-introduction of corticosteroid treatment for up to 12 months after the steroids are stopped.

Patients who have taken ≥10 mg prednisone daily within 3 months of surgery requiring a general anaesthetic are advised to tell their anaesthetist so that intraoperative intravenous hydrocortisone can be added.

Effects of reducing the dose of systemic steroids

No tapering is necessary if a course of prednisone has been for less than one to two weeks. Steroids should be withdrawn slowly after longer courses, to avoid acute adrenal insufficiency, particularly if the medication has been taken for several months or longer.

Side-effects from reducing prednisone may include:

- fever.
- hypotension.
- tiredness.
- headaches.
- muscle and joint aches.
- weight loss.
- depression.
- rhinitis.
- conjunctivitis.
- painful itchy skin nodules.

Hypothalamic–pituitary–adrenal (HPA) axis suppression can persist for months or years after steroids are stopped.

Monitoring during steroid treatment

Regular monitoring during treatment with systemic steroids may include:

- blood pressure.
- body weight.
- blood sugar.

Patients on prednisone or prednisolone should be advised to avoid NSAIDs and liquorice.

PREVENTION OF OSTEOPOROSIS

Bone density scans should be considered for patients that have taken or are expected to take 7.5 mg or more of prednisone each day for three months or longer. Baseline fracture risk can be estimated from T-scores. Current recommendations are:

- bisphosphonate therapy (alendronate, etidronate, zolidronic acid) for individuals with femoral T-scores <-2.5; it reduces fracture risk by half.
- smoking cessation.
- balanced diet, aiming for healthy body weight.
- minimal alcohol.
- regular weight-bearing exercise.
- consider risk of falling and its mitigation.

Calcium, vitamin D and oestrogen are no longer recommended for prophylaxis of osteoporosis, as adverse events outweigh benefit.

6.11 Other oral drugs

Antihistamines

Antihistamines are mainly used in dermatology to treat urticaria in its various forms. Histamine is rarely involved in the pathogenesis of other itchy skin disorders.

- Loratadine and cetirizine are the most commonly prescribed antihistamines and are remarkably safe medicines.
- Response often occurs within 30 minutes.
- If a once-daily dose of 10 mg is insufficient, in adults the dose can be gradually increased as required to a maximum of 40 mg daily in single or divided doses.
- First generation antihistamines are no longer recommended for urticaria.
- They cause sedation and are sometimes used for a few days to help an itchy patient sleep.
- Adverse effects of sedating antihistamines should be borne in mind, particularly in children and the elderly.

Oral antifungal agents

It is important that the antifungal chosen is appropriate for the disease. Dermatophytes (tinea; genus names are *Trichophyton*, *Microsporum* and *Epidermophyton*) respond best to oral terbinafine. Yeasts (candida, malassezia) respond best to oral azoles.

- The duration of a course of antifungal agents depends on the organism, the location and the severity of the infection.
- A single 150 mg dose of fluconazole is adequate for most women with acute vulvovaginal candida albicans infection.
- A 10-day course of itraconazole is recommended for widespread pityriasis versicolor.
- A 1–4 week course of terbinafine is effective for tinea except when involving nails, when 12 weeks is usually recommended.
- Seek advice from dermatologist or microbiologist for scalp infections and unusual organisms.

Aciclovir

Aciclovir is an antiviral used for treatment and prophylaxis of herpes simplex infections and in the treatment of herpes zoster.

- Dose ranges from 200–800 mg orally, taken 2–5 times per day.
- Intravenous treatment is rarely required and is expensive but is recommended in disseminated infection.
- Patients should be advised to drink plenty of fluids.
- Adverse reactions are uncommon.
- Prodrug valiclovir 500 mg – 1 g twice daily has better bioavailability and duration of action.

Hydroxychloroquine

Hydroxychloroquine is prescribed for cutaneous lupus erythematosus, polymorphous light eruption and rarely for other inflammatory skin diseases.

- It takes 6 weeks or so to start being effective and a usual trial is 6 months, at a dose of 200 mg once or twice daily.
- Monitoring is CBC/FBC, LFT at baseline and 3 months. Optometrist or ophthalmic review is advised early in the course of treatment, then every 1–5 years depending on patient risk of retinopathy.
- Potential adverse reactions are various and include pigmentation, lichenoid, and psoriasiform eruptions, gastrointestinal symptoms, visual disturbance, heart disease, cytopaenias and hepatitis.
- Check for drug interactions before treatment.

Acitretin

Acitretin is a retinoid, mainly used to treat psoriasis, ichthyosis, keratoderma, lichen planus, and for prophylaxis in skin cancer.

- **Acitretin is a teratogen and must not be taken during pregnancy or breast-feeding. A female must wait a minimum of 2 years in New Zealand and 3 years in UK and USA after the last dose of acitretin before conception. Strict contraception must be adhered to.**
- Dose ranges from 10 mg twice weekly to 1 mg/kg/day, taken after meals.
- Acitretin has many dose-limiting mucocutaneous side-effects including soft, peeling and sticky skin, skin fragility, mucosal erosions, sun sensitivity and thin hair (*Fig. 6.51*) and nails (*Fig. 6.52*).
- It can also cause headaches, tiredness, muscle and joint aches, and hyperlipidaemia.
- Monitoring is CBC, LFT, lipids at baseline and 3 months.

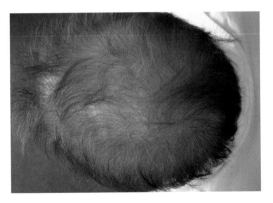

Figure 6.51. Severe diffuse alopecia due to acitretin.

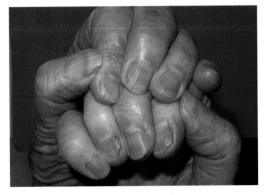

Figure 6.52. Thin brittle nails in patient on long-term acitretin.

Dapsone

Dapsone is the medicine of choice for leprosy, dermatitis herpetiformis and linear IgA bullous dermatosis. It is also used to treat acute neutrophilic disorders such as Sweet syndrome, leukocytoclastic vasculitis, pyoderma gangrenosum, aphthous ulcers and Behçet syndrome.

- Dose ranges from 25 mg to 300 mg daily.
- It causes inevitable haemolysis and carboxyhaemoglobinaemia, which can be severe and symptomatic.
- Other common and occasionally severe side-effects include rashes, hepatitis, neuropathy and psychosis.
- Baseline glucose 6-phosphate dehydrogenase screen/assay, CBC and LFT are recommended.

- Essential monitoring is with CBC, LFT after initial 5 days of treatment then monthly.

Colchicine

Colchicine is sometimes used for neutrophilic disorders such as Sweet syndrome, leukocytoclastic vasculitis, pyoderma gangrenosum, aphthous ulcers and Behçet syndrome.

- Dose is 500–600 mg 2–3 times daily.
- Therapeutic range is narrow. Colchicine is toxic and potentially dangerous in overdose.
- Most patients develop gastrointestinal side-effects.

6.12 Methotrexate, azathioprine, ciclosporin monitoring

Introduction

Second-line drugs commonly used in dermatology (on- or off-label) include:

- methotrexate.
  - dose is 5–30 mg once weekly
  - folic acid 5 mg is often also prescribed
- azathioprine.
  - dose is 0.5–3 mg/kg/day
  - taken 1 hour before or 3 hours after food
- ciclosporin.
  - dose is 2.5–5 mg/kg/day in 2 divided doses
  - caution if changing brand
- TNF-α inhibitors.
  - a loading dose is usual
  - maintenance dose of etanercept is 50 mg SC every week
  - maintenance dose of adalimumab is 40 mg SC every 2 weeks
  - maintenance dose of infliximab is 5 mg/kg IV every 8 weeks
  - maintenance dose of ustekinumab is 45 or 90 mg SC every 12 weeks.

These are prescribed by specialists, but other health professionals may be involved in the patient's care. They should be aware at least of indications, contraindications, adverse effects and monitoring requirements.

Indications for immune-modulating drugs

Immune-modulating drugs are used for diverse chronic inflammatory skin diseases that are not adequately controlled in other ways. The skin disease should be severe or have a severe functional or psychosocial impact on the patient.

EXAMPLES OF SUITABLE CONDITIONS

- Chronic plaque psoriasis.
- Atopic eczema.
- Hand dermatitis.
- Chronic photosensitivity dermatitis.
- Lichen planus.
- Bullous pemphigoid.
- Hidradenitis suppurativa.
- Chronic spontaneous urticaria.

Pre-treatment evaluation

The patient is assessed to determine the following.
- The disease is one that is expected to respond to the drug.

- The extent and severity of the disease is recorded.
  - PASI score for psoriasis
  - SCORAD or EASI for eczema
- The impact of the disease is recorded.
  - DLQI
- The patient wishes to receive the medication and can be expected to comply with monitoring instructions.
- Impact of patient comorbidities.
  - regular dental hygiene
- Potential contraindications to treatment.
- Vaccinations are up to date.
  - vaccinations may be less effective on immune suppressant.

CONTRAINDICATIONS TO TREATMENT

Pregnancy and breastfeeding:
- especially methotrexate, azathioprine.

Recent vaccination with live vaccine:
- e.g. yellow fever.

Non-immunity to varicella-zoster:
- consider immunisation before treatment.

Non-responsive disorder:
- azathioprine is not effective for chronic plaque psoriasis.
- TNF-α inhibitors are not effective for dermatitis or urticaria.

Co-morbidities:
- methotrexate may be unsuitable for patients with liver or haematological disease, or for people who drink excessive alcohol.

Hypersensitivity reactions:
- azathioprine hypersensitivity takes various forms.

Other medications – drug interactions are very common with these drugs and can be serious:
- caution if on another immunosuppressant.
- methotrexate should not be taken while on trimethoprim/cotrimoxasole.
- azathioprine should not be taken while on allopurinol.
- ciclosporin interacts with statins, erythromycin, azoles, dabigatran, grapefruit and many other drugs.

PRE-TREATMENT TESTS

- Weight, height, blood pressure.

- CBC, LFT, renal function.
- Hepatitis B and C serology.
- Sometimes: β-hCG, P3NP collagen (methotrexate), thiopurine methyl transferase (azathioprine), HIV and varicella serology, TB testing.
- Sometimes: chest X-ray, transient elastography scan (FibroScan) (methotrexate).
- Rarely: liver biopsy (methotrexate).

Follow-up visits

Follow-up visits are to determine the efficacy of treatment and any adverse events and to monitor safety.

EFFICACY OF TREATMENT
The extent and severity of the disease is recorded.
- PASI score for psoriasis.
- SCORAD or EASI for eczema.

The impact of the disease is recorded.
- DLQI.

Compliance with treatment and monitoring are discussed.
    Drug interactions are checked before prescribing.

ADVERSE EVENTS
The possible adverse events from drugs are numerous. Common ones are listed here. They may require reduction in dose or stopping treatment.

METHOTREXATE
- Nausea and other gastrointestinal symptoms.
- Mouth ulceration (*Fig. 6.53*).

- Haematological: especially thrombocytopenia, macrocytosis.
- Abnormal liver function: raised transaminases; hypoalbuminaemia is a late effect associated with cirrhosis.

AZATHIOPRINE
- Nausea and vomiting.
- Abnormal liver function: cholestasis or hepatitis.
- Hypersensitivity reactions: rash, lymphadenopathy (see *Fig. 6.54*).
- Bone marrow suppression.
- Susceptibility to infection including opportunistic infections.
- With long-term use, increased risk of skin cancer.

CICLOSPORIN
- Hypertension.
- Renal dysfunction.
- Nausea.
- Ankle oedema.
- Tremor.
- Paraesthesias.
- Susceptibility to infection including opportunistic infections.
- With long-term use:
  - increased risk of skin cancer
  - gum hypertrophy (*Fig. 6.55*)
  - hypertrichosis (*Fig. 6.56*).

BIOLOGICS
- Injection site or infusion reactions.
- Susceptibility to infection, especially during first year of treatment:
  - tuberculosis and opportunistic infections

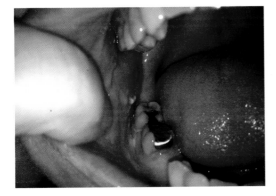

Figure 6.53. Mouth ulceration on methotrexate.

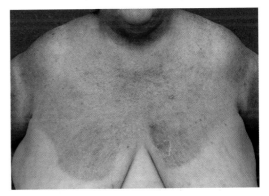

Figure 6.54. Photosensitive drug eruption due to azathioprine.

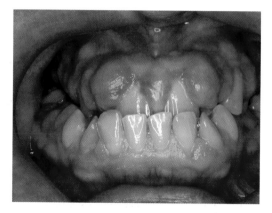

Figure 6.55. Gum hypertrophy on ciclosporin.

- Various autoimmune diseases are reported.
- Secondary failure after initial response.
- Increased risk of skin cancer.

SAFETY MONITORING
- Weight.
- Blood pressure (ciclosporin).
- CBC, LFT.
- Renal function (ciclosporin).
- Sometimes: βHCG, P3NP collagen (methotrexate).
- Sometimes: 6-thioguanine nucleotide (azathioprine).
- Sometimes: transient elastography scan (FibroScan) (methotrexate).
- Rarely: liver biopsy (methotrexate).

People on long-term treatment with immune-modulating drugs should undergo regular full body examination in case of skin cancer.

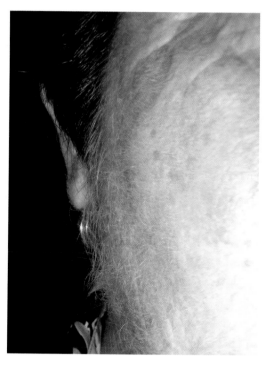

Figure 6.56. Hypertrichosis on ciclosporin.

Other immune-modulating drugs

Other drugs occasionally used in the treatment of severe and/or extensive skin diseases require similar monitoring. They include:
- mycophenolate mofetil.
- 6-mercaptopurine.
- hydroxyurea.

6.13 Isotretinoin

What is isotretinoin?

Isotretinoin (13-cis retinoic acid) is a vitamin A derivative (retinoid). The liver naturally makes small quantities of isotretinoin from vitamin A, but the drug we prescribe is made synthetically.

Isotretinoin was developed in the 1950s, but only started being used in the mid-1970s. The original brand names were Accutane and Roaccutane, but there are now many generic versions on the market, of varying potency.

What is isotretinoin used for?

Isotretinoin is a very effective medication for the treatment of acne. Originally licensed for use in severe disease, it is increasingly prescribed for all grades of acne.

Isotretinoin is also useful for other follicular conditions, such as:

- rosacea.
- seborrhoea.
- scalp folliculitis.

It is also prescribed for many other skin diseases. Examples include:

- discoid lupus erythematosus.
- granuloma annulare.
- transient acantholytic dermatosis.
- sarcoidosis.
- extensive actinic keratoses.
- prevention of squamous cell carcinoma.

Contraindications

Isotretinoin must not be taken in pregnancy, or if there is a significant risk of pregnancy.

Blood donation by males and females on isotretinoin is not allowed in case the blood is used for a pregnant woman.

Precautions

- Isotretinoin should be used with caution during breast-feeding.
- Commercial pilots may be subject to flying restrictions if they take isotretinoin.
- High dose isotretinoin in very young children has been associated with premature epiphyseal closure, leading to shorter stature (not seen in low dose for the treatment of acne).

How does isotretinoin work?

In acne, isotretinoin:

- reduces sebum production.
- shrinks the sebaceous glands.
- reduces follicular occlusion.
- inhibits growth of bacteria.
- has anti-inflammatory properties.

What is the usual dose of isotretinoin?

The range of doses used each day for acne is less than 0.1 to over 1 mg/kg body weight. Some patients may only need a small dose once or twice a week. A course of treatment may be completed in a few months or continue for several years. For acne, some prescribers have targeted a total cumulative dose of 120–140 mg/kg, in the hope of reducing relapse, but the evidence for this remains controversial. The general trend has been to use lower dosages, unrelated to body weight (e.g. 10 mg/day).

The individual dose prescribed by the dermatologist depends on:

- prescriber preference.
- patient body weight.
- the specific condition being treated.
- severity of the skin condition.
- response to treatment.
- other treatment used at the same time.
- side-effects experienced.

Isotretinoin is better taken with water or milk after food to help with its absorption. It may be taken on an empty stomach, but absorption may be halved. There is no particular advantage in splitting the dose over the day. A newer formulation (isotretinoin-lidose) can be taken without food.

For how long is isotretinoin taken?

Most patients should be treated until their skin condition clears and then for a further few months. However, courses have often been restricted to 16–30 weeks (4–7 months) to minimise risk of teratogenicity (risk of congenital abnormalities), and to comply with local regulatory authorities. Isotretinoin may be prescribed for years, usually in low dose or intermittently.

Drug interactions with isotretinoin

Care should be taken with the following
medications:

- vitamin A (retinoic acid) – side-effects are
  cumulative and could be severe; beta-
  carotene (provitamin A) is permitted.
- tetracyclines (including doxycycline,
  minocycline, and tetracycline) – these could
  increase the risk of headaches and blurred
  vision due to raised intracranial pressure.
- warfarin – monitor INR carefully.

What are the side-effects and risks of isotretinoin?

The side effects of isotretinoin are dose
dependent; at 1 mg/kg/day, nearly all
patients will have some side-effects, whereas at
0.1 mg/kg/day, most patients will not. The range
and severity of the side-effects also depends on
personal factors and the disease being treated.

Patients with significant liver or kidney
disease, high blood fats, diabetes and depression
may be advised not to take isotretinoin or to be
on a lower dose than usual and to have regular
follow-up visits.

CUTANEOUS AND MUCOCUTANEOUS SIDE-EFFECTS

Most of the side-effects due to isotretinoin
are cutaneous or mucocutaneous and relate
to the mode of action of the drug. The most
common are listed here. When side-effects
are troublesome, isotretinoin may need to be
withheld or the dose reduced.

- Acne flare-up (particularly if starting dose is
  >0.5 mg/kg/day); see *Fig. 6.57*.
- Dry lips, cheilitis (sore, cracked or scaly
  lips) (100% of patients on 1 mg/kg/day);
  see *Fig. 6.58*.
- Dry skin, fragile skin (*Fig. 6.59*), eczema/
  dermatitis (itchy, red patches of skin, see
  Fig. 6.60). Note: atopic eczema may improve.
- Increased sweating.
- Dry nostrils, epistaxis (nose bleeds).
- Dry, watery or irritable eyes (especially
  in contact lens wearers), conjunctivitis,
  keratitis.
- Dry anal mucosa, bleeding at the time of a
  bowel motion.
- Dry genitals, dyspareunia (discomfort during
  intercourse).
- Facial erythema.
- Sunburn on exposure to the sun.

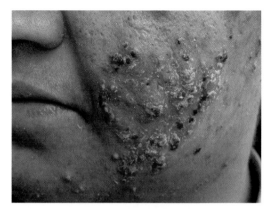

Figure 6.57. Acne flare-up on isotretinoin.

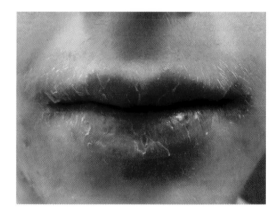

Figure 6.58. Cracked lips on isotretinoin.

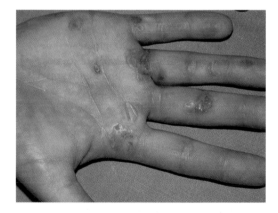

Figure 6.59. Friction blisters on isotretinoin.

- Temporary hair loss.
- Brittle nails.
- Skin infections: impetigo (*Fig. 6.61*), acute
  paronychia (*Fig. 6.62*), pyogenic granuloma.

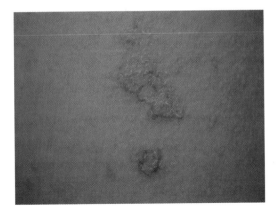

Figure 6.60. Dermatitis on isotretinoin.

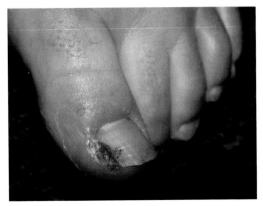

Figure 6.62. Acute paronychia.

OTHER COMMON DOSE-RELATED SIDE-EFFECTS OF ISOTRETINOIN

- Headache.
- Myalgia (muscle aches) and arthralgia (joint aches), especially after exercise.
- Tiredness (lethargy and drowsiness).
- Disturbed night vision and slow adaptation to the dark. Drivers may experience increased glare from car headlights at night.
- Hypertriglyceridaemia (high levels of triglyceride in the blood), usually of no clinical relevance.
- Irregular or heavy menstrual periods.

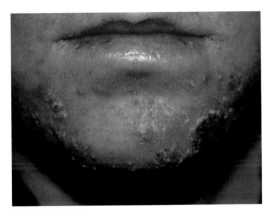

Figure 6.61. Impetigo on isotretinoin.

TREATMENT OF MUCOCUTANEOUS SIDE-EFFECTS

- Reduce the dosage (e.g. to 5–10 mg/day).
- Emollients, lip balm, petroleum jelly, sunscreen, eye drops and lubricants should be applied frequently and liberally when needed.
- Dermatitis can be treated with topical steroids.
- Take short, cool showers without using soap.
- Use mild or diluted shampoo.
- Do not start wearing contact lenses for the first time.
- Do not have elective eye surgery while on isotretinoin or for 6 months afterwards.
- Do not have ablative laser treatments (e.g. CO_2 resurfacing) while on isotretinoin or for 6 months afterwards. Other laser and light treatments may be performed with care.
- Shave rather than wax.
- Topical and/or oral antibiotics may be prescribed for impetigo.

RARE SIDE-EFFECTS OF ISOTRETINOIN

- Causality of the listed side-effects may not have been confirmed.
- Severe headache with blurred vision due to raised intracranial pressure.
- Mood changes and depression. Note: depression is more often related to the skin condition being treated or other health or psychosocial problems. Antidepressant medications may be helpful.
- Corneal opacities and cataracts.
- High-tone deafness.
- Accelerated diffuse interstitial skeletal hyperostosis (bony change).
- Abnormal liver function tests or symptomatic hepatitis.
- Diarrhoea or bleeding from the bowel.
- Pancreatitis.
- Allergy to isotretinoin causing liver disease and a febrile illness.

TREATMENT OF SYSTEMIC SIDE-EFFECTS

- Drink minimal alcohol.
- Take paracetamol for headache and for mild aches and pains.
- Seek medical attention early, if unwell.

Monitoring isotretinoin

Pregnancy must be excluded before and during treatment with isotretinoin. National or regional protocols may require other blood tests before and at intervals during treatment. The following tests should be undertaken if using high dose (1 mg/kg/day), prolonged courses (>12 months), or if patients have specific risk factors (e.g. family history of dyslipidaemia, higher risk of viral hepatitis, etc.):

- cholesterol and triglyceride levels.
- liver function tests.
- blood count.

Contraception in females considering isotretinoin

Isotretinoin must not be taken in pregnancy because of a very high risk of serious congenital abnormalities in the baby. Caution needs to be used during breast-feeding as it enters the breast milk and might affect the baby.

All females who could biologically have a child should take the following precautions during treatment with isotretinoin and for four weeks after the medication has been discontinued.

- Abstinence. The most reliable method of avoiding pregnancy is not to have sex. No method of contraception is completely reliable. "Natural" family planning is particularly risky.
- If sexually active, two reliable methods of contraception should be used. Discuss contraception with your doctor (general practitioner, family planning specialist, gynaecologist or dermatologist). The combined oral contraceptive, IUD (intrauterine device), progesterone implant or medroxyprogesterone injections may be suitable.
- The low-dose progesterone minipill on its own is not recommended.

A prescription for emergency contraception may be available from a medical practitioner (GP or family planning clinic) or accredited pharmacy. It prevents 85% of pregnancies if taken within 72 hours of unprotected sexual intercourse.

If contraception fails, termination of pregnancy (an abortion) may be advised if pregnancy arises during treatment with isotretinoin or within a month of discontinuing it.

WHAT HAPPENS IF A PREGNANT WOMAN TAKES ISOTRETINOIN?

Isotretinoin has a very high chance of resulting in a spontaneous miscarriage or a severe birth deformity if a fetus is exposed to it during the first half of pregnancy. The deformities affect the growth of tissues developing at the time of exposure to the drug:

- cranium (skull and brain).
- cardiac (heart).
- eye, ear.
- limbs.

NO CONTRACEPTIVE PRECAUTIONS ARE NECESSARY FOR MEN

Isotretinoin has no effect on sperm or male fertility and has not been shown to cause birth defects in children fathered by men taking it.

Does acne ever fail to clear on isotretinoin?

Although isotretinoin is usually very effective for acne, occasionally it responds unexpectedly slowly and incompletely. Poor response is associated with:

- macrocomedones (large whiteheads).
- nodules (large, deep inflammatory lesions).
- secondary infection.
- smoking.
- polycystic ovarian syndrome.
- younger age (<14 years).

Options available to slow responders include:

- cautery or diathermy of comedones.
- prolonged course of isotretinoin.
- additional treatment with oral antibiotics and corticosteroids.

Can isotretinoin be used again if acne recurs?

At least 50% of patients with acne have a long-lasting response after a single adequate course of isotretinoin. In others, acne may recur a few months to a few years after the medication has been discontinued. Relapse is more common in females than in males, and in patients >25 years of age. These patients may receive one or more further courses of isotretinoin.

Long-term treatment (>1 year) is often used for patients with:

- persistent acne.
- seborrhoea.
- rosacea.
- scalp folliculitis.
- skin cancer.

Special precautions for pilots considering isotretinoin

Good night vision is important for airline pilots and those flying after dark. Night vision may be affected by isotretinoin. Pilots taking isotretinoin or considering a course of isotretinoin must report to their national aviation authority to discuss how this treatment affects their flying privileges.

6.14 Physical treatments

Phototherapy

WHAT IS PHOTOTHERAPY?

Phototherapy is the use of sunlight or artificial sources of ultraviolet radiation or visible light as a form of treatment. These are non-ionising parts of the electromagnetic spectrum.

It includes:

- heliotherapy (natural sunlight therapy).
- blue light treatment used to treat neonatal jaundice and mild acne.
- home phototherapy.
- sunbeds and solaria when used therapeutically.
- ultraviolet B therapy (UVB, 290–320 nm).
- ultraviolet A therapy (UVA, 320–400 nm) including UVA1 (340–400 nm) used to treat atopic dermatitis, graft-versus-host disease and scleroderma.
- targeted phototherapy (UVB and/or UVA).
- photochemotherapy (PUVA) – the combination of oral or topical psoralen with UVA, used to treat inflammatory skin diseases.
- photodynamic therapy (PDT) – the combination of a porphyrin with visible light, used to treat superficial forms of skin cancer.

Narrowband UVB is the most common form of phototherapy offered by dermatologists. The term "narrowband" is used because the majority of spectral output is confined to a small band of the electromagnetic spectrum, 311–313 nm. This maximises therapeutic effect while minimising unnecessary exposure to non-therapeutic but potentially harmful radiation.

WHAT IS NARROWBAND UVB PHOTOTHERAPY USED FOR?

Narrowband UVB phototherapy is used to treat inflammatory skin diseases, most often psoriasis and eczema. It is also successful in the treatment of vitiligo, nonspecific generalised pruritus and cutaneous T-cell lymphoma.

THE PROCESS OF NARROWBAND UVB PHOTOTHERAPY

Typically, the patient attends three times weekly, removes clothing except underpants, dons eye protection and stands in a cabinet surrounded by fluorescent lamps.

- These are illuminated to deliver a calculated dose of UVB to the skin.
- The dose of UVB is steadily increased each week to a predetermined maximum (which depends on skin type).
- The course is completed once the skin disorder has cleared or typically after 20–40 treatments.

WHAT ARE THE ADVERSE EFFECTS OF PHOTOTHERAPY?

Short-term adverse effects of exposure to UV radiation include:

- erythema ("sunburn") (*Figs 6.63* and *6.64*).
- photokeratitis.
- polymorphous light eruption (*Fig. 6.65*).
- worsening skin disease.

Patients receiving multiple courses of phototherapy add to cumulative sun damage experienced over a

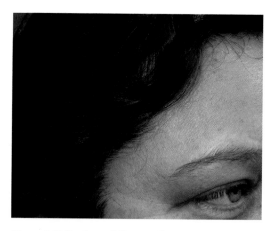

Figure 6.63. Erythema following phototherapy.

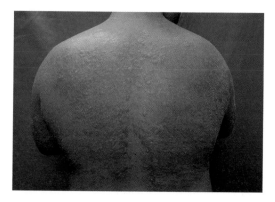

Figure 6.64. Erythema and blistering following phototherapy.

lifetime. Whole-body PUVA is rarely used because of significant incidence of later skin cancer.

Cryotherapy

WHAT IS CRYOTHERAPY?

In dermatology, cryotherapy refers to a treatment in which surface skin lesions are frozen. Cryotherapy is also called cryosurgery.

Cryogens used to freeze skin lesions include:
- liquid nitrogen (–196°C).
- carbon dioxide snow (–78.5°C).
- dimethyl ether and propane (DMEP, –57°C).

Liquid nitrogen is the most common cryogen found in a doctor's office.

WHAT IS LIQUID NITROGEN CRYOTHERAPY USED FOR?

Cryotherapy is mainly used to remove scaly skin lesions:
- viral warts.
- seborrhoeic keratoses.

- actinic keratoses.
- intraepidermal carcinoma.
- small superficial basal cell carcinomas.

THE PROCESS OF LIQUID NITROGEN CRYOTHERAPY

Liquid nitrogen can be applied to the skin for a few seconds using a cryospray, a cryoprobe or a cotton-tipped applicator.
- Time of application depends on the desired diameter and depth of freeze.
- The treatment is often repeated, once thawing has completed.
- The treated area may be gently washed once or twice daily, and should be kept clean.
- A dressing is optional.
- During healing phase, apply petroleum jelly.

WHAT ARE THE ADVERSE EFFECTS OF CRYOTHERAPY?

Cryotherapy damages the area of skin treated. The expected immediate effects are:
- stinging and pain.
- swelling (see *Fig. 6.66*).
- redness.

Within a few hours, effects at the treated site may include:
- clear or haemorrhagic blister (*Fig. 6.67*).
- oedema (most marked if cryotherapy is to a lesion near or on an eyelid).

Within a few days a scab forms and the blister gradually dries up (see *Fig. 6.68*). The scab peels off after 5–10 days on the face, after about 3 weeks on the hand, and after 6–12 weeks on the lower leg.

Undesirable effects may include:
- secondary wound infection (*Fig. 6.69*).
- ulceration and delayed healing.

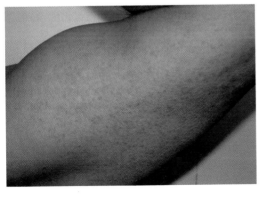

Figure 6.65. Polymorphous light eruption due to phototherapy with narrowband UVB.

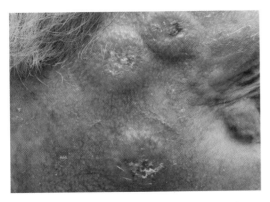

Figure 6.66. Unusually severe immediate swelling due to cryotherapy.

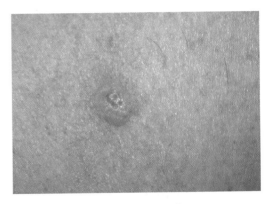

Figure 6.67. Blister the day after cryotherapy.

- local nerve damage (usually temporary).
- permanent hypopigmentation.
- persistent or recurrent skin lesions (*Fig. 6.70*).

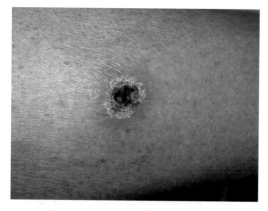

Figure 6.68. Scabbed blister following cryotherapy.

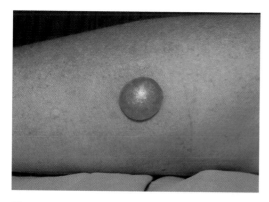

Figure 6.69. Secondary wound infection following cryotherapy.

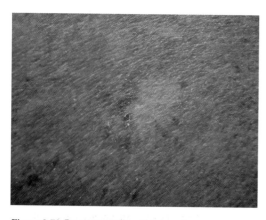

Figure 6.70. Recurrent BCC within cryotherapy scar.

Laser surgery

WHAT ARE LASERS?

'Laser' is an acronym: **l**ight **a**mplification by the **s**timulated **e**mission of **r**adiation. Lasers are sources of high intensity light with the following properties:

- monochromatic – the light is of a single wavelength.
- coherent – the light beam waves are in phase.
- collimated – the light beams travel in parallel.

Lasers used for dermatology (wavelength) include:

- carbon dioxide (10 600 nm).
- argon (488/514 nm).
- potassium–titanyl–phosphate (KTP) (532 nm).
- copper bromide/vapour (510/578 nm).
- argon-pumped tunable dye (APTD) (577/585 nm).
- krypton (568 nm).
- pulsed dye laser (PDL) (585–595 nm).
- QS ruby (694 nm).
- QS alexandrite (755 nm).
- excimer laser noble gas and halogen (308 nm).
- QS neodymium (Nd): yttrium–aluminium–garnet (YAG) (1064 nm).
- erbium: YAG (2940 nm).

WHAT ARE LASERS USED FOR IN DERMATOLOGY?

Laser light can be accurately focused into small spots with very high energy to destroy tissue. In dermatology, different wavelengths are used to remove:

- unsightly blood vessels and vascular proliferative lesions.
- pigmented lesions and tattoos.
- dark hairs.
- surface skin for facial rejuvenation.
- hypertrophic and keloid scars.
- small areas of inflammatory skin disease.
- neoplastic skin lesions.

THE LASER PROCESS

- The area to be treated is identified.
- Local anaesthetic may be used for deeper, more painful treatments.
- Staff and patient wear eye protection (see *Fig. 6.71*).
- The laser device is a box with a computer console.
- The laser light is emitted through a fine tube or wand-like instrument.

- The light is applied continuously or pulsed.
- The duration of treatment depends on the area to be treated.
- Dressings may be applied after treatment.

WHAT ARE THE ADVERSE EFFECTS OF LASERS?

Laser treatments are basically burns. The following adverse effects may occur.

- Short-term pain, redness, bleeding, bruising, blistering and/or crusting (*Figs 6.72* and *6.73*).
- Infection, including reactivation of herpes simplex.
- Temporary hyperpigmentation (*Fig. 6.74*) and/or permanent hypopigmentation (*Fig. 6.75*).
- Scarring.

Iontophoresis

WHAT IS IONTOPHORESIS?

Iontophoresis is a procedure in which an electrical current is passed through skin soaked in tap water or normal saline, allowing ionised (charged) particles to cross the normal skin barrier (*Fig. 6.76*).

WHAT IS IONTOPHORESIS USED FOR?

Iontophoresis is mainly used to treat focal hyperhidrosis, particularly on the palms or soles. Tap water iontophoresis is less effective in the axilla (armpit).

Iontophoresis has also been successfully used to deliver drugs to the skin, for example:

- reduce sweating using anticholinergic agents or botulinum toxin A.
- anaesthetise an area of skin with lidocaine.
- treat fungal infection of nail plate (onychomycosis).

THE PROCESS OF IONTOPHORESIS

Battery-powered direct current (DC) and mains-powered alternating current (AC) devices are available. Individual machines vary, and the

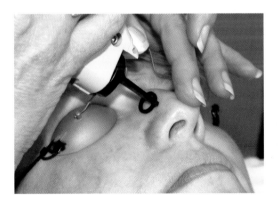

Figure 6.71. The laser process.

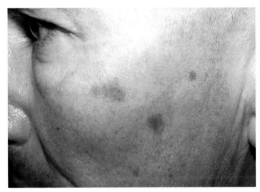

Figure 6.73. Purpura 24 hours after copper bromide laser to facial blood vessels.

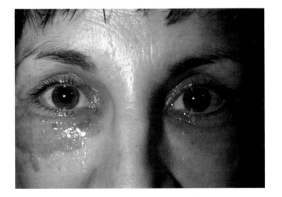

Figure 6.72. Immediate effect of CO_2 laser to lower eyelids.

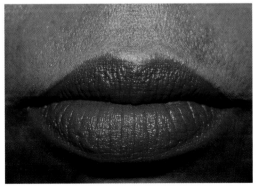

Figure 6.74. Temporary hyperpigmentation several weeks after laser hair removal to upper lip.

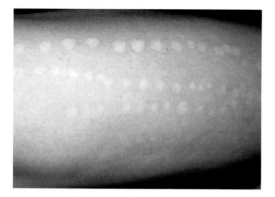

Figure 6.75. Hypopigmentation 1 year after ruby laser hair removal.

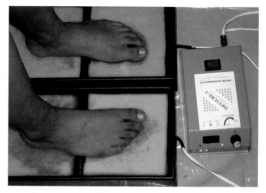

Figure 6.76. Iontophoresis.

instructions provided by the manufacturer should be followed carefully.

For palmar hyperhidrosis:
- petroleum jelly is applied to the skin at the water-line and to cuts or fissures.
- each hand is placed in a tray of water that contains the electrodes.
- the device is switched on so that current passes through the water between the electrodes.
- initial current should be very low, and adjusted according to tolerance.

Initially treatment is undertaken for 20–30 minutes every 1–3 days until the desired effect is achieved, and then reduced to once per week to maintain the result.

WHAT ARE THE ADVERSE EFFECTS OF IONTOPHORESIS?

Iontophoresis is generally a safe procedure. It is important to avoid direct contact with the electrodes during treatment, as it may cause a mild electric shock.

Paraesthesia (pins and needles) or burning sensation is usual. Adverse effects may include:
- redness of treated skin.
- vesicles or pompholyx.
- dry and cracked skin or dermatitis.

Emollients/moisturisers should be applied several times daily to reduce symptoms. Topical corticosteroids can be applied.

If anticholinergic drugs such as glycopyrronium are used, systemic side-effects may occur, such as dizziness, dry eyes and dry mouth.

Contraindications to iontophoresis include:
- epilepsy or history of seizures.
- heart conditions or pacemaker.
- metal implants.
- pregnancy.
- open wound.

6.15 Role of surgery in skin disease

What is dermatologic surgery?

Dermatologic surgery is the treatment of medically necessary and cosmetic skin, nail, and hair conditions by various surgical methods. It is also called dermatological surgery.

Dermatologists are all trained in basic dermatologic surgery. Some dermatologists undergo additional training in advanced dermatologic surgery procedures. Non-dermatologists who may also perform skin surgery include plastic and reconstructive surgeons, otolaryngologists, ophthalmic surgeons, general surgeons and general practitioners.

What is dermatologic surgery used for?

Surgery is essential for removal of skin cancers and suspected skin cancers, including:
- melanoma.
- squamous cell carcinoma.
- many basal cell carcinomas.
- rare skin tumours.

Mohs micrographic surgery is used to remove mid-facial skin cancers, especially if their margins are unclear or they are recurrent lesions.

Surgery is also used to remove benign growths that are causing a nuisance or are unsightly, such as large moles and seborrhoeic keratoses.

Cosmetic surgical procedures include:
- dermabrasion.
- eyelid surgery.
- scar treatments.
- hair restoration.
- liposuction.
- suction curettage for sweating.

Dermatologic surgeons also employ non-surgical cosmetic techniques, such as:
- laser resurfacing, tattoo removal, hair removal, and treatment of unwanted blood vessels.
- soft tissue augmentation (fillers).
- chemical peels.
- platelet-rich plasma treatments.
- sclerotherapy.

How is skin surgery carried out?

In most cases, dermatologic surgery can be undertaken using local anaesthetic in a side room at the doctor's office.

The most common procedure is a simple ellipse excision of a skin tumour, described here.
- A trolley is prepared with the instruments required for the procedure.
- The procedure is explained to the patient.
- The lesion may be photographed.
- Surgical lines are marked out in an ellipse around the lesion, attempting to choose the direction of least skin tension.
- Lidocaine/lignocaine is injected into the surrounding skin.
- The skin is cleaned with surgical antiseptic and surgical cloths are applied.
- The surgeon uses a scalpel to cut through the skin, following the marked lines.
- The skin sample is removed and put in a pot containing buffered formalin.
- Any bleeding is stopped using electrocautery.
- One or more layers of sutures (stitches) are applied to hold the edges of the wound together.
- A dressing is applied to the wound.
- The request form is completed and sent with the labelled sample to a dermatopathology laboratory for reporting.
- The patient is given instruction regarding care of the wound, removal of sutures, and follow-up.

Sometimes an additional procedure is necessary to close the wound, such as a skin flap (skin taken from an adjacent area and moved to fill the surgical defect) or skin graft (skin taken from a distant area and placed on the surgical defect).

What are the possible complications of skin surgery?

Immediate complications include:
- bleeding—especially in people with blood clotting abnormalities or on blood thinners.
- damage to important structures, such as sensory nerves, motor nerves or salivary glands.

- adverse reactions to medications used during surgery, such as local anaesthetics, non-steroidal anti-inflammatories.
- difficulty in closing the wound.

Delayed complications may include:
- wound infection (1%).
- wound breakdown.

- suture reactions.
- incomplete removal of skin lesion.
- delayed healing.
- persistent swelling.
- unsightly cosmetic result.
- diagnostic error.

Index

Major sections are highlighted in bold.